Complementary and Integrative Medicine and Nutrition in Otolaryngology

Editors

MICHAEL D. SEIDMAN
MARILENE B. WANG

OTOLARYNGOLOGIC CLINICS OF NORTH AMERICA

www.oto.theclinics.com

Consulting Editor
SUJANA S. CHANDRASEKHAR

October 2022 • Volume 55 • Number 5

ELSEVIER

1600 John F. Kennedy Boulevard • Suite 1800 • Philadelphia, Pennsylvania, 19103-2899

http://www.oto.theclinics.com

OTOLARYNGOLOGIC CLINICS OF NORTH AMERICA Volume 55, Number 5
October 2022 ISSN 0030-6665, ISBN-13: 978-0-323-93999-7

Editor: Stacy Eastman
Developmental Editor: Diana Grace Ang

Otolaryngologic Clinics of North America (ISSN 0030-6665) is published bimonthly by Elsevier, Inc., 360 Park Avenue South, New York, NY 10010-1710. Months of issue are February, April, June, August, October, and December. Business and Editorial Offices: 1600 John F. Kennedy Blvd., Suite 1800, Philadelphia, PA 19103-2899. Customer Service Office: 6277 Sea Harbor Drive, Orlando, FL 32887-4800. Periodicals postage paid at New York, NY and additional mailing offices. Subscription prices are $450.00 per year (US individuals), $1336.00 per year (US institutions), $100.00 per year (US & Canadian student/resident), $576.00 per year (Canadian individuals), $1396.00 per year (Canadian institutions), $628.00 per year (international individuals), $1396.00 per year (international institutions), $270.00 per year (international student/resident). Foreign air speed delivery is included in all *Clinics*' subscription prices. All prices are subject to change without notice. **POSTMASTER:** Send address changes to *Otolaryngologic Clinics of North America*, Elsevier Health Sciences Division, Subscription Customer Service, 3251 Riverport Lane, Maryland Heights, MO 63043. **Telephone: 1-800-654-2452 (U.S. and Canada); 314-447-8871 (outside U.S. and Canada). Fax: 314-447-8029. E-mail: journalscustomerservice-usa@elsevier.com (for print support); journalsonlinesupport-usa@elsevier.com (for online support).**

Reprints. For copies of 100 or more of articles in this publication, please contact the Commercial Reprints Department, Elsevier Inc., 360 Park Avenue South, New York, NY 10010-1710. Tel.: 212-633-3874; Fax: 212-633-3820; E-mail: reprints@elsevier.com.

Otolaryngologic Clinics of North America is also published in Spanish by McGraw-Hill Interamericana Editores S.A., P.O. Box 5-237, 06500 Mexico D.F., Mexico.

Otolaryngologic Clinics of North America is covered in *MEDLINE/PubMed (Index Medicus), Current Contents/Clinical Medicine, Excerpta Medica, BIOSIS, Science Citation Index,* and *ISI/BIOMED.*

Contributors

CONSULTING EDITOR

SUJANA S. CHANDRASEKHAR, MD, FACS, FAAOHNS
Past President, American Academy of Otolaryngology–Head and Neck Surgery, Secretary-Treasurer, American Otological Society, Partner, ENT & Allergy Associates, LLP, Clinical Professor, Department of Otolaryngology–Head and Neck Surgery, Donald and Barbara Zucker School of Medicine at Hofstra/Northwell, Hempstead, New York; Clinical Associate Professor, Department of Otolaryngology–Head and Neck Surgery, Icahn School of Medicine at Mount Sinai, New York, New York

EDITORS

MICHAEL D. SEIDMAN, MD, FACS
Director, Otologic/Neurotologic/Skull Base Surgery, Medical Director, Wellness and Integrative Medicine, Advent Health (Celebration and South Campuses), Professor, Otolaryngology–Head and Neck Surgery, University of Central Florida, Adjunct Professor, Otolaryngology–Head and Neck Surgery, University of South Florida, Past Board of Directors and Past Chair Board of Governors, American Academy of Otolaryngology–Head and Neck Surgery, AdventHealth Medical Group Otolaryngology–Head and Neck Surgery, Celebration, Florida; University of Central Florida College of Medicine, Orlando, Florida; University of South Florida Morsani College of Medicine, Tampa, Florida

MARILENE B. WANG, MD, FACS
Professor, Department of Head and Neck Surgery, UCLA David Geffen School of Medicine, Los Angeles, California

AUTHORS

MEHDI ABOUZARI, MD, PhD
Assistant Professor, Department of Otolaryngology–Head and Neck Surgery, University of California, Irvine, Irvine

BENJAMIN F. ASHER, MD, FACS
Private Practice, New York, New York; North Pomfret, Vermont

NATHALIE B. BENCIE, BS
Department of Otolaryngology, Hearing Research and Cochlear Implant Laboratory, University of Miami Miller School of Medicine, Miami, Florida

KATHLEEN R. BILLINGS, MD
Division of Pediatric Otolaryngology–Head and Neck Surgery, Ann & Robert H. Lurie Children's Hospital of Chicago, Department of Otolaryngology–Head and Neck Surgery, Northwestern University Feinberg School of Medicine, Chicago, Illinois

SETH M. BROWN, MD, MBA
Associate Clinical Professor, Division of Otolaryngology, Department of Surgery, University of Connecticut, Farmington, Connecticut

CAROLINE CASEY, BA
Medical Student, University of Central Florida College of Medicine, Orlando, Florida

AGNES CZIBULKA, MD, Fellow AAOA
Clinical Instructor, Yale University, Clinical Adjunct Assistant Professor, Quinnipiac University, Guilford

ALEXA J. DENTON, BS
Department of Otolaryngology, Hearing Research and Cochlear Implant Laboratory, University of Miami Miller School of Medicine, Miami, Florida

KARUNA DEWAN, MD
Assistant Professor, Department of Otolaryngology–Head and Neck Surgery, Louisiana State University Health Shreveport, Edinburg, Texas

HAMID R. DJALILIAN, MD
Professor of Otolaryngology and Biomedical Engineering, Director of Otology and Neurotology, Department of Otolaryngology–Head and Neck Surgery, University of California, Irvine, Irvine

LUKE EDELMAYER, MD
Advent Health Celebration, Kissimmee, Florida

ADRIEN A. ESHRAGHI, MD, MSc, FACS
Department of Otolaryngology, Hearing Research and Cochlear Implant Laboratory, Departments of Neurological Surgery and Pediatrics, University of Miami Miller School of Medicine, Miami, Florida; Department of Biomedical Engineering, University of Miami, Coral Gables, Florida

DIMITRI A. GODUR, MS
Department of Otolaryngology, Hearing Research and Cochlear Implant Laboratory, University of Miami Miller School of Medicine, Miami, Florida

JOSEPH F. GOODMAN, MD, FACS
Associate Professor, Otolaryngology–Head and Neck Surgery, George Washington University, Washington, DC

MICHAEL E. HOFFER, MD
Departments of Otolaryngology and Neurological Surgery, University of Miami Miller School of Medicine, Miami, Florida

HALEY HULLFISH, BS
Department of Otolaryngology, University of Miami Miller School of Medicine, Miami, Florida

NAUSHEEN JAMAL, MD
Associate Professor and Chair, Department of Otolaryngology–Head and Neck Surgery, Associate Dean of GME & DIO, The University of Texas Rio Grande Valley School of Medicine, Edinburg, Texas

WALTER M. JONGBLOED, MD
Resident Physician, Division of Otolaryngology, Department of Surgery, University of Connecticut, Farmington, Connecticut

HAILEY M. JUSZCZAK, MD
Department of Otolaryngology–Head and Neck Surgery, State University of New York Downstate Health Sciences University, Brooklyn, New York

DARLENE LEE, ND
Susan Samueli Integrative Health Institute, University of California, Irvine, Irvine

JESSICA R. LEVI, MD
Department of Otolaryngology–Head and Neck Surgery, Boston Medical Center, Boston, Massachusetts

CHARLENE S. LEVINE, LMT
Community Wellness Resources LLC, Florida

ROBERT A. LEVINE, PhD
Community Wellness Resources LLC, Florida

VANESSA LOPEZ, BA
The University of Texas Rio Grande Valley School of Medicine, Edinburg, Texas

JOHN MADDALOZZO, MD
Division of Pediatric Otolaryngology–Head and Neck Surgery, Ann & Robert H. Lurie Children's Hospital of Chicago, Department of Otolaryngology–Head and Neck Surgery, Northwestern University Feinberg School of Medicine, Chicago, Illinois

MATTHEW C. MILLER, MD, FACS
Associate Professor of Otolaryngology and Neurosurgery, Department of Otolaryngology–Head and Neck Surgery, University of Rochester Medical Center, Rochester, New York

JEENU MITTAL, MSc
Department of Otolaryngology, Hearing Research and Cochlear Implant Laboratory, University of Miami Miller School of Medicine, Miami, Florida

RAHUL MITTAL, PhD
Department of Otolaryngology, Hearing Research and Cochlear Implant Laboratory, University of Miami Miller School of Medicine, Miami, Florida

LAITH MUKDAD, MD
Department of Head and Neck Surgery, David Geffen School of Medicine at UCLA, Los Angeles, California

AJAY S. NATHAN, MS
Boston University School of Medicine, Boston, Massachusetts

CHAU T. NGUYEN, MD
Division of Otolaryngology–Head and Neck Surgery, Ventura County Medical Center, Ventura, California

ROBERT O'REILLY, MD
Perelman School of Medicine, University of Pennsylvania, Philadelphia, Pennsylvania

VARUN S. PATEL, MD
AdventHealth Medical Group Otolaryngology–Head and Neck Surgery, Celebration, Florida

LUIS P. ROLDAN, MD
Department of Otolaryngology, University of Miami Miller School of Medicine, Miami, Florida

RICHARD M. ROSENFELD, MD, MBA, MPH
Department of Otolaryngology–Head and Neck Surgery, State University of New York Downstate Health Sciences University, Brooklyn, New York

MICHAEL D. SEIDMAN, MD, FACS
Director, Otologic/Neurotologic/Skull Base Surgery, Medical Director, Wellness and Integrative Medicine, Advent Health (Celebration and South Campuses), Professor, Otolaryngology–Head and Neck Surgery, University of Central Florida, Adjunct Professor, Otolaryngology–Head and Neck Surgery, University of South Florida, Past Board of Directors and Past Chair Board of Governors, American Academy of Otolaryngology–Head and Neck Surgery, AdventHealth Medical Group Otolaryngology–Head and Neck Surgery, Celebration, Florida; University of Central Florida College of Medicine, Orlando, Florida; University of South Florida Morsani College of Medicine, Tampa, Florida

NINA L. SHAPIRO, MD
Department of Head and Neck Surgery, David Geffen School of Medicine at UCLA, Los Angeles, California

BRANDON TAPASAK, BS
University of Central Florida College of Medicine, Orlando, Florida

MALCOLM B. TAW, MD
UCLA Center for East-West Medicine, Westlake Village, California

KAREN TAWK, MD
Post-doctoral Fellow, Department of Otolaryngology–Head and Neck Surgery, University of California, Irvine, Irvine

MARILENE B. WANG, MD, FACS
Professor, Department of Head and Neck Surgery, UCLA David Geffen School of Medicine, Los Angeles, California

Contents

> This article is an introduction to the concepts of complementary, alternative, and integrative medicine. It discusses the scope and prevalence of complementary and integrative medicine (CIM) use among otolaryngology patients. Specific types of CIM are characterized in the context of their origins, philosophic and historical bases, scientific evidence, and applicability to the practice of otolaryngology. The author's intent is to provide a framework for discussing CIM with patients and integrate into treatment paradigms in an evidence-based manner.

> Aging, an ever-present process, is a part of every living organism's life cycle. Gerontology, the study of the biological, social, psychological aspects of aging, is a field that has been around since the 1930s, when the human inquiry into aging began to emerge. Aging can be characterized by the external changes, wrinkles, graying of the hair, among other changes, and lesser-seen but still important changes, presbycusis, arteriosclerosis, osteoporosis, cognitive decline, sarcopenia, and more. There is a strong drive to uncover as much as we can about the process of aging and the ways to delay its progression.

> Diet is essential to health and can modulate inflammatory markers, the microbiota, and epigenetic outcomes. Proper nutrition is also key to good postsurgical outcomes. Diet is challenging to study, resulting in a relative dearth of influential studies. There is substantial evidence regarding the benefits of a whole food plant-predominant diet on health and longevity, in general, but limited evidence regarding otolaryngologic disorders. Diet may be associated with the risk of head and neck cancer, hearing loss, laryngopharyngeal reflux, and sinonasal symptoms. Evidence, however, is heterogenous and often insufficient for treatment recommendations. Many opportunities exist for future research and expansion..

As of today, there are no therapeutic measures for the prevention or treatment of noise-induced hearing loss (NIHL). The current preventative measures, including avoidance and personal protective hearing equipment, do
not appear to be sufficient because there is an increasing number of people with NIHL, especially in the adolescent population. Therefore, we must
find a therapy that prevents the impact of noise on hearing. Antioxidants
are a promising option in preventing the damaging effects of noise by targeting free radicals but further studies are needed to confirm their efficacy
in humans.

Complementary/integrative medicine (CIM) is an evolving area of collaboration between oncology, patient and their beliefs, and practitioners of
complementary medicine. Evidence-informed decision-making is necessary to advise patients on which treatments may be incorporated into standard of care treatments for cancer. Patients use CIM for a variety of
reasons and often have unrealistic expectations of cure or disease modifications; on the other hand, there is increasing evidence that symptoms,
side effects, and dysfunction related to cancer and its treatment can be
ameliorated by CIM approaches to improve patient satisfaction and quality
of life. Open communication between patients and providers is paramount.

Dysphonia is a ubiquitous problem impacting a broad range of people. As
communication is central to the human experience, any perturbation of the
voice can be frustrating for the patient and the physician. Nutritional, psychological, and physical means of preventing and treating hoarseness
have been used by humans since the beginning of written record. Today,
we use a selection of these approaches, along with traditional medicine, to
alleviate problems of the vocal tract.

Migraine headaches frequently coexist with vestibular symptoms such as
vertigo, motion sickness, and gait instability. Migraine-related vasospasm
can also damage the inner ear, which results in symptoms such as sudden
sensorineural hearing loss and resultant tinnitus. The pathophysiology of
these symptoms is not yet fully understood, and despite their prevalence,
there is no universally approved management. This review summarizes the
data on complementary and integrative medicine in treating patients with
migrainous ear disorders.

OTOLARYNGOLOGIC CLINICS OF NORTH AMERICA

FORTHCOMING ISSUES

December 2022
Updates in Pediatric Otolaryngology
Romaine F. Johnson and Elton M. Lambert, *Editors*

February 2023
Unified Airway Disease
Devyani Lal, Angela Donaldson, David Jang, *Editors*

April 2023
Larynx Cancer
Karen M. Kost and Gina D. Jefferson, *Editors*

RECENT ISSUES

August 2022
Gender Affirmation Surgery in Otolaryngology
Regina Rodman and C. Michael Haben, *Editors*

June 2022
Comprehensive Management of Headache for the Otolaryngologist
Joni K. Doherty and Michael Setzen, *Editors*

April 2022
Pituitary Surgery
Jean Anderson Eloy, Christina H. Fang and Vijay Agarwal, *Editors*

SERIES OF RELATED INTEREST

Facial Plastic Surgery Clinics
Available at: https://www.facialplastic.theclinics.com/

THE CLINICS ARE AVAILABLE ONLINE!
Access your subscription at:
www.theclinics.com

Foreword

Physician, Educate Thyself: The Importance of Learning About Complementary and Integrative Medicine and Nutrition in Otolaryngology Practice

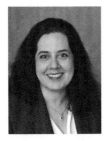

Sujana S. Chandrasekhar, MD, FACS, FAAOHNS
Consulting Editor

The other day a patient and her adult daughter came to see me. The patient is in her 70s and had been disabled by frequent episodes of severe vertigo accompanied with hearing loss, tinnitus, nausea, vomiting, diarrhea, and severe weakness necessitating hospital admission on a number of occasions. This had been going on for nearly one year, with the patient losing all of her independence as a result. She was unable to drive or be alone for fear of having another episode. Her quality of life had been demolished. But the past month was amazing, they related to me. She felt better than she had in ages. Her hearing was subjectively and objectively better. Her tinnitus was minimal. Most importantly, she had had no vertigo or disequilibrium and had been able to give up her cane and walker. She was hesitant to drive, still, but interested in starting again. "What made you better?," I asked. Sheepishly, they said she had gone to a naturopath who had put her on vitamin infusions and supplements and prescribed a significant dietary change that she was following. When I explained that she had Ménière's disease and I was pleased with the outcome of her naturopathic doctor's interventions, they jointly let out the breath they had been holding. They had anticipated that I, like many doctors she had seen before me, would pooh-pooh nonallopathic care and, in fact, dismiss her as a crackpot. They asked me why I reacted positively when others had not. I explained that much of the initial treatment for Ménière's involves dietary and lifestyle changes, which are effective a large majority of the time. I also explained

Otolaryngol Clin N Am 55 (2022) xiii–xv
https://doi.org/10.1016/j.otc.2022.07.016
0030-6665/22/© 2022 Published by Elsevier Inc.

that allopathic and even osteopathic physicians often do not know enough about, and feel there is inadequate evidence for, complementary health care interventions.

Only 55% of physicians suggest complementary and integrative medicine (CIM) to, and only 44% discuss CIM with, their patients, as reported in a large study out of Italy,[1] which also showed that academic and research physicians are better informed about CIM, particularly in the fields of oncology and chronic disease. Physicians everywhere understand the knowledge gap and wish for CIM education.[2] Practicing physicians are often bewildered by the various supplements taken by our patients, and how or why acupuncture, meditation, mindfulness, and other natural interventions work. We are even less likely to understand the mechanisms of action or benefits of cannabinoids or psychedelics. As far as knowledge in nutrition goes, although the Liaison Committee on Medical Education, the accrediting organization for US medical schools offering the MD degree, recommends at least 25 hours of nutrition education across the 4-year medical school curriculum, many schools fall short. Medical students and physicians report feeling "unprepared to counsel in nutrition" and having "insufficient nutrition knowledge and skills to effectively support dietary behavior change in their patients."[3]

Meanwhile, our patients are searching for treatments that will allow them to live healthy lives. As Dr Miller writes in his article, 60% of general Otolaryngology patients and a higher percentage of subspecialty ENT patients use CIM, while only 50% of those using CIM disclose this information to their physicians and other health care providers. The practicing otolaryngologist who chooses to hide their proverbial head in the sand and avoid learning about CIM and nutrition is doing themselves and their patients a disservice. Rather than decry the lack of Western or allopathic high levels of evidence, we should note that much of what we do pharmaceutically (such as giving systemic steroids for sudden sensorineural hearing loss), even though referred to as a "gold standard" of care, is based on quite flimsy evidence that is not necessarily reproducible. We should be aware of the existence of the National Center for Comprehensive and Integrative Health, a US National Institutes of Health–sponsored center whose mission is to facilitate the scientific study of nonconventional medical therapies. It is high time to eschew the artificial dichotomy between approaches to health care so that we can appreciate the areas of intersection to benefit our patients.

To get to the point where we can incorporate both allopathic and complementary/integrative medicine in our practices, we need to understand CIM and nutrition. Guest Editors Drs Michael Seidman and Marilene Wang have drawn upon their education and experience to compile this excellent issue of *Otolaryngologic Clinics of North America* for just that purpose. I encourage you to read and digest the information in detail. I hope this will allow you to help your patients navigate the world of CIM and nutrition and integrate that into your Otolaryngology care plan, to improve their overall health and quality of life.

Sujana S. Chandrasekhar, MD, FACS, FAAOHNS
Consulting Editor
Otolaryngologic Clinics of North America
Past President
American Academy of Otolaryngology–
Head and Neck Surgery
Secretary-Treasurer
American Otological Society
Partner, ENT & Allergy Associates LLP
18 East 48th Street, 2nd Floor
New York, NY 10017, USA

Clinical Professor, Department of Otolaryngology–
Head and Neck Surgery
Zucker School of Medicine at Hofstra–Northwell
Hempstead, NY, USA

Clinical Associate Professor
Department of Otolaryngology–
Head and Neck Surgery
Icahn School of Medicine at Mount Sinai
New York, NY, USA

Co-Executive Producer and Co-Host, She's On Call

E-mail address:
ssc@nyotology.com

Website:
http://www.ears.nyc

REFERENCES

1. Berretta M, Rinaldi L, Taibi R, et al. Physician attitudes and perceptions of complementary and alternative medicine (CAM): a multicentre Italian study. Front Oncol 2020;10:594. https://doi.org/10.3389/fonc.2020.00594. PMID: 32411599; PMCID: PMC7202223.
2. Patel SJ, Kemper KJ, Kitzmiller JP. Physician perspectives on education, training, and implementation of complementary and alternative medicine. Adv Med Educ Pract 2017;8:499–503. https://doi.org/10.2147/AMEP.S138572. PMID: 28794663; PMCID: PMC5536234.
3. Adams KM, Butsch WS, Kohlmeier M. The state of nutrition education at US medical schools. J Biomed Ed 2015. https://doi.org/10.1155/2015/357627.

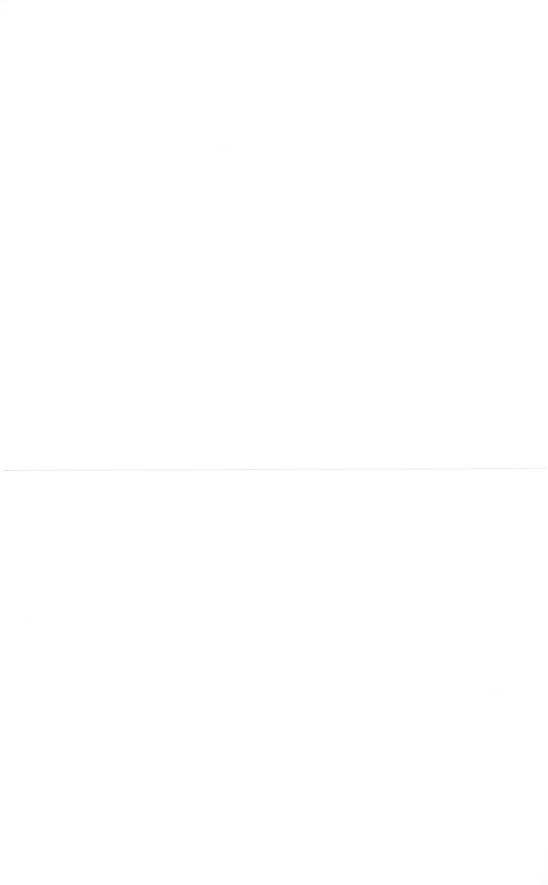

Preface

Complementary Integrative Medicine, Health, and Wellness: A Guide for the Otolaryngologist

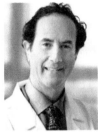   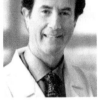

Michael D. Seidman, MD, FACS   Marilene B. Wang, MD
Editors

Complementary Integrative Medicine (CIM) treatments continue to gain in popularity and acceptance. While such treatments have been defined as modalities that have historically lacked scientific evidence, CIM is showing promise through both patient satisfaction surveys and research. The growing segment of the population utilizing complementary care has attracted national attention from the media, the medical community, and governmental agencies. Patients are increasing their use of complementary care to do the following:

- Improve the management of, or resolve, chronic disease conditions
- Be responsible for participating in achieving the highest quality of health
- Maintain an optimum state of wellness
- Assist in healing when conventional medical approaches have been exhausted
- Spend more quality time with a practitioner
- Receive more natural and noninvasive treatments
- Integrate care to utilize expertise in complementary medicine modalities that will enhance the likelihood of success of conventional care

CIM is further defined as any practice that can be used for the prevention and treatment of diseases, but not taught widely in medical schools, not generally available in hospitals, and not usually covered by health insurance. Similarly, Andrew Weil, MD, defines integrative medicine as a healing-oriented medicine that draws upon all therapeutic systems to form a comprehensive approach to the art and science of medicine.

Many CIM remedies have been in existence for thousands of years. However, given the general paucity of randomized, double-blind, placebo-controlled studies

Otolaryngol Clin N Am 55 (2022) xvii–xviii
https://doi.org/10.1016/j.otc.2022.07.015
0030-6665/22/© 2022 Published by Elsevier Inc.

oto.theclinics.com

supporting their efficacy, many health care professionals remain skeptical and hesitant to recommend CIM modalities. There is tremendous public interest in CIM, particularly in areas that are difficult to treat with conventional medicine. Statistics show that the amount of money being spent on CIM by the public is increasing rapidly each year. And, with increased funding now available from the NIH, preliminary research is showing that certain CIM remedies are appropriate for treating a number of acute and chronic health conditions. In view of this, it is imperative that medical professionals familiarize themselves with these options. In addition, we should be aware that modalities we may consider to be "alternative" are mainstream and accepted practices elsewhere in the world.

Hospitals and medical centers around the country are increasingly adding CIM to their repertoire.

Above all, as health care professionals, we need to remove our blinders and consider the options, without jeopardizing our patients' health. With both public interest and scientific research in CIM on the rise, our profession is certain to experience a further increase in the use of CIM therapies. For the sake of both our patients and our profession, it is essential that health care practitioners gain knowledge in this increasingly evolving field.

Michael D. Seidman, MD, FACS
Otologic/Neurotologic/Skull Base Surgery
Wellness and Integrative Medicine
Advent Health (Celebration and South Campuses)
AdventHealth Medical Group–
Otolaryngology–Head & Neck Surgery
410 Celebration Place, Suite 305
Celebration, FL 34747, USA

Marilene B. Wang, MD
Department of Head and Neck Surgery
UCLA David Geffen School of Medicine
200 Medical Plaza, Suite 550
Los Angeles, CA 90095, USA

E-mail addresses:
Michael.Seidman.md@adventhealth.com (M.D. Seidman)
mbwang@g.ucla.edu (M.B. Wang)

Complementary and Integrative Medicine
Origins and Expanding Horizons

Matthew C. Miller, MD*

KEYWORDS

- Complementary and integrative medicine • Nonconventional therapy
- Nonvitamin, nonmineral dietary supplement

KEY POINTS

- Many patients seeking care by an otolaryngologist will be using at least one form of complementary medical therapy.
- Most patients who use complementary therapies do not disclose this fact to their physicians.
- Education and training in complementary and integrative medicine are lacking in the United States.

DEFINITIONS AND RELATIVISM IN INTEGRATIVE MEDICAL PRACTICE

Historically, nonconventional therapies were collectively referred to as *Complementary and Alternative Medicines (CAM)*. These terms are by definition relative. That is to say, for something to be considered alternative and/or complementary, there must be a reference standard with which it is compared with. In medicine, cultural, historical, and scientific influences play a role in what is deemed to be conventional versus alternative. As such, the designations are somewhat fluid and can vary from place to place and over time.

For the purposes of this article, "conventional" medicine refers to what is typically known as *Western Medicine*, although the terms are often interchangeable. The National Institutes of Health (NIH) defines Western medicine as "a system in which medical doctors and other healthcare professionals (such as nurses, pharmacists, and therapists) treat symptoms and diseases using drugs, radiation, or surgery. This has also been called allopathic medicine, biomedicine, conventional medicine,

Department of Otolaryngology-Head and Neck Surgery, University of Rochester Medical Center, 601 Elmwood Avenue, Box 629, Rochester, NY 14642, USA
* Corresponding author.
E-mail address: Matthew_miller@urmc.rochester.edu
Twitter: @mcmmdoto1 (M.C.M.)

Otolaryngol Clin N Am 55 (2022) 891–898
https://doi.org/10.1016/j.otc.2022.06.015
0030-6665/22/© 2022 Elsevier Inc. All rights reserved.

oto.theclinics.com

mainstream medicine, and orthodox medicine."[1,2] In this context, complementary therapies are those which are used in conjunction with Western medicine, whereas *alternative* therapies are used in lieu of it. Integrative medicine, on the other hand, involves coordination between conventional and complementary approaches to patient care.[3] According to the National Center for Complementary and Integrative Health (NCCIH), complementary health can encompass a broad array of treatment modalities and approaches. These may be nutritional, psychological, physical, or any combination of the above. They may also involve traditional healers or whole-health systems that combine multiple facets of care.[3] In the United States, the most common complementary treatments include nonvitamin, nonmineral dietary supplements.[4,5] A comprehensive review of each of these complementary and alternative modalities is beyond the scope of this review. However, examples of complementary and alternative therapies are outlined in **Box 1**. Under this construct and in parts of the world where Western medicine predominates, the practice of medical treatment modalities and philosophies that fall outside of this mainstream would be considered either complementary or alternative to it.

Box 1
Categories and examples of complementary and alternative therapies

Nutritional approaches
- Botanicals (herbs)
- Vitamins and minerals
- Probiotics
- Dietary supplements
- Animal-derived extracts
- Special diets (eg, ketogenic, others)

Psychological
- Art therapy
- Music therapy
- Mindfulness
- Meditation
- Prayer
- Guided imagery
- Hypnotherapy
- Qigong

Physical
- Tai chi
- Yoga
- Acupuncture
- Massage therapy
- Osteopathic and chiropractic manipulation
- Pilates
- Rolfing
- Biofeedback
- Acupuncture

Traditional healers/shaman
  Whole medical systems
  - Ayurvedic medicine
  - Traditional Chinese medicine
  - Homeopathy
  - Naturopathy
  - Functional medicine

ESTABLISHMENT OF THE STATUS QUO

The dichotomy between mainstream Western medicine and its nonconventional counterparts likely traces its origins back to the latter half of the nineteenth century and the early half of the twentieth century. Medical training and practice up to this point were largely unregulated. Although the teachings of Hippocrates and Galen had largely been supplanted by empiric methods,[6] countless treatments and approaches (with varying degrees of credibility and efficacy) flourished without adequate checks and balances.[5,6] Around that same time, the United States (along with other Western nations) realized substantial advances in science and technology, which in turn solidified its position as a leader in industry, agriculture, and military might. These innovations spilled over into the medical profession, and as a result, the field of modern biomedical science was born. Around the turn of the twentieth century, the world saw the development of germ theory and antisepsis; diagnostic equipment, such as the stethoscope, electrocardiogram, and clinical microscopy; electric drills; radiography; drugs such as aspirin and anesthetics; and vaccination.[6] Each of these discoveries solidified medicine's position as less "art" and more "science."

Then, in 1910, Abraham Flexner, a noted proponent in educational reform, authored a report entitled, "Medical education in the United States and Canada: A report to the Carnegie Foundation for the advancement of teaching." In it, Flexner argued that scientific medicine necessitated "rigorous cross examination" through laboratory study and standardized clinical observation. Flexner believed that medical schools should be part of larger research universities as well. Moreover, he argued for more stringent oversight by government agencies and licensure boards.[7] Flexner's influence was far reaching, and public and governmental sentiment drove medical schools to comply. However, only around 20% were able to meet the rigorous standards set forth in the Flexner report. The remainder were forced to close. Federal and state regulatory and licensing agencies quickly followed suit, thereby creating a self-sustaining and dominant "medical oligarchy," which would ostensibly maintain the status quo.[8] The end result was the birth of modern-day institutionalized/academic medicine, but also the marginalization of those fields of study not explicitly covered in allopathic medical curricula.

SOCIAL REVOLUTION AND THE MAINSTREAMING OF NONCONVENTIONAL THERAPY

In the ensuing decades, scientific reductionism became the norm in medical education. Understanding physiology, anatomy, biochemistry, genetics, and ultimately molecular biology came to the forefront of what we now accept as fundamental health sciences. These disciplines became essential in understanding and treating disease processes. Their foundation was based on rigorous and reproducible testing of hypotheses and subsequent application of evidence derived thereof. "Fringe" practices (as characterized by Flexner and others) were not deemed worthy of being explored in the construct of evidence-based medicine.[9] However, the counterculture movement of the 1960s and 1970s resulted in many taking a more holistic approach to health care and prompted a renewed interest in complementary and alternative therapies.[8] "Mainstream" values and authority were being challenged at all levels of society. To many, the medical establishment became emblematic of a large dehumanizing patriarchy that suppressed free thinking and "natural" living. These beliefs were likely exacerbated by public disclosure and outcry over Nazi experimentation practices during World War II, the Tuskegee experiment, thalidomide-related birth defects, the

Willowbrook hepatitis experiments, and others. In addition, around this time, a growing portion of the population began to believe strongly in the concepts of self-help, holism, and mysticism. Coupled with these factors, globalization and the boom in marketing media during the middle and latter half of the twentieth century fostered a new wave of consumer-driven demand and marketplace for nontraditional therapies/practitioners.[5,8,10] In recent years, the explosion of Internet and social media–based interaction and marketing has also contributed to increases in the popularity of complementary and alternative therapies and skepticism of conventional Western medicine.[5,11,12]

MODERN-DAY SCOPE OF COMPLEMENTARY AND INTEGRATIVE MEDICINE

In keeping with this, the proportion of patients using complementary and integrative medicine (CIM) has been on the increase over the past few decades, both among the general population and for disease-specific reasons. According to the largest population-based study of its kind, nearly 40% of the US population uses some form of CIM.[13] The reasons patients use CIM are myriad. However, the top 3 reported reasons cited in a 2020 systematic review include a perceived benefit of CIM, a perceived safety of CIM, and a negative attitude toward conventional medicine[14] (**Box 2**). Others include market forces, a desire of patients to be more active participants in their care, and an impression that conventional therapies are not beneficial.[8] CIM use is most common among patients with chronic diseases, considering that conventional medicine rarely resolves their symptoms. Examples of these chronic disease are musculoskeletal pain and anxiety, but CIM is also frequently used for cardiovascular disorders, anxiety, headaches, upper respiratory symptoms, and cancer.[5,13] In general otolaryngologic practices, up to 60% of patients have been identified as users of complementary therapies.[15] Subspecialty clinics in rhinology and head and neck oncology have seen up to 65% and 92% of patients using CIM.[16–20] In 2012, approximately 59 million adults and children

---

Box 2
Reasons patients choose to use complementary therapies[13]

Perceived benefits
- Treatment of illness
- Alleviation of symptoms
- Reducing side effects of conventional medicine
- Maintenance of well-being
- Prevention of disease
- As a last resort

Perceived safety
Dissatisfaction with conventional medicine
- Ineffective in mitigating illness
- Treatments result in side effects
- Lack of trust in conventional medicine
- Avoid invasive care or aggressive treatment
- Lack of explanations and time spent by providers

Internal health locus of control/holistic approach
Social networks/social media influences
Affordability
Easy access

in the United States had a combined out-of-pocket expenditure of $30.2 billion (USD) for complementary and alternative therapies, with an average of $510 per person.[21]

INTEGRATIVE MEDICINE AS A FEDERALLY SPONSORED PUBLIC HEALTH INITIATIVE

In recognition of the expanding scope and penetrance of CIM usage, the National Center for Comprehensive and Alternative Medicine (NCCAM) was established by Congress in the 1990s. This began with $2 million in seed money to open an office within the NIH to "investigate and evaluate promising and unconventional medical practices." This office, the Office of Alternative Medicine (OAM), opened in 1992. The OAM was charged with facilitating study and evaluation of complementary and alternative medical practices and subsequently disseminating those results to the public. By the late 1990s, the OAM's scope and influence had grown substantially. It was officially renamed NCCAM and designated as an official NIH center. As one of 27 institutes and centers within the NIH, NCCAM's existence brought additional credibility to the study of nontraditional therapies. At the same time, it provided federal funding opportunities for CAM-related research that were previously unavailable, ostensibly holding researchers to a higher standard. In 2014, NCCAM was renamed the NCCIH as part of President Barack Obama's omnibus budget measure.[22] This was in part done to reflect the growing evidence that true "Alternative" medicine use was rare in the United States and that instead most patients were integrating complementary therapies with conventional treatments. Moreover, these integrative approaches to the patient experience and overall wellness were becoming central to a variety of different health care settings. The rebranding to NCCIH was intended to reflect both of these themes,[22] but also likely to combat continued skepticism and criticism from the scientific community and government watchdog agencies.[23]

Today, NCCIH has a congressionally funded budget of more than $154 million per year. Its stated mission is "to determine, through rigorous scientific investigation, the fundamental science, usefulness, and safety of complementary and integrative health approaches and their roles in improving health and health care."[3] For fiscal year 2022, the NCCIH will support 243 individual research project grants. A significant focus of these funding opportunities is on nonopioid pain management strategies; education and career development for underrepresented minorities; health disparities; and interventions aimed at mitigating the biological, behavioral, psychosocial, and socioeconomic impacts of the COVID-19 pandemic.[3]

BARRIERS AND OPPORTUNITIES

Despite the positive momentum and acceptance of CIM in the general population, obstacles to a truly integrated health care model remain widespread. Although government-sponsored research and NIH-endorsed status are firmly established at this point, the educational and clinical sectors continue to lag. To date, medical school and residency training curricula in the United States do not routinely provide CIM-related instruction. In a 2015 survey of 125 US medical schools, only 51% provided any CIM-specific didactic instruction, most of which was elective rather than part of the core curriculum. Only one of the schools required a clinical clerkship in complementary or integrative medicine.[24] The Accreditation Council for Graduate Medical Education does not support residency training programs specific to complementary/integrative medicine, nor does the American Board of Medical Specialties recognize integrative medicine as a distinct field of expertise. The bottom line is that US physicians are by and large undereducated and underprepared to discuss complementary medicine during routine patient encounters. The result is that practitioners of modern medicine may be seen by patients as ignorant, unenlightened, or uninformed with respect to CIM. This is likely reflected in the fact that only 30% to 60% of patients routinely disclose the use of complementary therapies during physician visits.[8,13,15,20,25,26]

At the same time, however, individual physicians are cognizant of their knowledge and credibility gap when it comes to discussing complementary therapies with patients. Moreover, when asked, most desire a more comprehensive fund of knowledge in this area. A 2006 survey of more than 200 practicing physicians found that nearly 60% of respondents believed that incorporation of CIM therapies would have a positive impact on their patients. This same group thought that they were not knowledgeable about complementary treatment options and that it was difficult or very difficult to find reliable information about CAM at their institution.[27] More than a decade later, another study revealed that there has not been substantial progress with respect to physician training in CIM and familiarity with evidence-based CIM resources for themselves or their patients.[28] Consequentially, physicians, feeling uncomfortable and unprepared to discuss CIM, do not broach the topic. Patients accordingly do not disclose owing to a perceived lack of interest on the part of their doctor. The net result is a missed opportunity to identify potential therapeutic benefits or harms related to CIM; to mitigate or avoid interactions between CIM and conventional therapies; to manage expectations; and to solidify the doctor-patient relationship by providing a truly holistic approach to the individual.[5,28]

SUMMARY

Complementary therapies are now enjoying widespread societal acceptance and usage in the United States. For physicians to truly provide "modern" medical care, we must first acknowledge the value of integrative care to our patients and practices. That an entire subspecialty journal volume such as this would be devoted to evidence-based CIM modalities underscores the fact that we are moving in the right direction. However, much work remains with respect to educating health care professionals about these treatments and engendering confidence to engage patients in frank discussions thereof.

Practicing integrative medicine necessitates an awareness that one's training in conventional Western medical doctrine and science is not all-encompassing or absolute. The ability to demarginalize and understand unfamiliar treatments will only serve to expand the opportunities for care and strengthen the bond between patient and physician. This has become increasingly important, as patients have evolved from being submissive and subordinate to "doctor's orders" to being active consumer participants in their health care decision making. Beyond respecting autonomy, integrative medicine also roots itself in the ethical principles of nonmaleficence and beneficence as well. In being knowledgeable of CIM, the physician can be better prepared to discuss potential risks of pursuing unproven, potentially dangerous, or counterproductive therapies. At the same time, they may identify new means of managing disease processes and promoting overall health and well-being.

In the end, understanding the history of how and why certain practices have been excluded from physician training; how and why our patients might seek out those options; and how they might ultimately benefit them should allow for more comprehensive and patient-centered care.

CLINICS CARE POINTS

- Approximately 60% of otolaryngology patients are users of complementary therapies.
- Approximately half of all patients routinely disclose complementary medicine use to their physicians.
- In the United States, the most frequently used form of complementary medicine is nonvitamin, nonmineral dietary supplements.
- The National Center for Comprehensive and Integrative Health is a National Institutes of Health–sponsored center whose mission is to facilitate the scientific study of nonconventional medical therapies.

DISCLOSURE

The author has nothing to disclose.

REFERENCES

1. Available at: https://www.cancer.gov/publications/dictionaries/cancer-terms/def/western-medicine. Accessed February 16, 2022..
2. Wiseman N. Designations of Medicines. Evid Based Complement Alternat Med 2004;1(3):327–9.
3. <NCCIH>. Available at: https://www.nccih.nih.gov/. Accessed March 2, 2022.
4. Clarke TC, Black LI, Stussman BJ, et al. Trends in the use of complementary health approaches among adults: United states 2002-2012. Natl Health Stat Rep 2015;79:1–16.
5. Ventola CL. Current issues regarding complementary and alternative medicine (CAM) in the United States. PT 2010;35(8):461–8.
6. Silvano G. A brief history of Western Medicine. J Traditional Chin Med Sci 2021;8: S10–6.
7. Stanisch FW, Verhoef M. The Flexner report of 1910 and its impact on complementary and alternative medicine and psychiatry in North America in the 20th Century. Evid Based Complement Alternat Med 2012;2012:1–10.
8. Saks M. Medicine and the Counter Culture. In: Cooter R, Pickston J, editors. Medicine in the twentieth century. New York: Taylor & Francis; 2000. p. 113–24.
9. Seidman MD, van Grinsven G. Complementary and integrative treatments: Integrative care centers and hospital: One center's perspective. Otolaryngol Clin North Am 2013;46(3):485–97.
10. Coulter ID, Willis EM. The rise and rise of complementary and alternative medicine: a sociological perspective. MJA 2004;180:587–9.
11. Bulmash B, Amar M, Ben-Assuli O, et al. Exploring the combined effects of social media use and medical skepticism tendency on recourse to complementary and alternative medicine. J Altern Complement Med 2021;27(8):710–2.
12. Sharma V, Holmes JH, Sarkar IN. Identifying Complementary and Alternative Medicine Usage Information from Internet Resources. A Systematic Review. Methods Inf Med 2016;55(4):322–32.
13. Barnes PM, Bloom B, Nahin RL. Complementary and alternative medicine use among adults and children: United States. Natl Health Stat Rep 2008;(12):1–23.
14. Tangkiatkumaji M, Boardman H, Walker DM. Potential factors that influence usage of complementary and alternative medicine worldwide: a systematic review. BMC Complement Med Ther 2020;20:363.

15. Shakeel M, Trinidade A, Jehan S, et al. The use of complementary and alternative medicine by patients attending a general otolaryngology clinic: can we afford to ignore it? Am J Otolaryngol 2010;31(4):252–60.
16. Newton JR, Santangeli L, Shakeel M, et al. Use of complementary and alternative medicine by patients attending a rhinology outpatient clinic. Am J Rhinol Allergy 2009;23(1):59–63.
17. Davis GE, Bryson CI, Yueh B. Treatment delay associated with alternative medicine among veterans with head and neck cancer. Head Neck 2006;28(10): 926–31.
18. Molassiotis A, Ozden G, Platin N, et al. Complementary and alternative medicine use in patients with head and neck cancers in Europe. Eur J Cancer Care 2005; 15:19–24.
19. Warrick PD, Irish JC, Monrningstar M, et al. Use of alternative medicine among patients with head and neck cancer. Arch Otolaryngol Head Neck Surrg 1999; 125:573–9.
20. Miller MC, Pribitkin EA, Difabio T, et al. Prevalence of complementary and alternative medicine use among a population of head and neck cancer patients: a survey-based study. Ear Nose Throat J 2010;89:E23–37.
21. Nahin RL, Barnes PM, Stussman BJ. Expenditures on complementary health approaches: United States, 2012. Natl Health Stat Rep 2016;95:1–11.
22. Available at: https://www.nih.gov/news-events/news-releases/nih-complementary-integrative-health-agency-gets-new-name. Accessed March 18, 2022.
23. Offit PA. Studying Complementary and alternative therapies. JAMA 2012;307(17): 1803–4.
24. Cowen VS, Cyr V. Complementary and alternative medicine in US medical schools. Adv Med Educ Pract 2015;6:113–7.
25. Tarn DM, Karlamangla A, Coulter ID, et al. Patient Educ Couns 2015;98(7):830–6.
26. Eisenberg DM, Kessler RC, Foster C, et al. Unconventional medicine in the United States: prevalence, costs, and patterns of use. N Engl J Med 1993;328: 246–52.
27. Wahner-Roedler DL, Vincent A, Elkin PL, et al. Physicians' attitudes toward complementary and alternative medicine and their knowledge of specific therapies: a survey at an academic medical center. Evid Based Complement Alternat Med 2006;3(4):495–501.
28. Patel SJ, Kemper KJ, Kitzmiller JP. Physician perspectives on education, training, and implementation of complementary and alternative medicine. Adv Med Educ Pract 2017;8:499–503.

Healthy Aging
Strategies to Slow the Process

Caroline Casey, BA[a], Michael Seidman, MD[b,c,d,e],*

KEYWORDS

- Healthy aging • Telomerase theory of aging • Gerontology

KEY POINTS

- There are several theories on aging; the leading ones are as follows: telomerase theory, mitochondrial DNA deletion theory, reactive oxygen species production, and the disdifferentiation hypothesis.
- There are many pharmacologic agents and supplements that have been shown to attenuate aging and presbycusis, including senolytics, mTOR inhibitors, resveratrol, N-acetyl-cysteine, alpha-lipoic acid, and lecithin, to name a few.
- Lifestyle modifications, such as calorie restriction and physical exercise, are associated with extension of lifespan.

PART I

Aging is an ever-present process that is a part of every living organism's life cycle. Gerontology or the study of the biological, social, psychological aspects of aging is a field that has been around since the 1930s, when the human inquiry into the field of aging began to emerge. Aging can be characterized by the external changes, such as wrinkles and graying of the hair, among other changes, as well as the lesser-seen but still important changes, such as presbycusis, arteriosclerosis, osteoporosis, cognitive decline, sarcopenia, and more. There is a strong drive to uncover as much as we can about the process of aging and the ways to delay its progression as we strive to live longer lives with a higher quality of life. We have made many advances in the field of gerontology, although there is much left to uncover. Many theories have emerged as to how aging begins in the body with an understanding that, as we learn more about how we age, we can then begin to look at strategies to delay those processes. Aging occurs gradually over time, and although there are many different manifestations of the process, there are a few leading theories that help us understand the

[a] University of Central Florida College of Medicine, Orlando, FL, USA; [b] Advent Health (Celebration and South Campuses); [c] University of Central Florida; [d] University of South Florida; [e] AdventHealth Medical Group-Otolaryngology-Head & Neck Surgery, 410 Celebration Place, Suite 305, Celebration, FL 34747, USA
* Corresponding author.
E-mail address: Michael.Seidman.md@adventhealth.com

Otolaryngol Clin N Am 55 (2022) 899–907
https://doi.org/10.1016/j.otc.2022.06.016
0030-6665/22/© 2022 Elsevier Inc. All rights reserved.

underlying pathophysiology and how aging occurs simultaneously in various systems throughout the body.

One of the leading theories of aging is the Telomerase theory of aging. It has long been known that telomeres exist as the endings of strands of DNA in that they serve as caps on each end so as to preserve the coding DNA and protect the genetic code when replication occurs. However, with each cell replication cycle, the telomeres shorten until the cell can no longer replicate, eventually leading to cell senescence.[1] There is an inverse relationship between age and telomere length, and specific findings, such as decreased leukocyte telomere length, has been associated with increased cardiovascular risk.[2] Telomerase is an enzyme that extends telomeres through adding repetitive sequences and is found in gametes, stem cells, and tumor cells.[3] The upregulation of telomerase is an active area of research in the field of gerontology.

Another leading theory of aging involves the mitochondria. Much research has been done over the past 30 years studying mitochondrial DNA deletions (mtDNA del) and alterations. Specific deletions have been associated with hypoxemia, cardiac diseases, maternally transmitted diabetes, deafness, and encephalomyopathy, among other findings.[4–6] A specific aging deletion called the common aging deletion or mtDNA(4834) in rats and mtDNA(4977) in humans has been found to be a molecular biomarker of aging.[7] Lifestyle has proven to be very influential in affecting mtDNA del associated with aging.[8] Take an example of two 50-year-old individuals. One individual lives in Florida, eats a healthy diet, has a body mass index (BMI) < 25, exercises daily, does not smoke, and drinks socially. Another individual lives in Basalt, Colorado and is exposed to more ionizing radiation living at 6500 feet above sea level, eats fast food 5 times per week, has a BMI of 45, never exercises, smokes 2 packs per day, and has 2 to 4 beers every evening. If the mtDNA del marker of aging was compared between these 2 individuals, there would be significantly higher amounts of the specific mtDNA del in the 50 year old with the unhealthy lifestyle living in Basalt as compared with the individual living in Florida. The 50 year old from Florida with the healthier lifestyle would be found to have an mtDNA del level comparable with most 30 year olds, and the 50 year old from Basalt would have an mtDNA del level comparable with most 85 year olds.[9]

Mitochondria, the fuel production centers of our cells, have thus proven to be very important in cell senescence and aging. The electron transport chain is a key aspect of the mitochondrial production of ATP. If there are any leaks present, electrons can leak and form reactive oxygen species (ROS) with surrounding water molecules. Low levels of ROS are constantly produced; however, at higher levels of production, ROS can lead to oxidative damage by oxidizing lipids, proteins, and even DNA. This puts mitochondrial DNA at a particularly increased risk of oxidation owing to the proximity to the site of ROS production.[10] Research has shown that the human body produces approximately 7 trillion free radicals per second at rest.[11] This then leads to a cycle of poor replication of electron transport chain proteins, leading to more ROS production and to more oxidative damage of the entire cell. Cross-linking of ROS species within the cell membrane has also been associated with cellular senescence.[12] Aberrant folding of proteins initiates the mitochondrial unfolded protein response; this stress response is sensed by the nucleus leading to protease and chaperone protein release in the cells. However, decreased protease levels are associated with aging leading to increased levels of misfolded proteins.[13] This has fueled the concept of ingesting higher amounts of fruits and vegetables that detoxify free radicals and has also led to an explosion of the use of antioxidant nutritional supplements. There are compelling, albeit controversial, data to suggest the importance of not only a healthy diet and lifestyle but also the supplementation of high-powered antioxidants.

The disdifferentiation hypothesis is another widely supported theory of aging that suggests there are protective and proapoptotic genes that support cell functioning or ensure malfunctioning cells become senescent. This is important for the overall protection and longevity of the organism. Bcl2 is a known gene that prevents oxidative damage and is found in high quantities in progenitor cells. Low levels of Bcl2 have been associated with early cell death and systemic damage in mouse models.[14] Another gene, Bax, has been found to be associated with the initiation of apoptosis in cells, and importantly, the ratio of Bcl2 to Bax in cells has been associated with survival or death.[15] Research over the past 5 years has also pointed to aberrant calcium signaling and its role in senescence. Increases in intracellular calcium levels have been associated with different types of stresses known to induce senescence, such as telomere shortening, oncogene activation, or oxidative stress.[16] Oxidative stress continues to be an important aspect of aging and one that is continually being investigated. Presbycusis, like many other aspects of aging, has been associated with oxidative damage to cells critical for hearing. Mitophagy and mitochondrial biogenesis are 2 pathways important in maintaining cellular homeostasis. These 2 pathways are often upregulated in aging leading to oxidative damage of the cochlear hair cells.[17] Markers of oxidative stress are being studied, as they can help reveal stress in advance of significant damage. The Ahl gene or adult hearing loss gene is one such marker and has been associated with increased oxidative stress within cells.[12] Aside from intracellular changes, another known concept of aging is that there are vascular alterations that lead to altered blood flow and altered oxygen delivery. This has been shown in the ear to cause damage to the hair cells. Noise has also been shown to induce changes in circulation of blood in the cochlea, indicating one possible source of presbycusis.[12] Certain compounds demonstrated the ability to protect against both noise and age-related hearing loss in an animal model.[18] The ingredients are now commonly found in supplements that report "antiaging" effects. It has been shown that using acetyl-l-carnitine, alpha-lipoic acid, glutathione, and coenzyme Q-10 is associated with statistically significant age-related hearing loss delay.[19] Although this does not necessarily translate to humans, it has since become "routine" for people to consider such nutrients.

PART II

The advancements in the field of gerontology do not stop at understanding different theories of aging, and there is also much research regarding different treatments that have been shown to delay aging. There is detailed literature covering different pharmacologic agents and supplements that have been shown in various studies to delay aging. Senolytics or agents that selectively eliminate senescent cells have been described and have shown promising results in delaying aging. Senescence is an important mechanism by which cells with damaged DNA are prevented from replicating. Dasatinib, a chemotherapeutic used to treat chronic myeloid leukemia, and quercetin, a flavonoid, are 2 well-studied pharmacologic agents known to help eliminate senescent cells.[20] Senescent cells release proinflammatory cytokines that lead to tissue dysfunction, so agents that can help eliminate these senescent cells can help preserve tissue function. In 1 study, mice with implanted senescent cells who were administered dasatinib with quercetin had decreased physical dysfunction and increased survival posttreatment by 36%.[20] Physical dysfunction has been associated with increased morbidity and increased impact of chronic conditions, so this is a significant finding.[21] The mTOR pathway is another known evolutionarily significant metabolic pathway important for cell senescence, apoptosis, and regulation of growth factors.[22] Literature suggests that the mTOR signaling pathway is important in aging; specifically, inhibiting mTOR complex 1 has been shown to increase lifespan owing to elimination of senescent cells.[22] Rapamycin, a macrolide with antitumor and immuno-suppressive effects, is 1 pharmacologic agent that has been shown to inhibit mTOR complex 1 and has proven effective in increasing lifespan in every organism studied.[22] Metformin, a commonly known type 2 diabetic medication and fisetin a type of flavo-noid polyphenol, also inhibits mTOR, through slightly different mechanisms.[23] In a mouse model, fisetin showed overwhelmingly positive effects on tissues, has been shown to improve memory, decrease aging-related pathologic conditions, and, as mentioned, increase lifespan.[24] Researchers were able to isolate geraldol as the major metabolite of fisetin that is responsible for its antiaging effects.[25] Apoptosis, or pro-grammed cell death, is an important mechanism by which damaged or senescent cells are removed from the body to prevent the replication of damaged DNA. The Bax gene is 1 important proapoptotic gene. Resveratrol is a nonflavonoid polyphenol found commonly in grapes, peanuts, and red wine and has been shown to promote the apoptosis pathway through translocation of Bax to the mitochondria.[26] In addition, resveratrol has been shown to increase neurogenesis of the hippocampus, an impor-tant brain region for long-term memory.[27]

Although the literature continues to expand on the topics of supplementation and pharmacologic management of aging, there are other antiaging protocols that have proven effective. Caloric restriction has long been studied as a lifespan-increasing protocol. It has been shown to promote autophagy, which is an important mechanism, by the body to eliminate damaged cells so that new cells can be generated.[28] Specif-ically, it has been found that a 30% reduction in caloric intake has been associated with improved lifespan.[29] Time-restricted eating, which is based on following the body's natural circadian rhythm and giving the body a true fasted period, involves eating in a 2- to 12-hour eating window each day and has been shown to decrease metabolic syndrome and chronic disease incidence.[30] In addition, plant-based diets high in polyphenols have been associated with improved long-term health outcomes, preventing age-related cognitive decline and preventing skin aging.[31,32] It is known that treatments for cancer, such as chemotherapy, although lifesaving, also put pa-tients with cancer at an increased risk for other pathologic conditions and is known to accelerate the aging process.[33] Dietary restriction, known as nutritional precondi-tioning, during cancer treatment can reduce DNA damage and protect from the DNA damage to healthy cells induced by treatments like chemotherapy and radio-therapy.[34] One study looked at a variety of clinical trials investigating nutritional pre-conditioning involving various dietary regimens, including the ketogenic diet, dietary restriction, and fasting, during chemotherapy, radiotherapy, or surgery and found a trend of decreased side effects and decreased DNA damage from chemotherapy in patients who fasted compared with those who did not.[34] Although often we are told there is no pill to mimic the effects of positive dietary changes, resveratrol has been shown to be a calorie-restriction mimetic in its positive antiaging effects.[35] Along with dietary changes, it is well known that physical exercise is important for overall well-being. It is commonly known to decrease cardiovascular risk, maintain bone strength, and increase metabolism. Interestingly, and not surprisingly, physical exer-cise also has antiaging benefits. Physical exercise has been shown to attenuate the production of ROS and, similarly to resveratrol, has been shown to enhance hippo-campal neurogenesis.[36] As discussed, telomeres have proven to play an important role in aging, and higher levels of physical exercise have been linked to longer lengths of telomeres, a theory with proven antiaging benefit.[36] Another interesting antiaging method is transfusion of young blood to the elderly. There are components of young blood that can aid with recovery of aging cells and tissue as was proven in a study on elderly patients with primary diffuse large B-cell lymphoma.[37]

Presbycusis is a component of aging that is being studied, as hearing loss presents a large health, economic, and social concern to the population. According to the National Institute of Aging, approximately 1 in 3 Americans between the ages of 65 and 74 have hearing loss and about half of Americans over the age of 75 years suffer from difficulty hearing. Similar to studying aging as a whole, significant research has investigated a variety of supplements and pharmacologic agents as well as other protocols that may prevent or attenuate presbycusis. Among different types of supplementation are a number of vitamins. Vitamin B complex has proven to be important, as a deficiency in one of the B vitamins can amplify tinnitus and cause hearing loss.[38] Vitamin B1 and B12 have proven to be particularly helpful, whereas vitamin B3 is still being studied because it is theorized the flushing effect could be accounting for the improvement in hearing.[38] Vitamin E and vitamin C are antioxidants that have been shown to attenuate hearing loss but do not seem to help at all frequencies.[39] High levels of zinc have been found in the inner ear; in fact, the cochlea has the highest concentration of zinc in the human body.[38] Tinnitus is a finding that can occur at any age; however, it is most common in the elderly. It was found that zinc, particularly in combination with vitamin B3, has been shown to reduce tinnitus.[38] Studies have shown that another mineral, magnesium, is excreted from cells under noise exposure as a stress response known as noise-induced permanent hearing threshold shifts.[40] In a study on human subjects who underwent basic military training, the group given magnesium supplementation had less hearing loss overall, and if subjects experienced hearing loss, it was to a lesser degree than the non–magnesium supplemented group.[40] Other minerals that have anecdotal and some scientific evidence of attenuating presbycusis include selenium, calcium, and manganese.

Vitamins and minerals are not the only supplementations proven effective in the fight against presbycusis. Phosphatidylcholine is one of the major phospholipids found in cellular membranes and has been shown to be important in aging. Specifically, lecithin, a specific type of phosphatidylcholine, has been found to be very important in presbycusis. Supplementation of lecithin in rats showed improved auditory sensitivity along with improved mitochondrial energy production.[41] In addition, an important mtDNA del sequence (mtDNA(4834) in rats and mtDNA(4977) in humans) that is associated with aging and found amplified in hearing loss was found less frequently when rats were treated with lecithin.[41]

As discussed previously, resveratrol has been shown to be an important antiaging polyphenol. It has also been shown to prevent noise-induced hearing loss through protecting the cochlea and preventing hair cell loss.[42] Cyclooxygenase-2 (COX-2) has been found to be an important marker of stress and ischemia throughout the body and is also found to be upregulated under noise-induced stress on the cochlea, much like ROS are also upregulated.[18] Resveratrol was found to decrease COX-2 expression and decrease ROS production when administered.[18] In addition, resveratrol has been shown to be important in restoring a balance between mitophagy and mitochondrial biogenesis, protecting cochlear hair cell damage from oxidation.[17] Alpha-lipoic acid is another supplement that in a mouse model has been shown to be otoprotective of outer hair cells and attenuate hearing loss.[43] N-acetyl cysteine is a potent antioxidant that has been shown to scavenge ROS after being transformed into glutathione.[44] This antioxidant, like alpha-lipoic acid, was proven to protect hair cells and delay age-related hearing loss in a mouse model.[44]

Herbal remedies have been used for centuries for the treatment of many different conditions, including anxiety, wound care, and skin care, to name a few. There are also a number of herbal treatments that anecdotally seem to be important in preventing and attenuating presbycusis. Although the research is sometimes limited in showing a scientifically proven benefit, there is a plethora of anecdotal support for these herbs. These include ginkgo extract, hydergine, mullein, and black cohosh.[38]

Although supplementation and pharmacologic agents have proven important in preventing presbycusis, there are other treatment protocols that have proven to be effective. Dietary restriction, particularly at about a 30% reduction in calories, has been proven to increase lifespan through promoting autophagy as discussed previously. Dietary restriction has also been shown to protect hearing through preventing build-up of harmful mtDNA deletions.[8] Another interesting treatment that has some efficacy in presbycusis is laser treatment of the cochlea. Particularly, soft-laser irradiation of the cochlea in combination with ginkgo extract supplementation showed an improvement in presbycusis and tinnitus in patients who experienced the treatment for 4 weeks.[45] Ginkgo extract has been shown to improve oxygen supply, and soft-laser irradiation is thought to increase ATP production as is seen in yeast fungus cultures that have undergone soft-laser irradiation.[38]

Combating aging has become a critical component of many different industries. People desire the magic pill that can allow them to live long lives with the same quality they enjoyed in their youth. Although there may not be 1 cure-all pill, there are many different supplements, medications, lifestyle changes, and treatment protocols that have shown some efficacy. Many resources have been dedicated to solving the aging problem, and strong evidence has emerged regarding beneficial treatments. Much research is dedicated to understanding how we age and how we can prevent the deleterious effects of aging, as well as how we can implement these findings into our daily lives. Although it may be hard to decipher what can be done in everyday life to prevent and prolong the aging process, 1 recipe for healthy aging that can be adapted by all follows the mnemonic "CREATION":

Choice: Make the right choices.

Rest: Humans need adequate rest.

Environment: Our natural environment where we find peace is critical to our health.

Activity: The gift of movement.

Trust: Trust that your life has a purpose; spiritual connection is imperative.

Intimacy: Interpersonal relationships, times you can truly be yourself.

Outlook: Positive outlook colors our perspective on life and influences our world view.

Nutrition: There is no secret pill that eliminates the need for healthy eating.

(Adapted from AdventHealth CREATION Life.)

DISCLOSURE

The senior author, Michael Seidman, MD has conflicts of interest as stated: A patent for compounds that in an animal model demonstrated the ability to protect against both noise and age-related hearing loss. The compounds are sold as supplements from body language vitamins and peak365nutrition which he founded and serves as Chief Science & Medical officer.

REFERENCES

1. Oeseburg H, de Boer RA, van Gilst WH, et al. Telomere biology in healthy aging and disease. Pflugers Arch 2010;459(2):259–68.

2. Dei Cas A, Spigoni V, Franzini L, et al. Lower endothelial progenitor cell number, family history of cardiovascular disease and reduced HDL-cholesterol levels are associated with shorter leukocyte telomere length in healthy young adults. Nutr Metab Cardiovasc Dis 2013;23(3):272–8.

3. Zvereva MI, Shcherbakova DM, Dontsova OA. Telomerase: structure, functions, and activity regulation. Biokhimiia. Biochemistry 2010;75(13):1563–83. https://doi-org.ezproxy.med.ucf.edu/10.1134/s0006297910130055. Accessed March 9, 2022.

4. Ballinger SW, Shoffner JM, Hedaya EV, et al. Maternally transmitted diabetes and deafness associated with a 10.4 kb mitochondrial DNA deletion. Nat Genet 1992; 1(1):11–5. Available at: https://doi-org.ezproxy.med.ucf.edu/10.1038/ng0492-11. Accessed March 9, 2022.

5. Corral-Debrinski M, Stepien G, Shoffner JM, et al. Hypoxemia is associated with mitochondrial DNA damage and gene induction. Implications for cardiac disease. JAMA 1991;266(13):1812–6.

6. Miyabayashi S, Hanamizu H, Endo H, et al. A new type of mitochondrial DNA deletion in patients with encephalomyopathy. J Inherit Metab Dis 1991;14(5): 805–12. Available at: https://doi-org.ezproxy.med.ucf.edu/10.1007/BF01799954. Accessed March 9, 2022.

7. Seidman MD. U.S. patent No. 6,933,120. Washington, DC: U.S. Patent and Trademark Office; 2005.

8. Seidman MD. Effects of dietary restriction and antioxidants on presbyacusis. Laryngoscope 2000;110(5 Pt 1):727–38. Available at: https://doi-org.ezproxy.med.ucf.edu/10.1097/00005537-200005000-00003. Accessed March 9, 2022.

9. "Method of Determining Biological Molecular Age". U.S. Serial 10/271,469. Patent 6,933,120 filed 10/15/02. Date of Patent Issue: August 23, 2005 issued to Michael Seidman MD.

10. Kowald A, Kirkwood T. Resolving the enigma of the clonal expansion of mtDNA deletions. Genes 2018;9(3):126. https://doi.org/10.3390/genes9030126.

11. Wallace DC. Mitochondrial DNA in aging and disease. Scientific Am 1997;277(2): 40–7. Available at: http://www.jstor.org/stable/24995869. Accessed March 9, 2022.

12. Seidman MD, Ahmad N, Joshi D, et al. Age-related hearing loss and its association with reactive oxygen species and mitochondrial DNA damage. Acta Otolaryngol Suppl 2004;(552):16–24. Available at: https://doi-org.ezproxy.med.ucf.edu/10.1080/03655230410017823.

13. Nargund AM, Fiorese CJ, Pellegrino MW, et al. Mitochondrial and nuclear accumulation of the transcription factor ATFS-1 promotes OXPHOS recovery during the UPR(mt). Mol Cell 2015;58(1):123–33. https://doi.org/10.1016/j.molcel.2015.02.008.

14. Korsmeyer SJ, Yin XM, Oltvai ZN, et al. Reactive oxygen species and regulation of cell death by the Bcl-2 gene family. Biochim Biophys Acta 1995;1271:63–6.

15. Oltvai ZN, Milliman CL, Korsmeyer SJ. Bcl-2 heterodimerizes in vivo with a conserved homolog, Bax, that accelerates programmed cell death. Cell 1993; 74:609–19.

16. Martin N, Bernard D. Calcium signaling and cellular senescence. Cell calcium 2018;70:16–23. Available at: https://doi-org.ezproxy.med.ucf.edu/10.1016/j.ceca.2017.04.001. Accessed March 9, 2022.

17. Xiong H, Chen S, Lai L, et al. Modulation of miR-34a/SIRT1 signaling protects cochlear hair cells against oxidative stress and delays age-related hearing loss through coordinated regulation of mitophagy and mitochondrial biogenesis.

Neurobiol Aging 2019;79:30–42. Available at: https://doi-org.ezproxy.med.ucf.edu/10.1016/j.neurobiolaging.2019.03.013. Accessed March 9, 2022.

18. Seidman MD, Tang W, Bai VU, et al. Resveratrol decreases noise-induced cyclooxygenase-2 expression in the rat cochlea. Otolaryngol Head Neck Surg 2013; 148(5):827–33. Available at: https://doi-org.ezproxy.med.ucf.edu/10.1177/0194599813475777. Accessed March 9, 2022.

19. Shirwany NA, Seidman MD. Antioxidants and their effect on stress-induced pathology in the inner ear. In: Miller J, Le Prell C, Rybak L, editors. Free radicals in ENT pathology. Cham: Humana Press; 2015. p. 57–89.

20. Xu M, Pirtskhalava T, Farr JN, et al. Senolytics improve physical function and increase lifespan in old age. Nat Med 2018;24(8):1246–56. Available at: https://doi-org.ezproxy.med.ucf.edu/10.1038/s41591-018-0092-9. Accessed March 9, 2022.

21. Xue QL. The frailty syndrome: definition and natural history. Clin Geriatr Med 2011;27(1):1–15. Available at: https://doi-org.ezproxy.med.ucf.edu/10.1016/j.cger.2010.08.009. Accessed March 9, 2022.

22. Weichhart T. mTOR as regulator of lifespan, aging, and cellular senescence: a mini-review. Gerontology 2018;64(2):127–34. Available at: https://doi-org.ezproxy.med.ucf.edu/10.1159/000484629. Accessed March 9, 2022.

23. Glossmann HH, Lutz O. Metformin and aging: a review. Gerontology 2019;65(6):581–90. Available at: https://doi-org.ezproxy.med.ucf.edu/10.1159/000502257. Accessed March 9, 2022.

24. Yousefzadeh MJ, Zhu Y, McGowan SJ, et al. Fisetin is a senotherapeutic that extends health and lifespan. EBioMedicine 2018;36:18–28. Available at: https://doi-org.ezproxy.med.ucf.edu/10.1016/j.ebiom.2018.09.015. Accessed March 9, 2022.

25. Schubert D, Currais A, Goldberg J, et al. Geroneuroprotectors: Effective Geroprotectors for the Brain. Trends Pharmacol Sci 2018;39(12):1004–7.

26. Jiang H, Zhang L, Kuo J, et al. Resveratrol-induced apoptotic death in human U251 glioma cells. Mol Cancer Ther 2005;4(4):554–61. Available at: https://doi-org.ezproxy.med.ucf.edu/10.1158/1535-7163.MCT-04-0056. Accessed March 9, 2022.

27. Kodali M, Parihar VK, Hattiangady B, et al. Resveratrol prevents age-related memory and mood dysfunction with increased hippocampal neurogenesis and microvasculature, and reduced glial activation. Sci Rep 2015;5:8075.

28. Madeo F, Zimmermann A, Maiuri MC, et al. Essential role for autophagy in life span extension. J Clin Invest 2015;125:85–93.

29. Hanjani NA, Vafa M. Protein restriction, epigenetic diet, intermittent fasting as new approaches for preventing age-associated diseases. Int J Prev Med 2018;9:58.

30. Manoogian E, Panda S. Circadian rhythms, time-restricted feeding, and healthy aging. Ageing Res Rev 2017;39:59–67. https://doi.org/10.1016/j.arr.2016.12.006.

31. Solway J, McBride M, Haq F, et al. Diet and dermatology: the role of a whole-food, plant-based diet in preventing and reversing skin aging—a review. J Clin Aesthet Dermatol 2020;13(5):38.

32. Rajaram S, Jones J, Lee GJ. Plant-based dietary patterns, plant foods, and age-related cognitive decline. Adv Nutr 2019;10(Supplement_4):S422–36.

33. Ness KK, Kirkland JL, Gramatges MM, et al. Premature physiologic aging as a paradigm for understanding increased risk of adverse health across the lifespan of survivors of childhood cancer. J Clin Oncol 2018;36(21):2206.

34. van den Boogaard W, van den Heuvel-Eibrink MM, Hoeijmakers J, et al. Nutritional preconditioning in cancer treatment in relation to DNA damage and aging.

Annu Rev Cancer Biol 2021;5:161–79. https://doi.org/10.1146/annurev-cancerbio-060820-090737. Available at: Accessed March 9, 2022.

35. Chung JH, Manganiello V, Dyck JR. Resveratrol as a calorie restriction mimetic: therapeutic implications. Trends Cell Biol 2012;22:546–54.

36. Arsenis NC, You T, Ogawa EF, et al. Physical activity and telomere length: Impact of aging and potential mechanisms of action. Oncotarget 2017;8(27):45008–19. Available at: https://doi-org.ezproxy.med.ucf.edu/10.18632/oncotarget.16726. Accessed March 9, 2022.

37. Fan L, Fu D, Hong J, et al. Prognostic significance of blood transfusion in elderly patients with primary diffuse large B-Cell lymphoma. Biomed Res Int 2018;2018: 6742646.

38. Seidman MD, Babu S. Alternative medications and other treatments for tinnitus: facts from fiction. Otolaryngol Clin North Am 2003;36(2):359–81. Available at: https://doi-org.ezproxy.med.ucf.edu/10.1016/s0030-6665(02)00167-6. Accessed March 9, 2022.

39. Darrat I, Ahmad N, Seidman K, et al. Auditory research involving antioxidants. Curr Opin Otolaryngol Head Neck Surg 2007;15(5):358–63. Available at: https://doi-org.ezproxy.med.ucf.edu/10.1097/MOO.0b013e3282efa641. Accessed March 9, 2022.

40. Attias J, Weisa G, Almog S, et al. Oral magnesium intake reduced permanent hearing loss induced by noise exposure. Am J Otolaryngol 1994;15:26–32.

41. Seidman MD, Khan MJ, Tang WX, et al. Influence of lecithin on mitochondrial DNA and age-related hearing loss. Otolaryngol Head Neck Surg 2002;127:138–44.

42. Seidman M, Babu S, Tang W, et al. Effects of resveratrol on acoustic trauma. Otolaryngol Head Neck Surg 2003;129(5):463–70. Available at: https://doi-org. ezproxy.med.ucf.edu/10.1016/s0194-5998(03)01586-9. Accessed March 9, 2022.

43. Huang S, Xu A, Sun X, et al. Otoprotective effects of α-lipoic Acid on A/J mice with age-related hearing loss. Otology & Neurotology 2020;41(6):e648–54. Available at: https://doi-org.ezproxy.med.ucf.edu/10.1097/MAO.0000000000002643. Accessed March 9, 2022.

44. Marie A, Meunier J, Brun E, et al. N-acetylcysteine treatment reduces age-related hearing loss and memory impairment in the senescence-accelerated prone 8 (SAMP8) mouse model. Aging Dis 2018;9(4):664–73. Available at: https://doi-org.ezproxy.med.ucf.edu/10.14336/AD.2017.0930. Accessed March 9, 2022.

45. Plath P, Olivier J. Results of combined low-power laser therapy and extracts of Ginkgo biloba in cases of sensorineural hearing loss and tinnitus. Adv Otorhinolaryngol 1995;49:101–4. Available at: https://doi-org.ezproxy.med.ucf.edu/10.1159/000424348. Accessed March 9, 2022.

Diet and Health in Otolaryngology

Hailey M. Juszczak, MD*, Richard M. Rosenfeld, MD, MBA, MPH

KEYWORDS

- Diet • Nutrition • Mediterranean diet • Diet score • Head and neck cancer
- Hearing loss • Plant-based

KEY POINTS

- Diet and nutrition are essential to human health and are important determinants of chronic disease incidence, prevalence, severity, and mortality.
- There is no single ideal diet but healthy diets contain high proportions of plant-based whole foods (eg, fruits, vegetables, whole grains, legumes, nuts, and seeds) with or without lean meat, and restrict consumption of salt, refined grains, added oil or sugar, and processed meats.
- Nutrition and diet should be part of the management plan of any patient undergoing major surgery to optimize recovery and surgical outcomes.
- Associations exist between diet and head and neck cancer, hearing loss, and laryngopharyngeal reflux; however, the evidence is mostly heterogenous and insufficient for treatment recommendations.

INTRODUCTION

It is well accepted and understood that diet influences human health. More than 2000 years ago, Hippocrates emphasized the fundamental role that nutrition plays in human health and disease.[1] One of the Hippocratic Aphorisms, for example, highlights how a nourishing diet can support an ill patient: "We must form a particular judgment of the patient, whether he will support the diet until the acme of the disease, and whether he will sink previously and not support the diet, or the disease will give way previously, and become less acute."[2]

Dietary factors are the leading determinant of mortality in 195 countries, responsible for 22% of deaths (11 million annually) from noncommunicable disease, based on a systematic review of global disease burden. The leading factors were high sodium intake (3 million deaths), low whole grain intake (3 million deaths), and low fruit intake (2 million deaths).[3] Dietary factors also rank substantially higher than tobacco smoking

Department of Otolaryngology-Head and Neck Surgery, State University of New York Downstate Health Sciences University, 450 Clarkson Avenue, Brooklyn, NY 11203, USA
* Corresponding author.
E-mail address: Hailey.juszczak@downstate.edu

Otolaryngol Clin N Am 55 (2022) 909–927
https://doi.org/10.1016/j.otc.2022.06.001
0030-6665/22/© 2022 Elsevier Inc. All rights reserved.
oto.theclinics.com

as the leading cause of death and disability-adjusted life-years in the United States from 1990 to 2010 for cardiovascular diseases, circulatory diseases, chronic respiratory disease, cirrhosis, and diabetes.[4] Many first-line treatments in medicine involve dietary changes (ie, decreased salt intake for hypertension[5] and decreased sugar intake for type II diabetes).[6] In otolaryngology, there are first-line treatments that involve changes in diet; for example, recommending low-salt diet for patients with Meniere disease.[7]

Diet and nutritional status affect surgical outcomes and factor into decisions regarding candidacy for elective surgery. The anatomic site of head and neck surgery can affect how a patient receives nutrition, whereas diet simultaneously can affect comorbid conditions that are often present. We have known for more than 30 years the power of food as medicine, whereby a low-fat vegetarian diet, plus other lifestyle interventions, substantially reduced cardiac events and coronary artery stenosis as compared with a control group with no lifestyle changes.[8] Yet, despite its importance, the amount of time dedicated to understanding nutrition and diet's impact on health, particularly in medical school, is limited.[9]

Reasons for limited knowledge of nutrition by clinicians include challenges in properly studying nutrition-based interventions and outcomes in a meaningful way without access to large cohorts, substantial funding, and reliable participants.[10] It is crucial to define baseline nutritional status and include appropriate control groups. Nutrient-specific studies do not account for absolute diet, and even when there is a proper study design, participant-specific factors, including individual diet inconsistency, recall bias, and confounding variables can muddy the validity of results. Moreover, the data that exist for nutrition-based interventions are clouded by fad diets, advertisements, personal anecdotes, and other flashy headlines meant to sell products.

Despite the challenge of studying diet, we cannot ignore its impact on human health and the powerful role it plays in the overall health of our patients. All clinicians should be familiar with diet and nutrition's impact on their patients' resilience and treatment outcomes. In this review, we will discuss current, evidence-based consensus on diet and health and what is currently understood about diet and its role in otolaryngologic-specific pathologic conditions.

"FOOD, NOT TOO MUCH, MOSTLY PLANTS"

Vast amounts of literature have been published regarding health and diet—ultimately, there is no one ideal diet with a strict set of rigid principles.[11] However, there are similarities that exist between diets considered to be healthy. Perhaps, the most succinct advice is Michael Pollan's suggestion to "Eat food. Not too much. Mostly plants. That, more or less, is the short answer to the supposedly incredibly complicated and confusing question of what we humans should eat in order to be maximally healthy."[12]

The national guidelines for healthy eating are regularly updated by the USDA in the United States,[13] which substituted MyPlate for the traditional Food Pyramid in 2011. Similar efforts occur in Canada under the auspices of Health Canada,[14] which last updated the Canadian Dietary Guidelines in 2019. There is general agreement that health-promoting eating patterns are high in fruits, vegetables, legumes, whole grains, nuts and seeds, and low in ultraprocessed foods, red meats, and processed meats. Similarly, a healthy diet is high in fibre, antioxidants, and phytonutrients, but low in trans-fat, saturated fat, cholesterol, and sodium. Although the US guidelines emphasize milk and dairy as a preferred beverage to ensure adequate calcium intake, the Canadian guidelines have water as the preferred beverage, with calcium from other whole food sources.

When comparing diets considered to be healthy, Katz and Meller found 3 overarching trends: (1) an emphasis on foods that are minimally processed and direct from nature, and foods that are made up of such ingredients, (2) an emphasis on foods comprised mostly of plants, and (3) animal foods that are the products of pure plant foods.[11] These overarching trends prove to be true when a diet is interpreted in a way that leads to consumption of foods following these principles. However, the actual foods consumed on an individual-to-individual basis can vary based on an individual's interpretation of the baseline principles.

Table 1 shows popular diet trends and highlights aspects of the diet interpretation that could lead to healthy eating or potentially unhealthy pitfalls. For example, a vegan diet could be interpreted as eating healthy whole plant foods (whole food plant-based diet) or it could include many plant-based, highly processed junk foods that are high in sugar and low in nutritional value; these interpretations will lead to different health effects. Moreover, putting all foods that fall into a specific category into one bucket of "healthy versus unhealthy" can lead to avoiding certain healthy foods or inclusion of unhealthy foods deemed to be healthy. For example, labeling all carbohydrates as potentially unhealthy and reducing their intake (ketogenic and paleolithic diets) fails to distinguish between healthy carbohydrates (high-fibre legumes and whole grains) and unhealthy carbohydrates (low-fibre refined grains and sugar-laden sweets and beverages). What is important, however, is the quality of the carbohydrate, not the volume; a diet high in whole grains—and the associated fibre—reduces overall mortality, cardiovascular mortality, stroke incidents, and rates of type II diabetes and colorectal cancer.[15]

The food industry is such a lucrative market that is heavily influenced by marketing. Hence, many diets that are built off the same fundamentals end up highlighting and exaggerating small differences and emphasizing mutual exclusivity to gain customers. This can lead to public confusion and to difficulty in guiding patients to more healthful eating. Ultimately, the emphasis is on limiting refined starches, added sugars, processed foods, and certain fats while emphasizing whole plant foods with or without lean meats, fish, poultry, and seafood.[11]

DIET AND SYSTEMIC PHYSIOLOGY

By understanding how diet affects the body at a physiologic level, we can better understand why diet plays an integral role in health. What we eat can affect our bodies in multiple ways that include producing proinflammatory or anti-inflammatory markers, altering our microbiota and microbiomes, triggering epigenetic mechanisms,[16] and providing the basic substrates for energy production, cell function, and reproduction.

Diet has been linked to proinflammatory markers, such as C-reactive protein, fibrinogen, white blood cell count, and homocysteine. A systematic review of 16 observational and 13 intervention studies found that plant-forward diets (Mediterranean, Dietary Approach to Stop Hypertension [DASH], vegetarian, USDA Health Eating Index) correlated with reduced oxidative stress and proinflammatory biomarkers; whereas, the opposite relationship was seen for Western and fast-food diets.[17] Of note, most of these studies were low-to-moderate quality, and the review presented individual study results with no data pooling. Another systematic review of 30 observational and 10 interventional studies of vegetarian versus nonvegetarian dietary patterns found that vegetarian-based dietary patterns had significantly lower C-reactive protein, fibrinogen, and total leukocytes.[18] An open-label trial with blinded study endpoint of 100 adults with angiographically defined coronary artery disease randomized patients to a vegan diet or a diet recommended by the American Heart

Table 1
Popular diets and aspects that promote health (pearls) or may detract from health (potential pitfalls)

Diet	Details	Pearls	Potential Pitfalls
Vegetarian	Plant-based diet that typically includes dairy and eggs; sometimes with selective inclusion of animal products (ie, fish and seafood)	Decreased meat intake High fiber from vegetables, fruits, whole grains, beans and legumes, and nuts and seeds	Not necessarily low in fat and does not necessarily comprise wholesome plant foods
Vegan	Vegetarian diet that may contain some animal products, such as fish (pescatarian) or dairy and eggs (lacto-ovo vegetarian)	High fiber from vegetables, fruits, whole grains, beans and legumes, and nuts and seeds Must be supplemented with vitamin B12	Eating only plant foods does not guarantee a healthy diet If poorly designed could result in plant-based junk foods leading to high sugar intake and nutrient deficiencies
Whole food, plant-based	Vegan diet that emphasizes healthy, whole or minimally processed plant foods: fruits, vegetables, whole grains, legumes, nuts, and seeds	Rich in fiber and complex carbohydrates that promote satiety Limited or no added oils, salt, or refined sugar	Reduces risk of deficiencies by eating a "rainbow" of foods Legumes essential for protein May need vitamin D supplement
Flexitarian	Plant-predominant diet that includes varying amounts of animal products	Emphasis on plant-foods while limiting animal foods Promotes transition to vegetarian diets	May include junk food, highly processed foods, refined grains and sugars May include significant meat and animal products, including processed meats
Mediterranean	Flexitarian diet that emphasizes olive oil, vegetables, fruits, nuts and seeds, and whole grains, seafood/fish; limited meat consumption	High intake of vegetables, fruits, nuts, olive oil, and legumes Moderate wine intake	High intake of cereal grains and fish, which have not specifically shown health benefits Increased fat intake (olive oil)
Paleolithic	Emphasis on avoiding processed foods, dairy, and grains; with favored intake of vegetables, fruits, nuts, seeds, and lean meat	Low in processed foods and added sugars High in vegetables, fruits, nuts and seeds, and lean meats	Can overemphasize meat and saturated fat, whereas true paleo diet emphasizes whole plant foods Emphasis on animal protein and fats has high caloric density
Mixed	Diets including both plants and animal products that conform to a particular authoritative dietary guideline (ie, Dietary Recommendations of the World Health Organization). Includes DASH diet	Minimizes highly processed foods with high caloric density Wholesome foods in moderate quantities	Can be high in dairy intake, in carbohydrate intake

Low carbohydrate	Restricts total carbohydrates to the lower limit of the recommended range established by the Institute of Medicine (45% of daily calories)	Decreased sugar intake (decreased refined starches and added sugars)	Low in all sources of carbohydrates, including: vegetables, fruits, whole grains, beans, and legumes
Low fat	Restricts total fat intake to the lower limit of the recommended range established by Institute of Medicine (20% of daily calories)	Avoidance of harmful fats Emphasize plant foods directly from nature	Could lead to increase in total caloric intake if lack of satiety or replacement of fats with high-starch, high-sugar, low-fat foods rather than plant foods direct from nature
Low glycemic	Limits the glycemic load of the overall diet by avoiding foods with high glycemic index or load	Decreased sugar intake by avoiding refined starches and added sugars High fiber intake if includes whole grains and legumes	Avoidance of certain vegetables and many fruits

Abbreviation: DASH, Dietary Approach to Stop Hypertension.

Association for 8 weeks. Results found that the vegan group had 32% lower (95% confidence interval [CI], 6%–51%) high-sensitivity C-reactive protein and had 13% reduction in LDL cholesterol (95% CI, 3%–22%).[19]

Diet can modify the body's microbiota,[20] which has significant health implications because the gut microbiome has been linked to chronic diseases that include hypertension and diabetes. The microbiota of the oral cavity, which can also be modulated by diet,[21] may affect pathologic condition of the head and neck, with burgeoning research suggesting a connection with head and neck cancer.[22–24] Currently, more research is required to understand exactly how different diets change the oral microbiome and how this might lead to head and neck pathologic conditions.

Gut microbes use ingested nutrients for biologic processes, which create metabolic outputs that affect human physiology.[25] More research is required to understand exactly what differences are created by adherence to different diets; however, preliminary data has suggested that the Mediterranean diet elicits favorable microbiota profiles and metabolite productions, with decreased ratio of *Firmicutes:Bacteroidetes* species and higher levels of fecal short-chain fatty acids (SFCAs). Vegan/vegetarian diets have also proven higher levels of SFCAs.[25]

DIET AND SURGICAL WOUND HEALING

Diet and nutrition play an uncontested role in the physiology of wound healing by providing energy and building substrates for the complex biochemical and cellular processes that comprise wound healing. These substrates include macronutrients (protein, carbohydrates, fat, amino acids) and micronutrients (vitamins and minerals). Energy required for building new cells is typically released from body stores and protein reserves; therefore, it is necessary to have sufficient stores, particularly when undergoing a major surgery.[26]

Malnutrition can lead to prolonged wound healing and complications, including infection. For example, insufficient protein can result in decreased wound tensile strength, decreased T-cell function, decreased phagocytic activity, and decreased complement and antibody levels.[27] Surgery can worsen undernutrition by causing a systemic inflammatory response leading to higher metabolic demands, increases in energy consumption, and impairment of organ function.[28] Preoperative malnutrition is associated with higher postoperative mortality, morbidity, hospital length of stay, readmission rates, and hospital costs.[29,30]

Guidelines have been created by the European Society for Clinical Nutrition and Metabolism with 37 recommendations regarding nutrition and surgery. One of the major themes of these guidelines is integrating nutrition into the overall management of the surgical patient. Recommendations include nutritional assessment[31–33] before and after any major surgery, and perioperative nutritional therapy in patients with malnutrition or at nutritional risk (including patients anticipated to be unable to eat for more than 5 days in the perioperative period and patients expected to have low oral intake and who cannot maintain >50% of recommended intake for more than 7 days). For patients with severe nutritional risk (**Table 2**), the guidelines recommend nutritional therapy (for a period of 7–14 days) before major surgery even if operations, including those for cancer, must be delayed.[34] There is currently no official recommendation from any health-care organization on micronutrient supplementation for optimal wound care.[35]

Nutritional supplementation has been studied in patients with head and neck cancer. A recent systematic review found that oral supplementation of arginine with omega-3 improved surgical wound healing in patients with head and neck cancer

Table 2
Nutritional assessment. Severe nutritional risk is defined as one of the following criteria listed below

Component of Nutritional Assessment	Severe nutritional Risk as Defined by ESPEN	Rationale[31–34]
Weight loss	Weight loss of more than 10% of body weight in <6 mo or 5% loss during 1 mo	GLIM criteria for diagnosis of malnutrition
BMI	BMI <18.5 kg/m^2	GLIM criteria for diagnosis of malnutrition
SGA	SGA score of grade C	Validated tool for assessing malnutrition using history of recent intake, weight change, gastrointestinal symptoms, and clinical evaluation
NRS	NRS >5	Four question prescreening tool (BMI, weight loss, recent intake, acute illness)
Serum albumin concentration	Serum albumin concentration of <30 g/L (with no evidence of hepatic or renal dysfunction)	Hypoalbuminemia reflects disease-associated catabolism and disease severity rather than undernutrition

Abbreviations: BMI, body mass index, GLIM, Global Leadership Initiative on Malnutrition; NRS, nutritional risk screening, SGA, subjective global assessment; ESPEN, European Society for Clinical Nutrition and Metabolism.

by decreasing the incidence of postoperative complications and decreasing the length of hospital stay.[36]

DIET AND OTOLARYNGOLOGY

There is a large gap in evidence-based knowledge surrounding diet and health in relation to otolaryngologic pathologic condition. The following sections describe associations that have been recognized in relation to preventing, treating, or mitigating otolaryngologic disease with diet and nutrition. We also highlight areas where further research may be worth pursuing.

Poor Diet Associated with Increased Risk of Developing Head and Neck Cancer

Diet likely plays a role as a risk factor in the etiology of head and neck cancers. Papadimitriou and colleagues completed a meta-analysis of 860 studies associating diet and cancers of 11 different anatomic sites. For head and neck cancer, 38 meta-analyses were found, noting an association between higher fruit consumption and lower risk of pharyngeal cancer and an association between higher vegetable consumption and lower risk of oral cancer.[37] Chen and colleagues completed a meta-analysis of 8 studies finding an odds ratio of 2.5 (95% CI, 1.9–3.4) for esophageal cancer in patients with the highest dietary inflammatory index compared with those with the lowest dietary inflammatory index.[38] In a meta-analysis of 117 studies, Morze and colleagues found that the adherence to a Mediterranean diet reduced the incidence of head and neck cancer by 44% (95% CI, 28%–56%) but with a low certainty of evidence.[39]

Some other large studies looking at head and neck cancer's relationship with diet have analyzed data from the Carolina Head and Neck Cancer (CHANCE) study,[40] from the International Head and Neck Cancer Epidemiology (INHANCE) consortium,[41] and from the National Institute of Health–American Association of Retired Persons (NIH-AARP) Diet and Health Study.[42] The CHANCE study was a population-based case-control study, using food frequency questionnaires, of 1389 cases and 1396 controls, in which cases had a first primary squamous cell carcinoma of the oral cavity, hypopharynx, oropharynx, or larynx diagnosed between 2002 and 2006. The INHANCE consortium is a collaboration of research groups leading large molecular epidemiology case-control studies of head and neck cancer across the globe, including populations from Europe, North America, Latin America, India, Japan, and Australia. The NIH-AARP Diet and Health Study collected surveys on demographic characteristics, diet, and lifestyle practices of a total of 566,398 AARP members, aged 50 to 71 years, residing in 6 US states.

- Mazul and colleagues used data from the CHANCE food frequency questionnaires to calculate an energy-adjusted diet inflammatory index (E-DII) for individual participants as a proxy for proinflammatory diets. They found an odds ratio of 2.91 (95% CI, 2.16–3.95) for head and neck cancer in patients with the highest quartile of E-DII as compared with those in the lowest quartile of E-DII, suggesting an association between proinflammatory diet with increased risk of head and neck squamous cell carcinoma (HNSCC).[43]
- Bradshaw and colleagues had previously used the CHANCE data to study food intake patterns with HNSCC. Based on food frequency questionnaires, patients were split into 2 patterns of food intake: (1) high consumption of fruits, vegetables, and lean proteins and (2) high consumption of fried foods, high-fats, processed meats, and sweets. They found that a higher consumption of fruits, vegetables, and lean meats reduced the odds of HNSCC (for highest quartile vs lowest quartile, odds ratio = 0.53; 95% CI, 0.39–0.71). The fried, fatty food group had increased odds of laryngeal cancer (odds ratio = 2.12, 95% CI, 1.21–3.72).[44]
- Saraiya and colleagues recently used the data from CHANCE to categorize patient's diets based on the following dietary quality scores: Healthy Eating Index 2005 (HEI-2005), Mediterranean diet score (MDS), and Mediterranean diet score - head and neck cancer (MDS-HNC). A one standard deviation summary decrement found a consistent inverse association with all 3 diet quality scores.[45]
- Chuang and colleagues used data from the INHANCE consortium, including 22 of 26 case-control studies to assess the relationship between head and neck cancer with consumption of fruit and vegetables and with consumption of red meat. They used food frequency questionnaires to determine participant quartiles for fruit and vegetable intake and for red meat intake. Higher frequency of fruit (OR = 0.52; 95% CI, 0.43–0.62) and vegetable intake (OR = 0.66; 95% CI, 0.49–0.90) was found to be inversely associated with head and neck cancer, whereas red meat (OR = 1.40; 95% CI, 1.13–1.74) and processed meat intake (OR = 1.37; 95% CI, 1.14–1.65) was positively associated with head and neck cancer.[46]
- Li and colleagues used the food frequency questionnaires collected by the NIH-AARP Diet and Health Study to give participants diet indices scores, including a HEI-2005 score and an alternate Mediterranean diet score (aMED). Higher HEI-

2005 and aMED scores were both associated with lower HNSCC risk. For men with higher HEI-2005 scores, the hazard ratio (HR) was 0.74 (95% CI, 0.61–0.89) and for women, the HR was 0.48 (95% CI, 0.33–0.70).[47]
- Lam and colleagues used data from the NIH-AARP Diet and Health Study and found intake of total fibre and grain foods was inversely associated with head and neck cancer incidence among women but not men.[48]
- Freedman and colleagues used data from the NIH-AARP Diet and Health Study and found an inverse association between total fruit and vegetable intake and head and neck cancer risk.[49]

Table 3 summaries the studies mentioned above.

In addition to the above cited studies and databases, various other large case-control and cohort studies have associated aspects of poor nutrition and dietary habits with increased risk of head and neck cancer. These studies vary in dietary factors studied and subsites of head and neck cancer, creating challenges in quantitative data pooling in large meta-analyses.

Diet and Potential Connections to Hearing Loss and Tinnitus

Many studies have investigated the relationship between single-nutrient intake and hearing loss in animal and translational studies.[50] These studies have reported that lack of certain single micronutrients, including vitamins A, B, C, D and E, zinc, Mg, Se, iron and iodine, are associated with increased incidence of hearing loss. Higher intake of carbohydrates, fats, and cholesterol, and lower protein intake correspond to poorer hearing status. Higher consumption of polyunsaturated fatty acids corresponded to better hearing status.[51,52]

More recently, studies have attempted to assess the relationship between overall dietary health with hearing loss through population-based studies. Curhan and colleagues completed a prospective study evaluating hearing loss and diet adherence scores in women participating in the Nurses' Health Study II. Diet adherence scores were calculated using food frequency questionnaires for the DASH diet, AMED diet, and the Alternative Healthy Eating Index 2010 (AHEI-2010). Hearing was evaluated with pure tone audiometry at baseline and at a 3-year follow-up. Higher adherence scores to DASH, AMED, and AHEI-2010 were associated with lower risk of midfrequency hearing loss.[53]

Other studies have looked at diet and hearing loss using data from the National Health and Nutrition Examination Survey (NHANES). Spankovich and Prell completed a cross-sectional analysis of NHANES data from 1999 to 2002 evaluating healthy eating index and high-frequency and low-frequency hearing loss, finding an association between higher healthy eating indexes and better high-frequency hearing thresholds.[54] Huang and colleagues completed a similar cross-sectional analysis of NHANES data, using surveys from 2000 to 2006 and 2009 to 2012 to evaluate MDS and hearing loss. Their findings indicated an association between higher MDS scores with decreased high frequency hearing loss in both men and women, and with decreased low frequency hearing loss in men but not in women.[55]

Spankovich used NHANES data to look for associations between diet and tinnitus. Again, looking at NHANES data from 1999 to 2002, higher healthy eating index scores were found to be associated with decreased odds of reported persistent tinnitus.[56] In all of the studies using NHANES data, dietary data was based off of a single, 24 hour dietary recall questionnaire. Other studies have looked at markers of nutrition, including BMI, waist-circumference, serum albumin, and found various

Table 3
Meta-analyses and large case-control/cohort studies finding associations between diet and head and neck cancer as addressed in this article

Study	Year	Type of Study	Participants or Sources	Nutritional Index/ Diet Categorization	Head and Neck Cancer	Results	Conclusion
Papadimitriou et al.	2021	Meta-analysis	860 studies total; 38 included HNC Of 38, one highly suggestive for fruits and one highly suggestive for vegetables	Dietary factors: fruit consumption (high vs low) Vegetable consumption (high vs low)	HNC: oral, pharyngeal, laryngeal, upper aerodigestive tract	Certainty of evidence: highly suggestive Decreased RR of pharyngeal cancer with higher fruit consumption (RR: 0.60; 95% CI: 0.52–0.70) and decreased RR of oral cancer with vegetable consumption (RR: 0.68; 95% CI: 0.60–0.77)	Increased fruit consumption lowers risk of pharyngeal cancer Increased vegetable intake lowers risk of oral cancer
Chen et al.	2020	Meta-analysis	8 studies	DII calculated from FFQ	Esophageal cancer	Highest DII category OR: 2.54 (95% CI: 1.90–3.40) when compared with lowest DII category	Higher odds of esophageal cancer in patients with proinflammatory diets
Morze et al.	2018	Meta-analysis	117 studies; 9 studies for HNC (1 cohort, 8 case-controls)	Highest vs lowest adherence to Mediterranean diet	HNC	Certainty of evidence: Very low Adherence to Mediterranean diet RR: 0.56 (95% CI: 0.44–0.72) decrease in HNC	High adherence to Mediterranean diet reduces risk of HNC

Author	Year	Study type	Data source	Exposure/Methods	Cancer type	Results	Conclusions
Saraiya et al.	2020	Case-control	CHANCE data	HEI-2005; MDS; MDS-HNC	HNSCC (oral cavity, pharynx, larynx)	HEI-2005 For 1 SD unit change, relative odds for HNC, OR: 1.35 (95% CI: 1.21–1.50) MDS For 1 SD unit change, relative odds for HNC, OR: 1.13 (95% CI: 1.02–1.25) MDS-HNC For 1 SD unit change, relative odds for HNC, OR: 1.17 (1.06–1.31)	Poorer diets as defined by HEI-2005, MDS, and MDS-HNC are associated with higher incidence of HNC
Mazul et al.	2018	Case-control	CHANCE data (Cases: 1389; Controls: 1396)	E-DII calculated from FFQ; divided participants into quartiles	HNSCC (oral cavity, oropharynx, hypopharynx, or larynx)	Highest quartile E-DII had odds of developing HNSCC. OR: 2.91 (95% CI: 2.16–3.95)	Increased odds of HNSCC with proinflammatory index
Bradshaw et al.	2012	Case-control	CHANCE data	Food frequency questionnaires to split into 2 groups: (1): High consumption fruits, vegetables, lean proteins (2): High consumption fried foods, high-fats, processed meats, sweets	HNSCC (oral cavity, oropharynx, hypopharynx, or larynx)	Group (1) lower odds of HNSCC. OR: 0.53 (95% CI: 0.39–0.71) Group (2) increased odds laryngeal cancer. OR: 2.12 (95% CI: 1.21–3.72)	Lower odds of HNSCC associated with diets high in fruits, vegetables, and lean proteins Increased odds of laryngeal cancer in diets higher in fried food, fats, processed meats, and sweets

(continued on next page)

Table 3
(continued)

Study	Year	Type of Study	Participants or Sources	Nutritional Index/ Diet Categorization	Head and Neck Cancer	Results	Conclusion
Chuang et al.	2011	Case-Control	INHANCE data (22 of 26 studies; Cases: 14,520; controls: 22,737)	Food frequency questionnaires to determine quartiles for fruit and vegetable intake and for red meat intake	HNC (oral, pharyngeal, laryngeal)	Increased fruit intake OR:0.52 (95%CI: 0.43–0.63) Increased vegetable intake OR: 0.66 (95% CI: 0.49–0.90) Increased red meat: OR 1.40 (95%CI: 1.13–1.74) Increased processed meat: OR 1.47 (95% CI: 1.14–1.65)	Increased fruit and vegetable intake decreased odds of HNC Increased red meat and processed meat intake increased risk HNC
Li et al.	2014	Cohort Study	NIH-AARP	Food frequency questionnaires to calculate: HEI-2005 score and aMED score	HNC (oral cavity, orohypopharynx, larynx)	HEI-2005: For men, higher HEI-2005 h 0.74 (95% CI: 0.61–0.89) Women higher HEI-2005 h 0.48 (95% CI: 0.33–0.70) aMED: For men, higher aMED associated with lower HNC risk (HR: 0.80; 95% CI: 0.64–1.01) and women (HR: 0.42; 95% CI: 0.24–0.74)	Higher HEI-2005 and aMED scores associated with lower risk of HNC

	Year	Study type	Cohort	Method	Cancer	Results	Conclusion
Lam et al.	2011	Cohort study	NIH-AARP	Food frequency questionnaires to calculate dietary fiber and grain intake	HNC (oral cavity, orohypopharynx, larynx)	Higher intake total fiber and total grains decreased HNC risk (HR: 0.77; 95% CI: 0.64–0.93; HR: 0.89; 95% CI: 0.80–0.99)	Total fiber and grain food intake inversely associated with HNC in women but not men
Freedman et al.	2008	Cohort study	NIH-AARP	Food frequency questionnaire to calculate portion sizes for fruits and vegetables and place in quintiles based on fruit and vegetable intake	HNC (oral cavity, orohypophayrnx, larynx, and squamous cell carcinomas of other anatomic head and neck sites)	Inverse association between total fruit and vegetable intake and HNC risk (HR: 0.94; 95% CI: 0.89–0.99)	Inverse association between total fruit and vegetable intake and HNC risk

Abbreviations: aMED, alternate Mediterranean diet; CHANCE, Carolina Head and Neck Cancer study; CI, confidence interval; E-DII, energy-adjusted diet inflammatory index; FFQ, food frequency questionnaire; HEI-2005, Health Eating Index-2005; HNC, head and neck cancer; HNSCC, head and neck squamous cell carcinoma; INHANCE, International Head and Neck Cancer Epidemiology consortium; MDS, Mediterranean diet score; MDS-HNC, Mediterranean diet score – head and neck cancer; NIH-AARP, National Institute of Health – American Association of Retired Persons; OR, odds ratio; RR, relative risk; SD, standard deviation.

associations with hearing loss.[51] No systematic reviews or meta-analyses exist evaluating current data linking diet to hearing loss in humans.

One of the first-line guideline recommendations for treating Meniere disease, as written in the International Consensus on the treatment of Meniere disease, is adopting a low salt diet[7]; however, a 2018 Cochrane review found that there is no evidence from randomized control trials to support or refute that these dietary changes would affect outcomes.[57] This further suggests how difficult diet is to study, especially in relationship to uncommon diseases or disorders in smaller medical specialties; yet the importance of diet is still presumed.

Diet and Laryngopharyngeal Reflux

Laryngopharyngeal reflux (LPR) is thought to be related to the direct and indirect effect of gastric content reflux causing morphologic changes in the upper aerodigestive tract.[58] The study of diet in relation to reflux has mostly been studied in the context of gastroesophageal reflux rather than LPR; however, due to the similarities in etiology, it has been suggested that diet may also play a role in LPR. The antireflux induction diet for LPR, first introduced by Koufman in 2011,[59] is defined as a low-acid, low-fat food diet for a minimum of 2 weeks. The purpose was to provide a basis for a long-term lifestyle change to potentially alter the mechanism and minimize the effects of LPR.

A systematic review of dietary modifications for LPR included 1 randomized control trial and 6 observational studies assessing the effect of LPR outcomes based on diet or dietary behavior. Dietary modifications, such as fasting, avoiding eating or drinking 2 to 3 hours before sleeping, consuming low-acid drink and food (including alkaline water and a plant-based, Mediterranean-style diet), and reduced consumption of fat, chocolate, and coffee were found to improve LPR symptoms. However, heterogeneity of studies and low certainty of evidence did not provide sufficient evidence for dietary recommendations in LPR patients.[60]

A group of 26 experts reviewed 72 studies to develop the Refluxogenic diet score (RDS), basing the final score on protective effects of raw and high-fibre vegetables and harmful effects of beverages high in sugar, caffeine, or alcohol.[61] These scores remain theoretic and require future studies for validation. Further research will provide guidance of using RDS in practice and its possible effects on patient outcomes.

Diet and Sinonasal Symptoms

A few, small studies have explored diet change and alteration of sinonasal symptoms. The studies mentioned below do not have the level of evidence to alter care guidelines but rather present areas where further research could prove enlightening.

In a small, randomized, double-blind control study in which subjects were studied for 8 days, Frosh and colleagues found subjective improvement in nasopharyngeal mucus production in patients randomized to a nondairy supplement when compared with patients randomized to a dairy supplement.[62] In a pilot, prospective case-control study, evaluating the effects of sugar intake on sinonasal symptoms in a pediatric population, Sawani and colleagues found that a 2 week decrease in sugar intake resulted in significant decrease in sinus infection and nasal obstruction scores (as defined by the Sinus and nasal quality of life survey; SN-5).[63]

A systematic review of 20 observational studies evaluating the relationship of dietary fibre intake with asthma, rhinitis, and lung function impairment found probable evidence for an inverse association between dietary fibre and chronic obstructive pulmonary disease but evidence regarding rhinitis and asthma were inconsistent.[64]

SUMMARY

Diet is one of the most important influences of human health and should be considered in the evaluating the health of otolaryngology patients. Although there is no consensus on the specific aspects of an optimal diet, there is strong agreement that an optimal eating pattern is plant-predominant and includes healthy, whole foods, whereas minimizing animal products and highly processed or ultraprocessed foods. Diet is understood to be an important factor in wound healing and surgical outcomes.

Associations have been recognized and documented between diet and otolaryngologic diseases and disorders; however, there are not overwhelmingly strong levels of evidence that exist for the associations mentioned and described in this article. Few to no systematic reviews that pool quantitative data are feasible because of inconsistencies across studies in how diet is defined and studied. Despite the lack of existing evidence, the complexity of how diet influences systemic physiology lends to the plausibility of its involvement in systems of the head and neck and should continue to be studied in a methodologically sound manner.

CLINICS CARE POINTS

- Healthy diets have similar underlying fundamental properties: high in fruits, vegetables, legumes, whole grains, nuts and seeds, and low in salt, ultraprocessed foods, red meats, and processed meats.

- Current guidelines suggest treating preoperative malnutrition in patients undergoing major surgeries. Oral supplementation of arginine with omega-3 may improve surgical wound healing in patients with head and neck cancer by decreasing incidence of postoperative complications and decreasing the length of hospital stay.

- Evidence is highly suggestive that higher fruit consumption decreases the risk of pharyngeal cancer and that higher vegetable consumption decreases the risk of oral cancer. Healthier diets, low in proinflammatory foods and high in fruit and vegetable consumption, may have a protective effect against developing certain types of head and neck cancer.

- Evidence suggests healthy diet may play a protective role in hearing loss; however, data are insufficient for definitive recommendations.

DISCLOSURE

H. Juszczak: Nothing to disclose. R. Rosenfeld: (1) Chief Medical Office for the American Board of Lifestyle Medicine, and (2) Sr. Liaison for Medical Society Relations for the American College of Lifestyle Medicine.

REFERENCES

1. Hippocrates. The genuine works of Hippocrates. London: Sydenham Society; 1849.
2. Hippocrates, Sprengell CJ. Aphorisms of Hippocrates: and the sentences of celsus; with explanations and references to the most considerable writers in physick and philosophy, both ancient and modern. London: R. Bonwick; 1708.
3. GBD 2017 Diet Collaborators. Health effects of dietary risks in 195 countries, 1990-2017: a systematic analysis for the Global Burden of Disease Study 2017. Lancet 2019;393(10184):1958–72.

4. Murray CJL, Atkinson C, Bhalla K, et al. The state of US health, 1990-2010: burden of diseases, injuries, and risk factors. JAMA 2013;310(6):591–608.
5. Unger T, Borghi C, Charchar F, et al. 2020 International society of hypertension global hypertension practice guidelines. Hypertension 2020;75(6):1334–57.
6. Gregg EW, Chen H, Wagenknecht LE, et al. Association of an intensive lifestyle intervention with remission of type 2 diabetes. JAMA 2012;308(23):2489–96.
7. Nevoux J, Barbara M, Dornhoffer J, et al. International consensus (ICON) on treatment of Ménière's disease. Eur Ann Otorhinolaryngol Head Neck Dis 2018; 135(1S):S29–32.
8. Ornish D, Scherwitz LW, Billings JH, et al. Intensive lifestyle changes for reversal of coronary heart disease. JAMA 1998;280(23):2001–7.
9. Bassin SR, Al-Nimr RI, Allen K, et al. The state of nutrition in medical education in the United States. Nutr Rev 2020;78(9):764–80.
10. Weaver CM, Miller JW. Challenges in conducting clinical nutrition research. Nutr Rev 2017;75(7):491–9.
11. Katz DL, Meller S. Can we say what diet is best for health? Annu Rev Public Health 2014;35:83–103.
12. Pollan M. In defense of food: an eater's manifesto. New York: Penguin Press; 2008.
13. MyPlate | U.S. Department of Agriculture. Available at: https://www.myplate.gov/. Accessed February 20, 2022.
14. Canada H. Welcome to Canada's food guide. 2021. Available at: https://food-guide.canada.ca/en/. Accessed February 20, 2022.
15. Reynolds A, Mann J, Cummings J, et al. Carbohydrate quality and human health: a series of systematic reviews and meta-analyses. Lancet 2019;393(10170): 434–45.
16. Katz DL. Lifestyle is medicine. Virtual Mentor 2013;15(4):286–92.
17. Aleksandrova K, Koelman L, Rodrigues CE. Dietary patterns and biomarkers of oxidative stress and inflammation: A systematic review of observational and intervention studies. Redox Biol 2021;42:101869.
18. Craddock JC, Neale EP, Peoples GE, et al. Vegetarian-Based Dietary Patterns and their Relation with Inflammatory and Immune Biomarkers: A Systematic Review and Meta-Analysis. Adv Nutr 2019;10(3):433–51.
19. Shah B, Newman JD, Woolf K, et al. Anti-Inflammatory Effects of a Vegan Diet Versus the American Heart Association-Recommended Diet in Coronary Artery Disease Trial. J Am Heart Assoc 2018;7(23):e011367.
20. Graf D, Di Cagno R, Fåk F, et al. Contribution of diet to the composition of the human gut microbiota. Microb Ecol Health Dis 2015;26. https://doi.org/10.3402/mehd.v26.26164.
21. Adler CJ, Dobney K, Weyrich LS, et al. Sequencing ancient calcified dental plaque shows changes in oral microbiota with dietary shifts of the Neolithic and Industrial revolutions. Nat Genet 2013;45(4):450–455e1.
22. Galvão-Moreira LV, da Cruz MCFN. Oral microbiome, periodontitis and risk of head and neck cancer. Oral Oncol 2016;53:17–9.
23. Wang L, Ganly I. The oral microbiome and oral cancer. Clin Lab Med 2014;34(4): 711–9.
24. Gong H, Shi Y, Zhou X, et al. Microbiota in the Throat and Risk Factors for Laryngeal Carcinoma. Appl Environ Microbiol 2014;80(23):7356–63.
25. Gentile CL, Weir TL. The gut microbiota at the intersection of diet and human health. Science 2018;362(6416):776–80.

26. Wild T, Rahbarnia A, Kellner M, et al. Basics in nutrition and wound healing. Nutrition 2010;26(9):862–6.
27. Arnold M, Barbul A. Nutrition and wound healing. Plast Reconstr Surg 2006;117(7 Suppl):42S–58S.
28. Ralph N, Brown L, McKillop KL, et al. Oral nutritional supplements for preventing surgical site infections: protocol for a systematic review and meta-analysis. Syst Rev 2020;9(1):37.
29. Wischmeyer PE, Carli F, Evans DC, et al. American society for enhanced recovery and perioperative quality initiative joint consensus statement on nutrition screening and therapy within a surgical enhanced recovery pathway. Anesth Analg 2018;126(6):1883–95.
30. Barker LA, Gout BS, Crowe TC. Hospital malnutrition: prevalence, identification and impact on patients and the healthcare system. Int J Environ Res Public Health 2011;8(2):514–27.
31. Jensen GL, Cederholm T, Correia MITD, et al. GLIM Criteria for the Diagnosis of Malnutrition: A Consensus Report From the Global Clinical Nutrition Community. JPEN J Parenter Enteral Nutr 2019;43(1):32–40.
32. Detsky AS, Baker JP, O'Rourke K, et al. Predicting nutrition-associated complications for patients undergoing gastrointestinal surgery. JPEN J Parenter Enteral Nutr 1987;11(5):440–6.
33. Kondrup J, Johansen N, Plum LM, et al. Incidence of nutritional risk and causes of inadequate nutritional care in hospitals. Clin Nutr 2002;21(6):461–8.
34. Weimann A, Braga M, Carli F, et al. ESPEN guideline: clinical nutrition in surgery. Clin Nutr 2017;36(3):623–50.
35. Saeg F, Orazi R, Bowers GM, et al. Evidence-based nutritional interventions in wound care. Plast Reconstr Surg 2021;148(1):226–38.
36. Daher GS, Choi KY, Wells JW, et al. A systematic review of oral nutritional supplement and wound healing. Ann Otol Rhinol Laryngol 2022;19. 34894211069437.
37. Papadimitriou N, Markozannes G, Kanellopoulou A, et al. An umbrella review of the evidence associating diet and cancer risk at 11 anatomical sites. Nat Commun 2021;12(1):4579.
38. Chen QJ, Ou L, Li K, et al. Meta-analysis of the relationship between Dietary Inflammatory Index and esophageal cancer risk. Medicine (Baltimore) 2020;99(49):e23539.
39. Morze J, Danielewicz A, Przybyłowicz K, et al. An updated systematic review and meta-analysis on adherence to mediterranean diet and risk of cancer. Eur J Nutr 2021;60(3):1561–86.
40. Divaris K, Olshan AF, Smith J, et al. Oral health and risk for head and neck squamous cell carcinoma: the Carolina Head and Neck Cancer Study. Cancer Causes Control 2010;21(4):567–75.
41. Winn DM, Lee YCA, Hashibe M, et al. Inhance consortium. the Inhance consortium: toward a better understanding of the causes and mechanisms of head and neck cancer. Oral Dis 2015;21(6):685–93.
42. Schatzkin A, Subar AF, Thompson FE, et al. Design and serendipity in establishing a large cohort with wide dietary intake distributions : the National Institutes of Health-American Association of Retired Persons Diet and Health Study. Am J Epidemiol 2001;154(12):1119–25.
43. Mazul AL, Shivappa N, Hébert JR, et al. Proinflammatory diet is associated with increased risk of squamous cell head and neck cancer. Int J Cancer 2018;143(7):1604–10.

44. Bradshaw PT, Siega-Riz AM, Campbell M, et al. Associations between dietary patterns and head and neck cancer: the Carolina head and neck cancer epidemiology study. Am J Epidemiol 2012;175(12):1225–33.

45. Saraiya V, Bradshaw P, Meyer K, et al. The association between diet quality and cancer incidence of the head and neck. Cancer Causes Control 2020;31(2): 193–202.

46. Chuang SC, Jenab M, Heck JE, et al. Diet and the risk of head and neck cancer: a pooled analysis in the INHANCE consortium. Cancer Causes Control 2012; 23(1):69–88.

47. Li WQ, Park Y, Wu JW, et al. Index-based dietary patterns and risk of head and neck cancer in a large prospective study. Am J Clin Nutr 2014;99(3):559–66.

48. Lam TK, Cross AJ, Freedman N, et al. Dietary fibre and grain consumption in relation to head and neck cancer in the NIH-AARP Diet and Health Study. Cancer Causes Control 2011;22(10):1405–14.

49. Freedman ND, Park Y, Subar AF, et al. Fruit and vegetable intake and head and neck cancer risk in a large United States prospective cohort study. Int J Cancer 2008;122(10):2330–6.

50. Spankovich C, Le Prell CG. The role of diet in vulnerability to noise-induced cochlear injury and hearing loss. J Acoust Soc Am 2019;146(5):4033.

51. Jung SY, Kim SH, Yeo SG. Association of nutritional factors with hearing loss. Nutrients 2019;11(2):307.

52. Rodrigo L, Campos-Asensio C, Rodríguez MÁ, et al. Role of nutrition in the development and prevention of age-related hearing loss: A scoping review. J Formos Med Assoc 2021;120(1 Pt 1):107–20.

53. Curhan SG, Halpin C, Wang M, et al. Prospective study of dietary patterns and hearing threshold elevation. Am J Epidemiol 2020;189(3):204–14.

54. Spankovich C, Le Prell CG. Healthy diets, healthy hearing: National Health and Nutrition Examination Survey, 1999-2002. Int J Audiol 2013;52(6):369–76.

55. Huang Q, Jin Y, Reed NS, et al. Diet quality and hearing loss among middle-older aged adults in the USA: findings from National Health and Nutrition Examination Survey. Public Health Nutr 2020;23(5):812–20.

56. Spankovich C, Bishop C, Johnson MF, et al. Relationship between dietary quality, tinnitus and hearing level: data from the national health and nutrition examination survey, 1999-2002. Int J Audiol 2017;56(10):716–22.

57. Hussain K, Murdin L, Schilder AG. Restriction of salt, caffeine and alcohol intake for the treatment of Ménière's disease or syndrome. Cochrane Database Syst Rev 2018;12:CD012173.

58. Lechien JR, Akst LM, Hamdan AL, et al. Evaluation and management of laryngopharyngeal reflux disease: state of the art review. Otolaryngol Head Neck Surg 2019;160(5):762–82.

59. Koufman JA. Low-acid diet for recalcitrant laryngopharyngeal reflux: therapeutic benefits and their implications. Ann Otol Rhinol Laryngol 2011; 120(5):281–7.

60. Min C, Park B, Sim S, et al. Dietary modification for laryngopharyngeal reflux: systematic review. J Laryngol Otol 2019;133(2):80–6.

61. Lechien JR, Bobin F, Mouawad F, et al. Development of scores assessing the refluxogenic potential of diet of patients with laryngopharyngeal reflux. Eur Arch Otorhinolaryngol 2019;276(12):3389–404.

62. Frosh A, Cruz C, Wellsted D, et al. Effect of a dairy diet on nasopharyngeal mucus secretion. Laryngoscope 2019;129(1):13–7.

63. Sawani A, Farhangi M, CA N, et al. Limiting dietary sugar improves pediatric sinonasal symptoms and reduces inflammation. J Med Food 2018;21(6): 527–34.
64. Sdona E, Georgakou AV, Ekström S, et al. Dietary fibre intake in relation to asthma, rhinitis and lung function impairment-a systematic review of observational studies. Nutrients 2021;13(10):3594.

Why Otolaryngologists Should Be Interested in Psychedelic Medicine

Benjamin F. Asher, MD

KEYWORDS

- Psychedelic • Ketamine • MDMA • Psilocybin

KEY POINTS

- Psychedelic medicine is on the leading edge in the mental health field.
- 3,4-Methylenedioxymethamphetamine-assisted psychotherapy is highly curative for post-traumatic stress disorder.
- Ketamine therapy is effective for treatment-resistant depression.
- Psilocybin therapy is highly effective for patients who have terminal cancer with end-of-life anxiety.
- The potential for new frontiers of research with these medicines is enormous.

INTRODUCTION

One only has to look at the mainstream media to realize that a psychedelic renaissance is upon us. Almost weekly magazine covers and bestselling books on the subject as well as countless articles on the Internet are showing up almost daily.[1,2] This intense public interest in the subject is not just a random phenomenon but is fueled by an outpouring of well designed, promising, clinical trials using legal (ketamine) and Schedule 1 drugs (3,4-methylenedioxymethamphetamine [MDMA], psilocybin, ayahuasca, and lysergic acid diethylamide [LSD]) for a number of challenging mental health-related issues. MDMA and psilocybin have been fast-tracked by the FDA for legalization pending phase 3 clinical trials which are underway. Once they are available and legal, clinical research using these powerful compounds will be much easier and clinicians from all medical disciplines might be interested in researching areas where these medicines could apply to their specialty. Ketamine, which is already legal, is currently being reexamined for potential uses in many new areas. The purpose of this article is to introduce the reader to what these molecules are, the clinical research and to discuss current applications and areas of future research for Otolaryngology–Head and Neck Surgery.

Private Practice, 174 West 4th Street, #163, New York, NY 10014, USA
E-mail address: drasher@asherent.com

Otolaryngol Clin N Am 55 (2022) 929–938
https://doi.org/10.1016/j.otc.2022.06.002
0030-6665/22/© 2022 Elsevier Inc. All rights reserved.

oto.theclinics.com

A BRIEF HISTORY OF PSYCHEDELICS

Humans throughout the world for thousands of years have used psychoactive plants for rituals and mystical experiences.[3] Although mescaline was identified in 1897 from peyote, a small cactus, by Arthur Heffter, a German pharmacologist, the most famous psychedelic chemical, LSD, was synthesized and then tested on himself in 1943 by the Swiss Chemist Albert Hoffman.[4]

Psychedelic mushrooms were introduced into popular culture by the amateur mycologist R. Gordon Wasson in 1955 who received them from the Mazatec shaman Maria Sabina. His trip to Mexico was documented in Life magazine.[3] (The term psychedelic was coined Dr Humphry Osmond, a British psychiatrist in 1957, meaning "manifesting the mind".)[5] Before the FDA rescheduling these compounds as Schedule 1, as having no medical value and high addiction potential, under the Nixon administration, a large amount of research was done on them in the 1950s and 1960s. Thousands of patients and research subjects received these psychedelic compounds, and hundreds of research articles were published in medical journals. Although some psychedelic research was done in the 1990s after it was determined that the FDA would allow such research, it was not until the early 2000s that researchers at Johns Hopkins University began doing well-controlled clinical research on high-dose psilocybin.[6] As I will discuss shortly, MDMA is not truly a psychedelic and ketamine was synthesized in 1962 by Calvin Stevens at Parke-Davis as an anesthetic agent, but it is being used at sub-anesthetic doses that can be psychedelic.

THE COMPOUNDS
3,4-Methylenedioxymethamphetamine

MDMA stimulates the release and inhibits the reuptake most potently of serotonin but also dopamine and norepinephrine.[7] It was initially synthesized in 1912 and patented in 1914 by the German pharmaceutical company Merk without any human studies.[8] In the late 1970s, the chemist Alexander Shulgin synthesized it for the purposes of supporting patients undergoing psychotherapy. Even though it was used underground at this time by psychotherapists, it was still legal but it was classed as a Schedule 1 drug in 1985 by the FDA.[9] MDMA also known as ecstasy is more properly categorized as an empathogen rather than a psychedelic.[8] It rarely induces hallucinations, but rather creates a sense of well-being, a lifting of fear and anxiety, and an ability to face difficult aspects of oneself with an openness to criticism.[8] These qualities that the drug induces allow it to be an ideal drug to be used during a psychotherapy session. In 1986, Rick Doblin founded the Multidisciplinary Association for Psychedelic Studies (MAPS) to promote further research into MDMA. MAPS, a nonprofit organization, has funded phase 2 and phase 3 clinical trials using MDMA-assisted psychotherapy for post-traumatic stress disorder (PTSD). In 2011, the first phase 2 placebo-controlled clinical trial was published, establishing that MDMA was safe and effective for patients with PTSD. Twenty patients were randomized into treatment and control groups, and both groups received psychotherapy. The treatment group had an 83% positive response to treatment with a reduction in their PTSD symptoms versus a 25% response in the placebo group. There were no significant side effects in the treatment group.[10] In a pooled analysis of six phase 2 clinical trials using MDMA-assisted psychotherapy for PTSD after two experimental treatment sessions, 54% of the treatment groups no longer fit the diagnostic criterion for PTSD versus only 22% of the control groups.[11] Because of its tremendous potential to be an effective treatment of PTSD, the FDA gave it "breakthrough therapy" status. The significance of this new treatment modality for PTSD, a condition that has evaded effective treatments to date cannot be underestimated. PTSD affects 7% to 8% of the population of the United States or about 31.3 million people at an estimated cost of $23 billion dollars a year.[12] As physicians, we see many of these people in our offices with somaticized anxiety disorders and are often uncomfortable with these conditions because of our lack of mental health training. The potential of this therapy to cure PTSD after a few treatment sessions and requiring no long-term psychotropic medications is promising.

Psilocybin

Psilocybin is the psychedelic compound found in "magic mushrooms." These mushrooms are members of the genus *Psilocybe* and grow throughout the world. *Psilocybe* mushrooms were known to the Aztecs as teonanacatl, translated as "flesh of the gods." Psilocybin (4-phosphoryloxy-N,N-dimethyltryptamine [DMT]) gets rapidly dephosphorylated in the intestinal mucosa to psilocin (N,N-DMT), which is the psychoactive psychedelic ingredient. Psilocin has a high affinity for the serotonin receptors 5-HT_{2A}, 5-HT_{2C}, and 5-HT_{1A} in the brain. Psilocybin also interacts with some non-serotoninergic receptors in the brain including dopaminergic and glutamatergic receptors. Psilocybin is considered a classical psychedelic based on the brain receptors that it acts upon.[4,6] Most of the clinical research studies that were done on the compound before it becoming Schedule 1 in the 1970s and in the past decade used or are using a chemically synthesized compound identical to the molecule in mushrooms. This allows for absolute control of dosing. The main significant research to date has focused on the following areas: the safety profile, treatment-resistant depression, alcohol and nicotine addiction, end-of-life depression and anxiety in patients with terminal cancer, and mystical experiences among religious leaders.

There have been 10 peer-reviewed published clinical trials from 1964 to the present on the treatment of patients who have advanced–terminal cancer with existential anxiety with a classical psychedelic. Three of those trials used psilocybin. The two most compelling randomized, double-blind, crossover trials included a total of 80 patients who have cancer with existential anxiety and they were treated with low-dose and high-dose psilocybin. At 6-month follow-up, both studies found that approximately 80% of the participants showed a decrease in depressed mood and anxiety. The apparent reduction in symptoms was attributed to the mystical experiences achieved with the high-dose psilocybin.[13]

Psilocybin combined with behavioral interventions has shown promise in the treatment of major depressive disorder. A meta-analysis of four small clinical trials, three of which were randomized, showed that the effects were large and statistically significant.[14] In an fMRI study of depressed patients dosed with psilocybin, there were unique alterations in cerebral blood flow and resting-state functional connectivity in various parts of the brain which were long lasting (5 weeks) and thought that related to the mood improvement from the medicine.[15] A phase 2 randomized double-blind controlled trial of 59 patients comparing psilocybin to escitalopram showed no difference between the two at 6 weeks. Secondary measures favored the psilocybin group but lacked correction for multiple comparisons. The psilocybin group received two doses of 25 mg psilocybin 6 weeks apart plus daily placebo and the escitaloprim group 1 mg of psilocybin 3 weeks apart and daily escitalprim.[16] There was a follow-up article in Nature describing the above study and an open-label trial of psilocybin 10 mg followed by 25 mg 7 days later in patients with treatment-resistant depression. Both trials resulted in a reduction in depressive symptoms in the psilocybin-treated patients with decreases in fMRI brain network modularity. The antidepressant response to escitalopram was milder, and there were no changes in brain network organization.[17]

Regarding tobacco and alcohol addiction, a small open-label trial of high-dose psilocybin of 15 patients with tobacco addiction found that 12/15 patients were tobacco free at 6 months. The mystical experience brought on by psilocybin was the basis for the effectiveness of the treatment. There are currently studies underway looking at psilocybin as a treatment for alcohol addiction.[18]

Ketamine

Ketamine is in the class of compounds called arylcyclohexylamines. It predominantly targets the excitatory neurotransmitter glutamate. Ketamine opposes this excitatory action by blocking the N-methyl-D-aspartate receptor (NMDA) and preventing it from being activated by glutamate. Ketamine also has effects either directly or indirectly on other receptors in the brain including μ-opioid, dopamine, serotonin. acetylcholine, and cannabinoid receptors.[19]

Ketamine was initially developed as an agent for general anesthesia that did not suppress respiration. The first article was published on the use of ketamine for treatment-resistant depression in 2006.[20] Since then more than 2000 articles have been published on the psychiatric uses of ketamine.[19] Ketamine can be administered orally, via a nasal spray, intramuscularly and intravenously. When used for depression it is given in sub-anesthetic doses, .5 to 2 mg/kg. At doses of .9 mg/kg and above, the patient can have a psychedelic experience (ego dissolving). Ketamine is also used in conjunction with psychotherapy, ketamine-assisted psychotherapy where the individual undergoes psychotherapy under the influence of the medicine.[19,21] Although the psychiatric use of ketamine remains off-label because no large RCTs have been done to satisfy the FDA standard for clinical indication, the prevailing evidence would appear that it will become an important tool in the armamentarium for some mood disorders.

OTHER PSYCHEDELICS

Although there are other psychedelic compounds, none of the following have undergone enough research to potentially get the FDA to reschedule them for clinical use: LSD, ayahuasca, N,N-DMT, 5-Meo-DMT, peyote, and ibogaine. I have included brief descriptions of each.

Lysergic Acid Diethylamide

LSD is derived from ergotamine which is produced by a fungus. It is well absorbed orally and has a potent affinity for serotonin and dopamine receptors especially the 5-HT$_{2A}$ receptor as is seen with other psychedelic compounds.[4] In spite of much research being done on it in the 1950s and 60s, it was moved to a Schedule 1 drug during the Nixon administration.

Ayahuasca

Ayahuasca is an ancient brew from the Amazon and has been used for thousands of years by the indigenous peoples who live there. There are no ethnographic data as to when people started using it. It is a combination of two plants, but not always the same ones. The psychedelic component comes from the stems of the vine *Banisteriopsis caapi* which contains N,N-DMT. The other component that is used can be from the leaves of the *Psychotria viridis* (chacruna) plant or *Diplopterys cabrerana* (chaliponga) plant. These plants provide beta-carboline alkaloids such as harmine and tetrahydroharmine. These compounds function as an MAO inhibitor, which allows the N,N-DMT to be active orally. These two plants are cooked together for several days to produce the psychoactive liquid.[22] N,N-DMT occurs widely in nature and is not just limited to the ayahuasca brew. It is found in other plants and also in the animal kingdom. Humans produce their own DMT.[23]

N,N-Dimethyltryptamine and 5-MeO-Dimethyltryptamine

These are fast-acting tryptamines that are both naturally occurring in the plant kingdom and produced in mammals and they have also been synthesized. The 5-MeO-DMT is also found in the poisonous secretions of a Sonoran Desert toad Bufo alvarius. They both act on the $5 HT_{2A}$ receptors. They are not active orally and must be smoked or injected. Research in the early 1990s by Rick Strassman looking at IV infusion of DMT was the first psychedelic research to be conducted after the rescheduling of these psychedelic molecules. There are no significant research data to date on the use of these molecules for medical or psychiatric conditions.[23]

Peyote

Mescaline, 3,4,5-trimethoxy-phenylethylamine, is a psychoactive compound found in various species of cactus, peyote (*Lophophora williamsii*) and San Pedro (*Echinopsis pachanoi*). It has a centuries old tradition of usage among the native peoples of North America. Carbon-dated samples of peyote have been found in an archeological site along the Rio Grande, Texas, dating to 5700 years ago. Religious use of peyote in the Native American Church is legally protected in the United States. The peyote cactus has lost much of its natural habitat and it is becoming endangered. Its mechanism of action as with the other classic psychedelics is as an agonist of the $5-HT_{2A}$ receptor. It is more weakly bound and therefore requires a higher dose to produce a psychedelic effect. There is little research currently in terms of clinical applications.[24]

Iboga and Ibogaine

Ibogaine is a monoterpene indole alkaloid which is found in the root bark of the Tabernanthe Iboga Baill bush in Gabon and West Central Africa. Among the peoples in West Central Africa practicing the Bwiti religion, it is a psychoactive sacrament and has been used for several centuries. The contemporary interest in this medicine is in its capacity to treat substance use disorders, especially detoxification from opioids. It is legal in several countries where detoxification clinics use this substance quite successfully.[25]

FUTURE DIRECTIONS (PSYCHEDELICS AND THE OTOLARYNGOLOGIST)

At first blush, it would appear that these medicines while having a broad range of uses in the mental health fields would not be particularly useful for those in otolaryngology. Although it is true that there are no current studies that I was able to find pointing to a direct use of psychedelics for an otolaryngologic disorder, this emerging and nascent field has plenty offer researchers in our specialty. First and foremost is the conundrum of intractable tinnitus. These patients often have treatment-resistant depression. Intratympanic injection of esketamine gel has been recently studied for synaptopathic tinnitus because cochlear NMDA receptor activation has been postulated as an etiology. To date, there is no phase 3 clinical trial proving its efficacy.[26,27] Although systemic administration of ketamine may not relieve tinnitus, it may relieve the depression associated with it.

In the area of head and neck oncology, there are a few potential avenues for study. First and foremost would be in palliative care for patients with incurable disease. Head and neck surgeons should know that this type of therapy will soon be available to their patients. Also, some patients often embark on extensive, disfiguring, operations which result in loss of function and loss of quality of life. People often choose these procedures because they are so fearful of dying that they are willing to do anything to prolong life for even a few months. Perhaps the mystical experience provided by psilocybin could inform a patient about whether that is the approach that they truly want to take. A patient from the end-of-life anxiety study and psilocybin had the following experience on high-dose psilocybin:

> *From here on, love was the only consideration. Everything that happened, anything and everything that was seen or heard centered on love. It was and is the only purpose. Love seemed to emanate from a single point of light .... it was so pure. The sheer joy .... The bliss was indescribable. And in fact, there are no words to accurately capture my experience .... my state ... I know I've had no earthly pleasure that's ever come close to this feeling ... no sensation, no image of beauty, nothing during my time on earth has felt as pure and joyful and glorious as the height of this journey. I was beginning to wonder if men spent too much time and effort at things unimportant ... trying to accomplish so much ... When really, it was all so simple. No matter the subject it all came down to the same thing: love. Earthly matters such as food, music, architecture, anything, everything ... Aside from love, seemed silly and trivial. I thought about my cancer but only briefly. I took a tour of my lungs. I could see some things. But it was more a matter of feeling the inside of my lungs. I remember breathing deeply to help facilitate the seeing. There were nodules but they seemed rather unimportant ... I was being told (without words) to not worry about the cancer ... It's minor in the scheme of things ... Simply an imperfection of your humanity and that the more important matter... The real work to be done before you. Again love. Undoubtedly, my life has changed in ways I may never fully comprehend. But I now have an understanding... An awareness that goes beyond intellect ... That my life, that every life, and all that is the universe equals one thing . . . Love.[28]*

There is an emerging body of research looking at the effects of psychedelics on inflammation and immunity. Classic psychedelics exert effects on both the innate and adaptive aspects of the immune system. Some of this is through the interaction with the multiple subtypes of the 5-HT serotonin receptors resulting in a decrease in the production of inflammatory cytokines. Studies have shown that psychedelics inhibit TNF-α-mediated inflammatory pathways via the 5-HT$_{2A}$ subtype. In vivo studies have shown that one psychedelic, R-DOI (not mentioned in this article) through the inhibition of TNF and the inflammatory cytokines IL-1β and IL-6 had anti-allergic asthma effects in low doses in a mouse allergic asthma model. DMT and 5-MEO-DMT in the in vitro models markedly reduce the activation of T-lymphocytes into effector Th1 and Th17 subtypes which are known to be involved in autoimmune and autoinflammatory conditions.[29]

As mentioned previously, PTSD is a condition that affects millions of people. Forty-four percent of women and 25% of men in the United States have experienced some form of sexual violence.[30] Clinical studies are beginning to show that a history of trauma can result in increased risk for a physical disease. In a longitudinal study, women in midlife who had a history of being assaulted were found to have a three to fourfold increase in carotid plaque scores compared with their non-assaulted counter parts.[31] Although the epidemiology of physical and emotional trauma as an etiology for disease has not been well studied, the above carotid plaque study certainly makes one wonder what we are missing given the prevalence of violence in our society. It has been my clinical experience that most people underestimate the effect of trauma in their lives. I saw a patient who was repeatedly being seen in the emergency room because he felt like his throat was closing off. He wanted me to reassure him that nothing was wrong with his airway. After determining that his airway was fine, I discussed anxiety as a possible etiology of his symptoms and he was interested in trying ketamine to see if he could gain some insight into his condition. While under ketamine, he relived a childhood experience of watching a friend in his neighborhood being struck and killed by a moving vehicle. He had never spoken to anyone of this trauma before. Following the ketamine experience, all of his throat issues disappeared, and he has been symptom-free for a year. I would venture to say that many of our patients with globus symptoms that do not respond to reflux treatment fall into this category. Up to 96% of patients with globus symptoms report an exacerbation during times of high emotional intensity.[32] I would assume that there may be some connections to diseases in our specialty, including hand and neck cancer, which are so closely related to nicotine and alcohol addiction. Having a treatment protocol that so effectively treats PTSD like MDMA-assisted psychotherapy could potentially go a long way to preventing some illnesses. Given the fact that alcoholism and nicotine addiction are known contributors to diseases of the head and neck, if the current studies underway reveal that high dose psilocybin therapy helps these conditions, otolaryngologists should know about it.

At the time of this writing, we are two and a half years into the global Covid-19 pandemic and stress and burn out among health care practitioners would appear to be at an all-time high.[33] Symptoms of burnout include emotional exhaustion, depersonalization, and a sense of reduced personal accomplishment. Solutions for physician burnout include mindfulness-based stress reduction and developing organizational practice modifications.[34] Given the capacity for psychedelic medicines to provide deep insight into the human condition, perhaps, in the future, psychedelic therapy could be a tool for physicians to recover the joy of being in the healing arts.

SUMMARY

Although otolaryngologists are not mental health practitioners, the mental health of many patients has a large impact on their physical well-being as well as treatment-related outcomes. Psychedelic medicines represent a new horizon in mental health with the potential to treat some chronic mental health conditions that have previously not fared well with the current treatment options. Some understanding of these new medicines, their indications and contraindications, and their potential to serve patients in our specialty will be helpful to head and neck physicians as they become legalized and used in mainstream medicine.

DISCLOSURE

Investor in CaaMTech, Onsero, Noetic Psychedelic Fund.

REFERENCES

1. Depression: doctors are turning to ketamine for treatment | time. Available at: https://time.com/4876098/new-hope-for-depression/. Accessed December 28, 2021.
2. Pollan M. How to change your mind: what the new science of psychedelics teaches us about consciousness, dying, addiction, depression, and transcendence. New York, NY: Penguin Books; 2019.
3. McKenna D. Plants for the people: the future of psychedelic therapies in the age of biomedicine. In: Grob CS, Grigsby J, editors. Handbook of medical

hallucinogens. New York, NY: The Guilford Press; 2021. p. 29–45. Available at: http://public.eblib.com/choice/PublicFullRecord.aspx?p=6465149. Accessed February 23, 2022.

4. Nichols DE, Nichols CC. The pharmacology of psychedelics. In: Grob CS, Grigsby J, editors. Handbook of medical hallucinogens. New York, NY: The Guilford Press; 2021. p. 3–28.

5. Mangini M. A short strange trip: LSD politics, publicity, and mythology-from discovery to criminalization. In: Grob CS, Grigsby J, editors. Handbook of medical hallucinogens. New York, NY: The Guilford Press; 2021. Available at: http://public.eblib.com/choice/PublicFullRecord.aspx?p=6465149. Accessed February 23, 2022.

6. Ross S, Franco S, Reiff C, et al. Psilocybin. In: Grob CS, Grigsby J, editors. Handbook of medical hallucinognes. New York, NY: The Guilford Press; 2021. p. 181–214.

7. de la Torre R, Farré M, Ortuño J, et al. Non-linear pharmacokinetics of MDMA ('ecstasy') in humans. Br J Clin Pharmacol 2000;49(2):104–9.

8. Mithoefer Michael, Mithoefer Annie. MDMA. In: Grob CS, Grigsby J, editors. Handbook of medical hallucinogens. New York, NY: The Guilford Press; 2021. p. 233–63. Available at: http://public.eblib.com/choice/PublicFullRecord.aspx?p=6465149. Accessed February 28, 2022.

9. Passie T. History of the use of hallucinogens in psychiatric treatment. In: Grob CS, Grigsby J, editors. Handbook of medical hallucinogens. New York, NY: The Guilford Press; 2021. p. 95–118. Available at: http://public.eblib.com/choice/PublicFullRecord.aspx?p=6465149. Accessed February 28, 2022.

10. Mithoefer MC, Wagner MT, Mithoefer AT, et al. The safety and efficacy of {+/-}3,4-methylenedioxymethamphetamine-assisted psychotherapy in subjects with chronic, treatment-resistant posttraumatic stress disorder: the first randomized controlled pilot study. J Psychopharmacol 2011;25(4):439–52.

11. Mithoefer MC, Feduccia AA, Jerome L, et al. MDMA-assisted psychotherapy for treatment of PTSD: study design and rationale for phase 3 trials based on pooled analysis of six phase 2 randomized controlled trials. Psychopharmacology (Berl) 2019;236(9):2735–45.

12. Keane TM, Marshall AD, Taft CT. Posttraumatic stress disorder: etiology, epidemiology, and treatment outcome. Annu Rev Clin Psychol 2006;2:161–97.

13. Ross S, Bossis A, Guss J, et al. Rapid and sustained symptom reduction following psilocybin treatment for anxiety and depression in patients with life-threatening cancer: a randomized controlled trial. J Psychopharmacol 2016;30(12):1165–80.

14. Goldberg SB, Pace BT, Nicholas CR, et al. The experimental effects of psilocybin on symptoms of anxiety and depression: a meta-analysis. Psychiatry Res 2020;284:112749.

15. Carhart-Harris RL, Roseman L, Bolstridge M, et al. Psilocybin for treatment-resistant depression: fMRI-measured brain mechanisms. Sci Rep 2017;7(1):13187.

16. Carhart-Harris R, Giribaldi B, Watts R, et al. Trial of Psilocybin versus Escitalopram for Depression. N Engl J Med 2021;384(15):1402–11. https://doi.org/10.1056/NEJMoa2032994.

17. Daws RE, Timmermann C, Giribaldi B, et al. Increased global integration in the brain after psilocybin therapy for depression. Nat Med 2022;1–8. https://doi.org/10.1038/s41591-022-01744-z.

18. Garcia-Romeu A, Griffiths RR, Johnson MW. Psilocybin-occasioned mystical experiences in the treatment of tobacco addiction. Curr Drug Abuse Rev 2014;7(3): 157–64.

19. Kolp E, Friedman H. Ketamine psychedelic psychotherapy: Focus on its pharmacology, phenomenology, and clinical applications. In: Wolfson P, Hartelius G, Multidisciplinary Association for Psychedelic Studies, editors. The ketamine papers: science, therapy, and transformation. Santa Cruz, CA: Multidisciplinary Association for Psychedelic Studies; 2016. p. 97–197.

20. Zarate CA, Singh JB, Carlson PJ, et al. A randomized trial of an N-methyl-D-aspartate antagonist in treatment-resistant major depression. Arch Gen Psychiatry 2006;63(8):856–64.

21. Bravo G, Grant R, Bennett R. Ketamine. In: Grob CS, Grigsby J, editors. Handbook of medical hallucinogens. New York, NY: The Guilford Press; 2021. p. 327–44. Available at: http://public.eblib.com/choice/PublicFullRecord.aspx? p=6465149. Accessed February 28, 2022.

22. De Araujo DB, Tofoli LF, Rehen S, et al. Biological and psychological mechanisms underlying the therapeutic use of ayahuasca. In: Grob CS, Grigsby J, editors. Handbook of medical hallucinogens. New York, NY: The Guilford Press; 2021. p. 277–93. Available at: http://public.eblib.com/choice/PublicFullRecord.aspx? p=6465149. Accessed March 1, 2022.

23. Lancelotta R, Davis A. Therapeutic potential of fast-acting synthetic tryptamines. In: Grob CS, Grigsby J, editors. Handbook of medical hallucinogens. New York, NY: The Guilford Press; 2021. p. 215–32. Available at: http://public.eblib.com/ choice/PublicFullRecord.aspx?p=6465149. Accessed March 1, 2022.

24. Van Derveer W. Mescaline. In: Grob CS, Grigsby J, editors. Handbook of medical hallucinogens. New York, NY: The Guilford Press; 2021. p. 227–32. Available at: http://public.eblib.com/choice/PublicFullRecord.aspx?p=6465149.   Accessed March 1, 2022.

25. Alper K. The ibogaine project: urban ethnomedicine for opioid use disorder. In: Grob CS, Grigsby J, editors. Handbook of medical hallucinogens. New York, NY: The Guilford Press; 2021. p. 294–312. Available at: http://public.eblib.com/ choice/PublicFullRecord.aspx?p=6465149. Accessed March 1, 2022.

26. van de Heyning P, Muehlmeier G, Cox T, et al. Efficacy and safety of AM-101 in the treatment of acute inner ear tinnitus–a double-blind, randomized, placebo-controlled phase II study. Otol Neurotol 2014;35(4):589–97.

27. Bing D, Lee SC, Campanelli D, et al. Cochlear NMDA receptors as a therapeutic target of noise-induced tinnitus. Cell Physiol Biochem 2015;35(5):1905–23.

28. Bossis A. Utility of psychedelics in the treatment of psychospiritual and existential distress in palliative care: a promising therapeutic paradigm. In: Grob CS, Grigsby J, editors. Handbook of medical hallucinogens. New York, NY: The Guilford Press; 2021. p. 441–73. Available at: http://public.eblib.com/choice/ PublicFullRecord.aspx?p=6465149. Accessed February 28, 2022.

29. Szabo A. Effects of psychedelics on inflammation and immunity. In: Winkelman M, Sessa B, editors. Advances in psychedelic medicine: state-of-the-art therapeutic applications. Santa Barbara, CA: Praeger, an imprint of ABC-CLIO, LLC; 2019. Available at: http://search.ebscohost.com/ login.aspx?direct=true&scope=site&db=nlebk&db=nlabk&AN=2031907. Accessed February 23, 2022.

30. Smith: The national intimate partner and sexual violence... - Google Scholar. Available   at: https://scholar.google.com/scholar_lookup?title=The+National+Intim ate+Partner+And+Sexual+Violence+Survey+(NISVS):+2015+Data+Brief%E2

%80%94Updated+Release&publication_year=2018&. Accessed February 3, 2022.

31. Thurston RC, Jakubowski K, Chang Y, et al. Sexual assault and carotid plaque among midlife women. J Am Heart Assoc 2021;10(5):e017629.

32. Lee BE, Kim GH. Globus pharyngeus: a review of its etiology, diagnosis and treatment. World J Gastroenterol 2012;18(20):2462–71.

33. Amanullah S, Ramesh Shankar R. The impact of COVID-19 on physician burnout globally: a review. Healthcare (Basel) 2020;8(4):E421.

34. West CP, Dyrbye LN, Shanafelt TD. Physician burnout: contributors, consequences and solutions. J Intern Med 2018;283(6):516–29.

Probiotics for Otolaryngologic Disorders

Agnes Czibulka, MD*

KEYWORDS

- Probiotics • Microbiome • Laryngopharyngeal reflux • Sinusitis • Otitis media
- Microflora

KEY POINTS

- Understanding the microbiome and diet connection.
- The role of microbiota of the gastrointestinal system in human health.
- Probiotics used in specific otolaryngologic conditions such as laryngopharyngeal reflux, sinusitis, and otitis media.

INTRODUCTION

Many chronic conditions such as cardiovascular disease, neurodegenerative disease, and cancer, as well as chronic infections such as sinusitis and otitis media have one thing in common: they all have low level of chronic inflammation at their root. The standard Western diet contains an overabundance of processed foods that are high in saturated fatty acids, trans-fatty acids, refined carbohydrates, and sodium. The anti-inflammatory diet contains minimal processed foods and is full of monounsaturated and omega-3 polyunsaturated fatty acids. It is composed of nuts, vegetables, seeds, legumes, whole grains, and lean protein. Both the Mediterranean and the traditional Asian dietary patterns have combinations of foods that reduce chronic systemic inflammation. The Mediterranean diet is a plant-based diet with three to nine servings of vegetables, two servings of fruits, one to three servings of whole grains a day. Accumulating evidence indicates that the five most important adaptations induced by the Mediterranean dietary pattern are:

1. Lipid-lowering effect
2. Protection against oxidative stress, inflammation, and platelet aggregation
3. Modification of hormones and growth factors involved in the pathogenesis of cancer
4. Inhibition of nutrient-sensing pathways by specific amino acid restriction
5. Gut microbiota-mediated production of metabolites influencing metabolic health.[1]

Yale University, Quinnipiac University, 6 Burgis Lane, Guilford 06437, USA
* Corresponding author. North Haven, ENT Medical and Surgical Group, 31 Broadway, North Haven, CT 06437
E-mail address: aczibulka@gmail.com

Otolaryngol Clin N Am 55 (2022) 939–946
https://doi.org/10.1016/j.otc.2022.06.003
0030-6665/22/© 2022 Elsevier Inc. All rights reserved.

Research on the association between diet and inflammatory markers has studied many components of the Mediterranean diet, finding a decrease of numerous inflammatory markers such as decreased C-reactive protein (CRP), Interleukin (IL)-6, IL-1B, and reduced low-density lipoprotein (LDL) and tumor necrosis factor (TNF)-α.[2]

There is no single Asian diet, but generalizations can be made. Similar to the Mediterranean diet, Asian diets are composed of unprocessed, nutrient-dense foods. A variety of seeds, nuts, soy, whole grains, vegetables, and lean proteins like fish are included. Whole soy products such as edamame, tofu, and tempeh are consumed daily, providing a variety of nutrients and phytochemicals including vitamin C, magnesium, calcium, and potassium. *Fermented vegetables such as kimchi enrich this diet with probiotic lactic acid bacteria.* An inverse association was found between soy food consumption and interleukin-6, TNF-α, and soluble TNF receptors 1 and 2.[3] Another staple of the Asian diet are mushrooms. They are rich in anti-inflammatory components, such as polysaccharides, phenolic and indolic compounds, mycosteroids, fatty acids, and vitamins.[4] *Mushrooms act as prebiotics to foster the growth of healthy gut microbiota.* Mushrooms are one of the few natural food sources of vitamin D that is important for vegetarians. Traditionally, shiitake mushrooms are used for diseases that involve depressed immune function such as environmental allergies, fungal infections, frequent flu and colds, bronchial inflammation, infectious diseases, heart disease, and hypertension. Antibiotic, anticarcinogenic, antiviral, and immunogenic compounds have been isolated both intracellularly and extracellularly from shiitake mushrooms. In a study after 4 weeks of shiitake mushroom consumption, increased T-cell and natural killer (NK) T-cell proliferation and activity and increased IL-4, IL-10, and TNF-α was found. *An increase in serum (IgA) implies improved gut immunity.*[5]

The Human Microbiome

The term "microbiome" refers to the community of fungi, viruses, and bacteria in a location, the latter being the most prominent. Today, it is known that 50% of all cells within the human body are not of human origin, and over 90% of microorganisms do not routinely cause disease. These microorganisms are understood to play essential roles in maintaining the health and normal physiologic function of the human body. These microorganisms are found throughout the body, from the oral cavity to the stomach, lung, intestinal, and urogenital tracts. Each of these locations has its own unique set of microbes that is influenced by many factors including age, sex, genetics, environment, diet, and lifestyle.

The microbiota of the gastrointestinal (GI) tract is essential for the proper functioning of several physiologic systems, including the immune, digestive, and nervous systems. The microflora participates in the digestive system by supporting the breakdown of complex carbohydrates and by producing vitamins and nutrients, including vitamin K and B12, niacin, pyridoxine, and others.[6] It also functions as the first line of defense in the digestive tract and participates in the training of the developing immune system. Microflora takes part in detoxification and in the modulation of the nervous system through the gut-brain axis.[7–10]

In 2008, the National Institute of Health funded the Human Microbiome Project to analyze the human microbiome and determine its role in human health and disease. As a result, the taxonomic distribution, prevalence, and abundance of microbial taxa that inhabit a healthy human body sites were codified.[11] The project concluded that the microbiome begins at birth, whether via cesarean section or vaginal delivery. Unlike the human genome, the human microbiome does not seem to be passed down through generations but may be genetically influenced. There is no evidence for a core microbiome either within an individual or within a population. However, 40% of the microbiome genes are shared by 50% of the population. It changes as an individual ages but stays remarkably constant from childhood through middle adulthood. Bacterial cells are seen in a 1:1 ratio with human cells. There is a close association between the human microbiome and the external environment, including the lifestyle factors. There is evidence for a close association and interaction between the mucosal immune system and the human microbiome. *Antibiotic usage greatly affects the human microbiome on a short term and permanent basis through selection of resistant organisms, horizontal gene transfer, and by long-term alteration of the microbiota.*

The human intestines contain more than 100 trillion microorganisms that maintain a symbiotic relationship with the host. The upper portion of the digestive tract has low quantities of bacteria, most of that are aerobes, whereas the lower portion of the GI system contains high densities of microbes most of that are anaerobes. The quality and quantity of microflora and their metabolites are constantly altered by host's dietary choices, stress, and antibiotic exposure to name only a few.

Probiotics are used for the prevention and in some instances for the treatment of specific diseases because appropriate probiotic therapy can optimize systemic and local immune system activity. The data specific to respiratory tract infections are relatively sparse but point to potential benefits in duration and severity of illness. Most studies do not support a role for probiotic therapy as a preventive measure against respiratory tract infections. As antibiotic administration often alters the gut microflora balance, there can be an important role for a course of probiotic therapy to prevent antibiotic-associated diarrhea and the alteration of the microbiome.

Recent research is expanding toward disease-specific use of probiotics. Intestinal bacteria have been shown to participate in the regulation of psychological processes. Two studies from 2016 showed the importance of *Lactobacillus* and *Bifidobacterium* families in depression and anxiety.[7,8] *Lactobacillus sp* are shown to prevent diarrhea associated with antibiotics. *Bifidobacterium infantis* has been successfully used in the treatment of irritable bowel syndrome. *Clostridium difficile* colitis is treated with *Saccharomyces boulardii*. Transfer of intestinal flora through fecal bacterial therapy from one individual to another was first studied in 1958. The cure rate for chronic and recurrent *C difficile* is 90% with fecal bacterial therapy. Studies have shown that *Lactobacillus reuteri* can accelerate gastric emptying time and decrease regurgitation episodes in infants. *Bifidobacterium lactis* has been found to decrease whole gut transit time in a dose-dependent manner and also decrease functional GI symptoms, including vomiting, regurgitation, abdominal pain, nausea, and gurgling. The above-mentioned studies support the efficacy of probiotics in maintaining healthy gut microbiota with potential beneficial effects on reflux.[12–20]

Manufacturers differ in their recommendations on best probiotic therapy, but most agree that to minimize exposure to gastric acid, probiotics should be taken on an empty stomach. Some brands pasteurize products, which kills the bacteria. This unfortunately nullifies their medicinal powers, so it is crucial to find brands that are labeled raw or unpasteurized. Daily dosage for infants is 1 to 10 billion CFU and 10 to 20 billion CFU for older children and adults. Caution should be taken when considering probiotic therapy in immunocompromised patients and premature infants.

Regular consumption of foods that support diverse microorganisms can be simple. Prebiotic and probiotic foods are becoming more widely available in supermarkets. Prebiotics are indigestible food components (dietary fibers) that support the growth of beneficial gut microbiota in the colon. Foods rich in prebiotics are onions, garlic, leeks, bananas, artichokes, soybeans, asparagus, and whole wheat foods. Fermented foods rich in probiotics include sauerkraut, miso, kombucha, kimchi, pickled vegetables, tempeh, and cultured dairy foods that contain live bacteria such as bifido-bacteria and lactobacilli.

Some of the most interesting new areas of research are the interplay of our environment, diet, and genetics to modulate the risk of common diseases. Recent research shows that healthy fat intake with increased mono and polyunsaturated fat and decreased saturated fat over 2 years partially restores a healthy gut microbiome in obese patients with coronary heart disease, depending on the degree of metabolic dysfunction.[21] Studies also suggest that genetically susceptible individuals develop intolerance to dysregulated gut microflora and chronic inflammation develops as a result of environmental triggers, resulting in inflammatory bowel disease. Nutritional interventions such as the specific carbohydrate diet, the low fermentable oligosaccharides, disaccharides, monosaccharides, polyol diet, and the Mediterranean diet have shown strong anti-inflammatory properties and great promise for improving disease symptoms in inflammatory bowel disease.

We have begun to rethink our view on the trillions of microorganisms that inhabit the human body. Instead of invaders, one can view the microbiota as part of a very efficient mutualistic ecosystem.

Laryngopharyngeal Reflux

Gastroesophageal reflux disease (GERD) and laryngopharyngeal reflux (LPR) are largely driven by Western lifestyle. Poor diet, being overweight, and chronic stress are all contributing factors. Dietary advice and proton-pump inhibitors (PPIs) are the mainstream treatment plan. Unfortunately, prolonged PPI therapy can result in poor absorption of essential nutrients, including calcium, iron, magnesium, and vitamins.[22] Long-term use is associated with multiple diseases. PPIs double the rates of *C difficile* colitis and bacterial colonization with resistant microbes in intensive care unit settings. Chronic acid inhibition may lead to bacterial overgrowth of the stomach and proximal small intestine. Research shows that patients treated with PPIs carry an increased load of intragastric bacteria.[23] PPIs reduce gastric acidity and in fact current use of PPIs is associated with an increased risk of bacterial gastroenteritis.[24] PPIs are also associated with an increased risk of community-acquired pneumonia.[25] PPIs are one of the most frequent causes of drug-induced acute interstitial nephritis.[26]

Other means to treat LPR are lifestyle modifications, diet, weight loss, exercise, positional sleep, and alternative treatments with herbal therapies. Most of these data are based on studies done for GERD. Multiple small meals throughout the day are preferred. The evening meal should be 3 to 6 hours before planned nighttime sleep. Avoidance of late meals has shown decreased gastric and esophageal acidity.[27] Koufman and colleagues showed the advantage of a strict low-acid diet in PPI-resistant LPR patients.[28] This temporary 2-week-long diet avoids foods with pH less than 4 as well as chocolate, caffeine, citrus and spicy and acidic foods.

Plants that assist the diet are demulcent herbs containing mucilaginous materials to directly coat and soothe the lining of the GI tract. They are ingested before meals to coat and protect the mucosa. Commonly used demulcent plants include aloe vera, marshmallow root, slippery elm root, and licorice root. Licorice root has long been used for gastric inflammation because of its muco-protective effect. The deglycyrrhizinated licorice (DGL) is recommended for long-term use to avoid side effects from its mineralocorticoid properties. DGL is taken in a chewable tablet before meals and at bedtime, in dosage ranging from 700 to 1200 mg, with a maximum daily dose of 5000 mg. Another herbal product is Iberogast that contains the following herbs: lemon balm, licorice, peppermint, chamomile flower, milk thistle, caraway, celandine, candytuft, and angelica root. It is fast-acting and effectively relieves stomach pain, bloating, gas, heartburn, and diarrhea. It also increases gastric motility.[29]

Otitis Media, Sinusitis, and Allergic Rhinitis

Infections (viral, bacterial or fungal) and allergies are the most common causes of sinusitis and otitis media. Otitis media is one of the most common health problems in children. The cause of otitis media is unclear, but it is frequently associated with eustachian tube dysfunction. Similarly, sinusitis will develop when the normal drainage passageway of the sinuses is obstructed either by inflammation or by anatomic abnormalities. Dietary factors in both cases are related to the consumption of large amounts of refined sugar and have been shown to impair immune function. Ingestion of 100 g of sucrose, fructose, or glucose caused a transient decrease in the ability of neutrophils to phagocytose bacteria.[30]

Acute and Secretory Otitis Media

Seventeen randomized controlled trials (RCTs) of children with acute otitis media (AOM) were analyzed to compare with the effect of probiotics with placebo to groups of usual care. The probiotic strains used in the studies varied; 11 of them used *Lactobacillus*-containing probiotics and 6 RCTs used *Streptococcus*-containing probiotics. It was found that one-third of children not prone to AOM, taking probiotics experienced acute middle ear infections as compared with children not taking probiotics. Unfortunately, probiotics did not help children prone to AOM episodes. Probiotics also decreased the proportion of children taking antibiotics for any infection.[31]

A few smaller sample size studies showed promising results with *Streptococcus* strains either taken orally or in a nasal spray form to prevent or treat secretory otitis media (SOM).[32]

A double-blind pilot study with 60 children using *Streptococcus sanguinis* significantly increased spontaneous recovery from SOM.[32]

In a double-blind randomized placebo-controlled study, 108 children were given streptococcal or placebo nasal spray. The results proved a significant improvement in the probiotic group to be protected against recurrent AOM and SOM.[33]

In an uncontrolled pilot study of 22 children prone to AOM in 2015, those used oral *Streptococcus salivarius* tablets were found to have reduced frequency of recurrent AOM episodes.[34]

Chronic Rhinosinusitis and Allergic Rhinitis

Emre and colleagues reviewed 33 RCTs to assess the effect of probiotics on upper respiratory infections (URIs) and found decreasing incidence of URIs and severity of symptoms when probiotics were used.[35]

Chronic rhinosinusitis (CRS) patients show reductions in markers of biodiversity. The sinonasal microbiota is altered by medical and surgical treatments. The presence of dysbiosis in CRS was studied by Psaltis and Wormald.[36] A 6-month course of bacterial immunostimulant comprised cells and autolysate of human *Enterococcus faecalis* bacteria-reduced acute exacerbation in CRS in an RCT was reported by Habermann and colleagues[37]

Other studies demonstrated that a short-term administration of a 2 or 4 weeks regimen with probiotic *E faecalis* as adjuvant therapy or topical lactic acid did not result in a significant benefit.[38,39]

In allergic rhinitis multiple studies have found some benefits of adjuvant probiotics therapy either added to steroid nasal sprays[40] or oral antihistamines.[41] Coadministration of *Clostridium butyricum* with immunotherapy improved symptoms and medication scores but suppressed serum-specific Immunoglobulin E (IgE) and T help-er type 2 (Th2) levels.[42]

Oral Cavity

The oral microbiota is frequently altered by antibiotics, poor oral hygiene, and a high-sugar diet, as well as medical conditions including diabetes, radiation therapy, immu-nocompromised status, bacterial, and yeast infections.

Probiotics were found to be superior as compared with placebo in both preventing and treating oral candidiasis in the elderly and denture wearers.[43]

Even a 1-week course of a probiotic mouth rinse was as effective as chlorhexidine for candidiasis in children.[44]

Promising results for conservative management of recurrent chronic adenoid and tonsillar inflammation in children were found after a 3-month course of a twice daily oral spray probiotic suspension. The spray contained S salivarius and Streptococcus oralis and was compared with placebo in group A beta-hemolytic Streptococcus-infected children.[45]

SUMMARY

Probiotics have potential benefits on otolaryngologic diseases, including laryngophar-yngeal reflux, allergic rhinitis, chronic sinusitis, and upper respiratory tract infections.

They have an important role to prevent antibiotic-associated diarrhea and alteration of the microbiome when antibiotics are administered. Prebiotics and probiotics rich foods with healthy fat intake support a healthy gut and help to prevent inflammatory processes.

REFERENCES

1. Tosti V, Bertozzi B, Fontana L. Health benefits of the Mediterranean Diet: meta-bolic and molecular mechanisms. J Gerontol A Biol Sci Med Sci 2018;73(3):318–26.
2. Mazzocchi A, Leone L, Agostoni C, et al. The Secrets of the Mediterranean Diet. Does [Only] Olive Oil Matter? Nutrients 2019;11(12):2941.
3. Wu SH, Shu XO, Chow WH, et al. Soy food intake and circulating levels of inflam-matory markers in Chinese women. J Acad Nutr Diet 2012;112(7):996–1004.
4. Muszyńska B, Grzywacz-Kisielewska A, Kała K, et al. Anti-inflammatory proper-ties of edible mushrooms: A review. Food Chem 2018;243:373–81.
5. Dai X, Stanilka JM, Rowe CA, et al. Consuming Lentinula edodes (Shiitake) mush-rooms daily improves human immunity: A randomized dietary intervention in healthy young adults. J Am Coll Nutr 2015;34(6):478–87.
6. LeBlanc JG, Milani C, de Giori GS, et al. Bacteria as vitamin suppliers to their host: a gut microbiota perspective. Curr Opin Biotechnol 2013;24(2):160–8.
7. Sarkar A, Lehto SM, Harty S, et al. Psychobiotics and the manipulation of bacteria-gut-brain signals. Trends Neurosci 2016;39(11):763–81.
8. Sherwin E, Sandhu KV, Dinan TG, et al. May the force be with you: the light and dark sides of the microbiota-gut-brain axis in neuropsychiatry. CNS Drugs 2016;30(11):1019–41.
9. Rhee SH, Pothoulakis C, Mayer EA. Principles and clinical implications of the brain-gut-enteric microbiota axis. Nat Rev Gastroenterol Hepatol 2009;6(5):306–14.
10. Foster JA, McVey Neufeld K-A. Gut-brain axis: how the microbiome influences anxiety and depression. Trends Neurosci 2013;36(5):305–12.

11. Belizário JE, Napolitano M. Human microbiomes and their roles in dysbiosis, common diseases, and novel therapeutic approaches. Front. Microbiol 2015;6: 1050. https://doi.org/10.3389/fmicb.2015.01050.

12. Hempel S, Newberry SJ, Maher AR, et al. Probiotics for the prevention and treatment of antibiotic-associated diarrhea. J Am Med Assoc 2012;307(18):1959–69.

13. Yuan F, Ni H, Asche CV, et al. Efficacy of Bifidobacterium infantis 35624 in patients with irritable bowel syndrome: a meta-analysis. Curr Med Res Opin 2017; 33(7):1191–7.

14. Aroniadis OC, Brandt LJ, Greenberg A, et al. Long-term follow-up study of fecal microbiota transplantation for severe and/or complicated clostridium difficile infection. J Clin Gastroenterol 2016;50(5):398–402.

15. Francavilla R, Miniello V, Magista AM, et al. A randomized controlled trial of lactobacillus GG in children with functional abdominal pain. Pediatrics 2010;126(6): e1445–52.

16. Ait-Belgnaoui A, Durand H, Cartier C, et al. Prevention of gut leakiness by a probiotic treatment leads to attenuated HPA response to an acute psychological stress in rats. Psychoneuroendocrinology 2012;37(11):1885–95.

17. Qin H-L, Shen T-Y, Gao Z-G, et al. Effect of lactobacillus on the gut microflora and barrier function of the rats with abdominal infection. World J Gastroenterol 2005; 11(17):2591–6.

18. Indrio F, Riezzo G, Raimondi F, et al. Lactobacillus reuteri accelerates gastric emptying and improves regurgitation in infants. Eur J Clin Invest 2011;41(4): 417–22.

19. Garofoli F, Civardi E, Indrio F, et al. The early administration of lactobacillus reuteri DSM 17938 controls regurgitation episodes in full-term breastfed infants. Int J Food Sci Nutr 2014;65(5):646–8.

20. Waller PA, Gopal PK, Leyer GJ, et al. Dose-response effect of Bifidobacterium lactis HN019 on whole gut transit time and functional gastrointestinal symptoms in adults. Scand J Gastroenterol 2011;46(9):1057–64.

21. Haro C, García-Carpintero S, Rangel-Zúñiga OA, et al. Consumption of two healthy dietary patterns restores microbiota dysbiosis in obese patients with metabolic dysfunction. Mol Nutr Food Res 2017;61(12). https://doi.org/10.1002/mnfr.201700300.

22. Malfertheiner P, Megraud F, O'Morain C, et al. Current concepts in the management of Helicobacter pylori infection: the Maastricht III Consensus Report. Gut 2007;56(6):772–81.

23. Gregor JC. Acid suppression and pneumonia: a clinical indication for rational prescribing. J Am Med Assoc 2004;292(16):2012–3.

24. Hassing RJ, Verbon A, de Visser H, et al. Proton pump inhibitors and gastroenteritis. Eur J Epidemiol 2016;31(10):1057–63.

25. Zedtwitz-Liebenstein K, Wenisch C, Patruta S, et al. Omeprazole treatment diminishes intra- and extracellular neutrophil reactive oxygen production and bactericidal activity. Crit Care Med 2002;30(5):1118–22.

26. Sierra F, Suarez M, Rey M, Vela MF. Systematic review: Proton pump inhibitor-associated acute interstitial nephritis. Aliment Pharmacol Ther 2007;26(4): 545–53.

27. Duroux P, Bauerfeind P, Emde C, et al. Early dinner reduces nocturnal gastric acidity. Gut 1989;30(8):1063–7.

28. Koufman JA. Low-acid diet for recalcitrant laryngopharyngeal reflux: therapeutic benefits and their implications. Ann Otol Rhinol Laryngol 2011;120(5):281–7.

29. Pilichiewicz AN, Horowitz M, Russo A, et al. Effects of Iberogast on proximal gastric volume, antropyloroduodenal motility and gastric emptying in healthy men. Am J Gastroenterol 2007;102(6):1276–83.
30. Sanchez A, Reeser JL, Lau HS, et al. Role of sugars in human neutrophilic phagocytosis. Am J Clin Nutr 1973;26(11):1180–4.
31. Scott AM, Clark J, Julien B, et al. Probiotics for preventing acute otitis media in children. Cochrane Database Syst Rev 2019;6(6):CD012941.
32. Skovbjerg S, Roos K, Holm SE, et al. Spray bacteriotherapy decreases middle ear fluid in children with secretory otitis media. Arch Dis Child 2009;94(2):92–8.
33. Roos K, Håkansson EG, Holm S. Effect of recolonisation with "interfering" alpha streptococci on recurrences of acute and secretory otitis media in children: randomised placebo controlled trial. BMJ 2001;322(7280):210–2.
34. Di Pierro F, Di Pasquale D, Di Cico M. Oral use of Streptococcus salivarius K12 in children with secretory otitis media: preliminary results of a pilot, uncontrolled study. Int J Gen Med 2015;8:303–8.
35. Emre IE, Eroğly Y, Kara A, et al. The effect of probiotics on prevention of upper respiratory tract infections in the paediatric community - a systematic review. Benef Microbes 2020;11(3):201–11.
36. Psaltis AJ, Wormald P-J. Therapy of Sinonasal Microbiome in CRS: A Critical Approach. Curr Allergy Asthma Rep 2017;17(9):59.
37. Habermann W, Zimmermann K, Skarabis H, et al. [Reduction of acute recurrence in patients with chronic recurrent hypertrophic sinusitis by treatment with a bacterial immunostimulant (Enterococcus faecalis Bacteriae of human origin]. Arzneimittelforschung 2002;52(8):622–7.
38. Kitz R, Martens U, Zieseniß E, et al. Probiotic E.faecalis - adjuvant therapy in children with recurrent rhinosinusitis. Open Med 2012;7(3):362–5.
39. Mårtensson A, Abolhalaj M, Lindstedt M, et al. Clinical efficacy of a topical lactic acid bacterial microbiome in chronic rhinosinusitis: A randomized controlled trial. Laryngoscope Investig Otolaryngol 2017;2(6):410–6.
40. Jalali MM, Soleimani R, Foumani AA, et al. Add-on probiotics in patients with persistent allergic rhinitis: A randomized crossover clinical trial. Laryngoscope 2019;129(8):1744–50.
41. Lue K-H, Sun H-L, Lu K-H, et al. A trial of adding Lactobacillus johnsonii EM1 to levocetirizine for treatment of perennial allergic rhinitis in children aged 7-12years. Int J Pediatr Otorhinolaryngol 2012;76(7):994–1001.
42. Xu L-Z, Yang L-T, Qiu S-Q, et al. Combination of specific allergen and probiotics induces specific regulatory B cells and enhances specific immunotherapy effect on allergic rhinitis. Oncotarget 2016;7(34):54360–9.
43. Hu L, Zhou M, Young A, et al. In vivo effectiveness and safety of probiotics on prophylaxis and treatment of oral candidiasis: a systematic review and meta-analysis. BMC Oral Health 2019;19(1):140.
44. Mishra R, Tandon S, Rathore M, et al. Antimicrobial Efficacy of Probiotic and Herbal Oral Rinses against Candida albicans in ChildrenL A Randomized Clinical Trial. Int J Clin Pediatr Dent 2016;9(1):25–30.
45. Andaloro C, Santagati M, Stefani S, et al. Bacteriotherapy with Streptococcus salivarius 24SMB and Streptococcus oralis 89a oral spray for children with recurrent streptococcal pharyngotonsillitis: a randomized placebo-controlled clinical study. Eur Arch Otorhinolaryngol 2019;276(3):879–87.

Integrative Approach to Rhinosinusitis: An Update

Malcolm B. Taw, MD[a],*, Chau T. Nguyen, MD[b],
Marilene B. Wang, MD[c]

KEYWORDS

- Rhinosinusitis • Sinusitis • Integrative medicine • Traditional Chinese medicine
- Complementary medicine • Herbal medicine • Acupuncture

KEY POINTS

- Dietary recommendations for RS: ginger, quercetin, green tea, horseradish.
- Herbal supplements: Pelargonium sidoides, Sinupret, Sinfrontal, Bromelain, Cineole, and others- Traditional Chinese Medicine: acupuncture, acupressure, Chinese herbal medicine.
- Lifestyle recommendations: minimize exposure to environmental toxins, adequate hydration, steam inhalation, avoidance of dairy/refined sugars/processed food, regular exercise, good sleep quality, stress management.

OVERVIEW

The causes of rhinosinusitis (RS) include infectious and allergic components, and environmental, general host, and local anatomic factors. Psychiatric conditions, such as depression, are also significant factors in the outcomes of patients with chronic RS.[1,2] Current standard conventional management of RS commonly uses multiple therapeutic modalities to break the cycle of chronic disease. However, to date, there is no consensus as to the optimal treatment algorithm for patients with chronic RS.[3] Success in the treatment of chronic RS, unlike in acute RS, is variable and prone to relapse. Therefore, it is important to find other safe and effective treatments for RS.

Although there has been an explosion in the use of complementary medicine over the last few decades,[4–6] surveys have also demonstrated that there is a parallel amount of interest in the use of such modalities specifically for the treatment of RS in the United States[7–11] and internationally.[12–14] This seems to be true along the entire continuum of care for RS, whether before seeing an otolaryngologist or after

[a] UCLA Center for East-West Medicine, 1250 La Venta Drive, Suite 101A, Westlake Village, CA 91361, USA; [b] Division of Otolaryngology-Head & Neck Surgery, Ventura County Medical Center, 300 Hillmont Avenue, Suite 401, Ventura, CA 93003, USA; [c] UCLA Department of Head and Neck Surgery, 200 UCLA Medical Plaza, Suite 550, Los Angeles, CA 90095, USA
* Corresponding author.
E-mail address: mtaw@mednet.ucla.edu

Otolaryngol Clin N Am 55 (2022) 947–963
https://doi.org/10.1016/j.otc.2022.06.004
0030-6665/22/© 2022 Elsevier Inc. All rights reserved.

oto.theclinics.com

aggressive medical and surgical therapy. There is also a wide range of therapies sought, including acupuncture, herbal medicine, and various supplements.

This article focuses on an integrative approach to RS and serves as an update to our original article published in 2013.[15]

DIAGNOSIS

RS is categorized by duration of symptoms: acute (up to 4 weeks), subacute (4–12 weeks), and chronic (more than 12 weeks). Acute RS is further categorized into viral RS or acute bacterial RS, with four or more episodes per year described as recurrent acute bacterial RS.[16–19]

INTEGRATIVE TREATMENT APPROACHES
Pelargonium sidoides EPs 7630

In South Africa, *Pelargonium sidoides* has historically been used to treat a variety of ailments including upper respiratory tract infections, such as bronchitis.[20] *P sidoides*, traditionally known as Umckaloabo, is rich in phenols and flavonoids.[21–23] It has been standardized in Germany as an aqueous ethanolic extract of its root known as EPs 7630 and has been shown to have antibacterial, antiviral, and immunomodulatory effects.[24–27]

Bachert and colleagues,[28] in a multicenter, double-blinded randomized controlled trial (DBRCT) comparing EPs 7630 with placebo involving 103 patients with sinonasal symptoms of at least 1 week and radiographically and clinically confirmed acute RS, demonstrated superior efficacy and tolerance of EPs 7630 based on changes in Sinusitis Severity Scores. A Cochrane review in 2013 concluded that *P sidoides* may be effective in alleviating symptoms of acute RS and the common cold in adults, although the overall quality of the evidence was considered to be low.[29] In 2020, another study randomized 50 patients with uncomplicated acute bacterial RS to receive either EPs 7630 or amoxicillin and found that EPs 7630 demonstrated better clinical and antimicrobial efficacy.[30]

Bromelain

Bromelain, a mixture of proteolytic enzymes extracted from pineapples (*Ananas comosus*), has demonstrated anti-inflammatory, antiedematous, antithrombotic, and fibrinolytic effects.[31] Three DBRCTs were conducted in the 1960s on patients with acute and chronic RS, using similar protocols of parallel treatment arms comparing bromelain with placebo, with each group also receiving conventional medical management consisting of antibiotics, decongestants, antihistamines, and analgesics.[32–34] A meta-analysis showed a small, but statistically significant difference in favor of adjunctive treatment with bromelain for nasal mucosal inflammation, nasal discomfort, breathing difficulty, and overall rating, but not for nasal discharge.[35]

A recent multicenter trial enrolling children younger than 11 years of age with acute sinusitis had three treatment groups (bromelain vs bromelain + standard therapy vs standard therapy) and showed a statistically significant recovery time with bromelain monotherapy compared with the other treatment groups.[36] Only one mild self-limiting allergic reaction was noted.

Bromelain has been shown to have excellent penetration into the blood and sinonasal mucosa in patients with chronic RS.[37] Caution must be used when prescribing bromelain for patients already on anticoagulants because of the increased risk of bleeding and various antibiotics, such as penicillin and tetracycline, because bromelain is also known to promote their absorption.[31] Moreover, bromelain strongly inhibits human cytochrome P-450 2C9 (CYP2C9) activity and can thereby affect metabolism of its substrates.[38] Recommended doses range from 500 to 2000 mg per day.[39]

Cineole

Cineole, or more specifically 1,8-cineole, is a monoterpene present in many plant-based essential oils and is commonly derived from *Eucalyptus globulus*. It has been shown to reduce mucus production, block inflammation through inhibiting cytokines tumor necrosis factor (TNF)-α and interleukin (IL)-1β, and produce antinociceptive effects.[40–42]

A prospective DBRCT comparing cineole (200 mg three times per day) with placebo in 152 patients with acute nonpurulent RS, showed a statistically significant difference in symptoms-sum-scores in the cineole group, in addition to a reduction in secondary symptoms, such as headache on bending, frontal headache, nasal obstruction, and nasal secretion.[43] Mild side effects included heartburn and exanthem. The authors concluded that cineole may serve as an alternative therapy during the first 4 days of acute RS, but antibiotics should be initiated if symptoms persist. In addition, another DBRCT demonstrated that cineole was more effective than an herbal preparation containing five different ingredients in the treatment of acute viral RS.[44]

Cod Liver Oil

Cod liver oil, which is rich in omega-3 fatty acids and vitamin D, has historically been used as a remedy for rickets in the 1800s.[45] There is limited evidence for use of cod liver oil for RS, including a 4-month, open-label study enrolling four children with recurrent chronic RS who were given escalating doses of cod liver oil and a multivitamin with selenium.[46,47] Three subjects demonstrated a positive response with decreased sinus symptoms, reduced episodes of acute sinusitis, and fewer physician visits.

Manuka Honey

Manuka honey is produced from the nectar of flowers native to Australia and New Zealand, particularly from species of *Leptospermum*, and may potentially modulate expression of multiple cytokines, including IL-6, IL-8, IL-13, and macrophage inflammatory protein-1β.[48] It was found to have bactericidal activity against biofilms formed by *Pseudomonas aeruginosa* and *Staphylococcus aureus*.[49–51]

Manuka honey may also help generate nitric oxide to produce a potent antibiofilm effect in patients with chronic RS.[52]

Thamboo and colleagues[53] studied the use of a topical combination of manuka honey and saline in 34 patients with allergic fungal RS who were treated for 1 month. Although there was symptomatic improvement on the Sino-Nasal Outcome Test (SNOT)-20 as an outcome measure, culture results from their ethmoid cavities were unchanged, as was their endoscopic staging.

A prospective randomized controlled trial (RCT) compared manuka honey with saline sinus irrigation for patients with active chronic RS and prior sinus surgery and did not find any significant difference between the two groups; however, among those who were not treated with antibiotics/steroids, manuka honey alone was found to be statistically better on culture negativity suggesting possible effectiveness for acute exacerbations of chronic RS.[54] Another RCT demonstrated that manuka honey with augmented methylglyoxal sinonasal rinses was not superior to culture-directed antibiotic therapy and twice-daily saline rinses.[55] For cystic fibrosis–associated chronic RS, a pilot study showed that manuka honey achieved a clinically important difference in quality of life (QoL) score and significantly better endoscopic outcome compared with saline sinus irrigation.[56]

Sinupret

Sinupret is comprised of *Gentianae radix*, *Primulae flos*, *Rumex herba*, *Sambuci flos*, and *Verbena herba*, and was approved by the German Commission E in 1994 for the treatment of acute and chronic inflammation of the paranasal sinuses.[57]

Sinupret has been shown to have in vitro antiviral activity and can strongly stimulate transepithelial Cl(−) secretion to maintain normal mucociliary clearance in sinonasal epithelium through hydration of the airway surface liquid.[58,59]

Three RCTs evaluated Sinupret as adjunctive therapy for acute RS and one RCT for chronic RS.[60–63] A systematic review demonstrated that Sinupret may be effective as an adjunctive therapy in acute RS.[35] In 2015, a prospective, multicenter study supported these findings for acute RS and determined that treatment with Sinupret was safe.[64] However, for chronic RS, an RCT in 2017 did not find a significant difference between Sinupret (BNO 1016) and placebo, although there were trends toward improvement for secondary end points.[65] Another study found no significant difference in olfactory function between patients treated with Sinupret versus placebo, although an initial therapy of oral prednisolone for 1 week had preceded the treatment intervention.[66] For children 6 to 11 years of age, a multicenter randomized trial published in 2020 found Sinupret (BNO 1012) to be effective for treating acute RS and reduced the need for antibiotics, when given in addition to standard therapy.[67]

Esberitox

Esberitox is an herbal extract containing *Thuja occidentalis* (white cedar), *Echinacea purpurea/pallida* (purple coneflower), and *Baptisia tinctoria* (wild indigo) with demonstrated immunomodulatory properties.[68] A placebo-controlled DBRCT showed a dose-dependent efficacy in the treatment of upper respiratory infections and, in particular, certain symptoms, such as rhinorrhea.[69] Another study that enrolled 90 patients with acute RS compared (1) Esberitox and doxycycline, (2) Sinupret and doxycycline, and (3) doxycycline alone, and found that both groups with combination therapies had a significantly higher rate of response.[35,63] Reported adverse events included photosensitivity and gastrointestinal symptoms, such as nausea.

Myrtol

Myrtol is a standardized phytotherapeutic extract (GeloMyrtol/GeloMyrtol Forte), taken from *Pinus* spp, *Citrus aurantiifolia*, and *E globulus*, and is mainly comprised of three monoterpenes: (+) alpha-pinene, D-limonene, and 1,8-cineole. It has been shown to inhibit 5-lipoxygenase activity, leukotriene C4, and prostaglandin E_2.[70]

In a multicenter DBRCT, 330 patients with acute sinusitis were enrolled into one of three arms: (1) Myrtol extract (300 mg per day), (2) other unidentified essential oil, or (3) placebo.[71] Myrtol and the other essential oil groups demonstrated superior efficacy to placebo based on the total symptom score, although there was insufficient statistical data to support this conclusion.[35] Another prospective, multicenter trial demonstrated that Myrtol (ELOM-080) led to a faster recovery of facial pain in patients with acute RS, when compared with Sinupret (BNO 1016).[72] Mild to moderate reported adverse events were mostly gastrointestinal in nature.

Cyclamen europaeum

Cyclamen europaeum is a member of the primrose family and has been used in southeastern Europe as a traditional remedy for acute RS. In 2019, a Cochrane review that included two placebo-controlled DBRCTs and a total of 147 adult patients with acute RS confirmed by radiology or nasal endoscopy, concluded that the effectiveness of *C europaeum* is unknown, but there was moderate-quality evidence of reported mild adverse effects (nasal/throat irritation, epistaxis, sneezing) in up to 50% of participants.[73-75]

Nasturtium and Horseradish Root

Nasturtium (*Tropaeoli majoris herba*) and horseradish root (*Armoraciae rusticanae radix*) have broad antimicrobial activities against multiple gram-positive and gram-negative bacteria, including *Haemophilus influenzae*, *Moraxella catarrhalis*, *P aeruginosa*, *S aureus*, and *Streptococcus pyogenes*.[76]

A prospective, multicenter study performed in children between 4 and 18 years of age with acute RS found that an herbal drug preparation, containing nasturtium and horseradish root, had similar efficacy and fewer adverse events compared with standard antibiotics.[77]

NUTRITION: GINGER, QUERCETIN, AND EPIGALLOCATECHIN GALLATE

Dietary polyphenols are widely available in food and well-known for their anti-inflammatory effects. Both ginger and quercetin, a polyphenolic bioflavonoid commonly found in apples and onions, have potent antioxidant and anti-inflammatory properties.[78,79] Quercetin has been shown to suppress the inflammatory mediator cyclooxygenase-2, inhibit histamine release through downregulation of mast cell activity and enhance mucociliary clearance through augmented transepithelial chloride secretion via the cystic fibrosis transmembrane conductance regulator anion channel.[80-82]

A combination of ginger extract and green tea (*Camellia sinensis*), which is rich in epigallocatechin gallate, demonstrated significant antiallergy effects through suppression of TNF-α and macrophage inflammatory protein-1α.[83] The dietary polyphenols of [6]-gingerol, quercetin, and epigallocatechin gallate were found to effectively inhibit excess mucus secretion of respiratory epithelial cells while maintaining normal nasal ciliary movement.[84]

HOMEOPATHY

Homeopathy is based on the principle of similars ("like cures like") whereby therapeutic effects are achieved by stimulating the body's homeostatic healing response via substances that have been serially diluted and shaken. There is evidence from RCTs that homeopathy may be effective for the treatment of influenza and allergies.[85] In a prospective observational trial from Germany, 134 adult patients with refractory chronic RS were treated with different homeopathic remedies and found to have sustained improvements in QoL outcomes (Short Form-36) with decreased use of conventional medications, especially during the first 3 months of follow-up.[86]

Sinfrontal

Sinfrontal is a homeopathic remedy (containing Cinnabaris D4, Ferrum phosphoricum D3, Mercurius solubilis D6) commonly used in Germany for a variety of upper respiratory tract infections. A multicenter DBRCT comparing Sinfrontal with placebo in 113 patients with radiography-confirmed acute maxillary sinusitis found that there was a significant difference in patients treated with Sinfrontal with no recurrence of symptoms 8 weeks posttreatment.[87] An economic analysis demonstrated that Sinfrontal can lead to substantial cost savings with markedly reduced absenteeism from work.[88]

TRADITIONAL CHINESE MEDICINE

Traditional Chinese medicine (TCM) is a whole medical system that has been used for several millennia and incorporates certain therapies, such as acupuncture and Chinese herbal medicine. Specifically, the use of TCM for the treatment of disorders involving the ears, nose, and throat is traced back as early as the fifth century BC with several therapies that may be beneficial for RS.[89]

Acupuncture

The therapeutic effects of acupuncture primarily involve modulation of several physiologic cascades, including the inflammatory response, immune system, autonomic nervous system, neuroendocrine axis, limbic system, or pain pathway.[90–95] Although acupuncture may regulate many of these cascades in patients with RS, specific effects of improved mucociliary clearance and airway surface liquid have also been demonstrated.[96] In a placebo-controlled DBRCT, acupuncture was used to treat patients with nasal congestion and hypertrophic inferior turbinates and was found to have significant improvement on visual analog scale and nasal airflow as measured by active anterior rhinomanometry.[97] Another study demonstrated a 60% reduction in sinus-related pain compared with only 30% in the placebo group.[98] Acupuncture also showed beneficial results among children who were treated for chronic maxillary sinusitis.[99]

A research team in Norway performed two different studies using a similar protocol, which included 65 patients with chronic RS who were randomized into three cohorts: (1) traditional Chinese acupuncture; (2) sham acupuncture; or (3) conventional management with antibiotics, steroids, nasal saline irrigation, and local decongestants.[100,101] In both studies, health-related QoL symptom scores improved in all three groups, although there was no statistically significant difference among them. In 2020, a systematic review found acupuncture to have a moderate to high GRADE (Grading of Recommendations, Assessment, Development and Evaluations) rating.[102]

Chinese Herbal Medicine

Xanthii fructus (Chinese herbal name: Cang Er Zi) and *Flos magnoliae* (Chinese herbal name: Xin Yi Hua) are commonly used herbs in TCM to treat RS. From a TCM perspective, *X fructus* "disperses wind and dampness" to remove thick, viscous nasal discharge and sinus-related headaches, whereas *F magnoliae* "expels wind-cold" to treat nasal discharge, hyposmia, sinus congestion, and headaches.[103] In fact, these two herbs are typically combined as key components of the Chinese herbal preparations, Cang Er Zi Wan and Cang Er Zi San, which are the pill and powder formulations, respectively.[104]

It is important to emphasize that Chinese herbs should be used according to TCM theory. If not, severe adverse events can occur. One notable example was the inappropriate use of Ephedra (Chinese name: Ma Huang) for weight loss, increased energy, and performance enhancement, which traditionally is taken only for brief amounts of time to treat upper respiratory infections, much like how pseudoephedrine is used only temporarily for such symptoms.[105]

Xanthii fructus (Chinese name: Cang Er Zi)

X fructus was found to exhibit (1) anti-inflammatory effects by inhibiting interferon-γ, TNF-α, and lipopolysaccharide-induced nitric oxide synthesis; (2) antiallergic effects via blocking mast cell–mediated histamine release; and (3) antioxidant effects through increased activities of catalase, superoxide dismutase, and glutathione peroxidase in the liver.[106–108] *X fructus* is also known as *Xanthium strumarium* because the former is the fruit of the latter. Specific components of *X strumarium* displayed antibacterial, antiviral, antifungal, anti-inflammatory, antioxidant, and antiallergic effects.[109]

A DBRCT divided 126 patients into equal cohorts receiving either Shi-Bi-Lin (a modified version of the Chinese herbal formula Cang Er Zi San) or placebo, and found that Shi-Bi-Lin significantly improved symptoms with a sustained response for at least 2 weeks.[110] However, caution must be exercised when using either *X fructus* or Cang Er Zi Wan, because they have been shown to lead to certain side effects, such as muscle spasm and hepato- and nephrotoxicity.[111,112]

Flos magnoliae (Chinese herbal name: Xin Yi Hua)

The primary bioactive components of *F magnoliae* include neolignans, epimagnolin, and fargesin.[113] Neolignans have been found to have anti-inflammatory effects through mechanisms of action different from steroids, whereas epimagnolin and fargesin decrease production of nitric oxide, a potent mediator in inflammation.[114,115] *F magnoliae* also demonstrates antiallergy activity through inhibition of immediate-type hypersensitivity reactions and blockade of mast cell degranulation.[116]

A study in Taiwan found that 29% of 14,806 patients with chronic RS had used TCM, in addition to conventional Western treatment, and found that a lower proportion of these patients underwent endoscopic sinus surgery compared with those who did not receive TCM. The most commonly used Chinese herbal formula was Xin-Yi-Qing-Fei-Tang, which contains *F magnoliae*.[117]

Chinese Herbal Supplements (Postoperative)

Bi Yuan Shu is a Chinese herbal liquid mixture composed of several herbs, including *Magnolia liliiflora*, *X strumarium*, *Astragalus membranaceus*, *Angelica dahurica*, and *Scutellaria baicalensis*. A multicenter RCT randomized 340 postoperative patients with chronic RS and nasal polyps who had undergone endoscopic sinus surgery into two groups with both receiving antibiotics and topical steroids, whereas the test group was also treated with Bi Yuan Shu.[118] Adjunctive treatment with Bi Yuan Shu was found to have significant improvement of purulent nasal discharge, breathing difficulty, pain, hyposmia, and halitosis for up to 2 months, with positive trends noted for fever and cough.[35]

Another study that examined the use of Chinese herbal medicine in patients who had received endoscopic sinus surgery, enrolled 97 patients into one of three treatment arms: (1) Tsang Erh San extract granules and Houttuynia extract powder, (2) oral amoxicillin, or (3) placebo; and found no benefit of either treatment group over placebo.[119]

A subsequent study by the same research group, however, showed that Tsang Erh San and Houttuynia had similar efficacy to erythromycin in the treatment of patients with chronic RS without nasal polyps.[120]

MULTIMODAL APPROACHES

A multicenter, nonrandomized study of 63 patients with acute RS compared multiple conventional (antibiotics, secretolytics, and sympathomimetics) versus combination complementary (Sinupret and homeopathic remedy, Cinnabaris 3X) therapies and demonstrated similar effectiveness based on patients' self-assessment score, physicians' score, and HCG-5 questionnaire.[121] However, the only validated outcome measure was the HCG-5 QoL instrument. Other limitations with this study included a small sample size and lack of randomization and blinding.

A pilot study at UCLA was conducted using integrative East-West medicine to treat patients with recalcitrant chronic RS.[122] Eleven patients received eight weekly sessions of acupuncture (**Table 1**) and therapeutic acupressure-style massage, along

Table 1
Acupuncture and acupressure point locations and indications

Name	Location	Purpose
	Acupuncture Point Locations and Indications	
Sinus specific		
LI-4 (He Gu)	On the dorsum of the hand, on the midpoint of the second metacarpal bone, near its radial border	Nasal congestion, rhinorrhea, headache, "wind-cold" TCM pattern, neck pain, facial pain, stress
GB-20 (Fang Chi)	Near the base of skull, in the depression between the origins of the sternocleidomastoid and trapezius muscles	Nasal congestion, rhinorrhea, headache, "wind-cold" TCM pattern
ST-3 (Ju Liao)	Lateral to the nasolabial groove, level with the lower border of the ala nasi, directly inferior to the midpoint of the eye	Pain and swelling involving the maxillary sinus
LI-20 (Ying Xiang)	In the nasolabial groove, at the level of the midpoint of the lateral border of the ala nasi	Nasal congestion, rhinorrhea, anosmia
UB-2 (Zan Zhu)	Superior to the inner canthus, in a depression at the medial border of the eyebrow	Rhinitis, pain and swelling of the frontal sinus, frontal headache, "wind" TCM pattern
DU-23 (Shang Xing)	At the top of the head on the midline, 1 finger breadth posterior to the anterior hairline	Nasal obstruction and discharge, headache, rhinitis
Quality-of-life improvement		
LI-11 (Qu Chi)	With the elbow flexed, at the lateral end of the transverse cubital crease	Loss of voice, sore throat, "heat" TCM pattern
SJ-5 (Wai Guan)	3 finger breadths proximal to the wrist crease, on the radial side of the extensor digitorum communis tendons	Headache, neck pain, "wind-heat" TCM pattern
GB-21 (Jian Jing)	Midway between the spinous process of C7 and the tip of the acromion, at the highest point trapezius muscle	Neck pain, cough, phlegm
P-6 (Nei Guan)	3 finger breadths proximal to the wrist crease in between the tendons of the palmaris longus and flexor carpi radialis	Anxiety, pain of the head and neck, cough
ST-36 (Zu San Li)	With the knee extended, 4 finger breadths below the patella, just lateral to the tibia within the tibialis anterior muscle	Fatigue, vitality
LIV-3 (Tai Chong)	On the dorsum of the foot, in the depression distal to the junction of the first and second metatarsal bones	Headache, insomnia, stress, irritability

Adapted from: Suh JD, Wu AW, Taw MB, Nguyen C, Wang MB. Treatment of Recalcitrant Chronic Rhinosinusitis with Integrative East-West Medicine: A Pilot Study. Arch Otolaryngol Head Neck Surg. 2012 Mar;138(3):294-300.

with dietary modification, lifestyle changes, and self-acupressure. Four items on the SNOT-20 (need to blow nose, runny nose, reduced concentration, and frustrated/restless/irritable) and three domains on the Short Form-36 (role physical, vitality, and social functioning) showed a statistically significant difference, whereas trends of improvement were noted in most other elements on both QoL instruments. Although the data look promising, this study was also limited by its small size, lack of randomization, and control group.

PATIENT SELF-TREATMENTS

Lifestyle modifications can also be conducive toward achieving optimal sinus health and function. These include regular aerobic exercise, adequate hydration, steam inhalation, stress management, and good sleep quality. Minimizing exposure to pollution, smoke, and environmental toxins and incorporating nutritional changes, such as consuming an anti-inflammatory diet and avoiding dairy products, refined sugars, and processed foods, are important.[123] A regular spiritual practice, such as prayer, is also beneficial along with anger management and attitudes of forgiveness, gratitude, and optimism.[124] Self-acupressure of certain acupoints can also be helpful to reduce sinus-related symptoms (see **Table 1**).

SUMMARY

As a greater understanding of the complex pathogenesis of RS is gained, what is becoming apparent is a shift in philosophic paradigm. Previous reductionistic models of disease and health are being replaced by holism, systems biology, and complex, nonlinear dynamics.[125–127] Holism is a central philosophic underpinning of complementary/integrative medicine and TCM.

This paradigm shift is now seen in the approach to RS. No longer is the medical community looking at the diagnosis of RS as solely an infectious process, but rather as complex and multifactorial.[128]

The therapeutic repertoire, likewise, has broadened significantly from antibiotics alone as the mainstay of treatment to the use of multiple therapies to act on different pathophysiologic facets of RS. Integrative medicine provides an expanded approach and armamentarium to help patients with RS, whether acute, chronic, or recalcitrant. Although numerous recent papers have been published since our original article in 2013, the evidence and recommendations remain the same.

CLINICS CARE POINTS

- Dietary recommendations for RS: ginger, quercetin, green tea, horseradish
- Herbal supplements: *Pelargonium sidoides*, Sinupret, Sinfrontal, Bromelain, Cineole, and others
- Traditional Chinese medicine: acupuncture, acupressure, Chinese herbal medicine
- Lifestyle recommendations: minimize exposure to environmental toxins, adequate hydration, steam inhalation, avoidance of dairy/refined sugars/processed food, regular exercise, good sleep quality, stress management

---

DISCLOSURE

The authors have no relevant financial interests pertaining to this article.

REFERENCES

1. Brandsted R, Sindwani R. Impact of depression on disease-specific symptoms and quality of life in patients with chronic rhinosinusitis. Am J Rhinol 2007; 21(1):50–4.
2. Davis GE, Yueh B, Walker E, et al. Psychiatric distress amplifies symptoms after surgery for chronic rhinosinusitis. Otolaryngol Head Neck Surg 2005;132(2): 189–96.
3. Bhattacharyya N. Clinical and symptom criteria for the accurate diagnosis of chronic rhinosinusitis. Laryngoscope 2006;116(7 Pt 2 Suppl 110):1–22.
4. Eisenberg DM, Davis RB, Ettner S, et al. Trends in alternative medicine use in the United States, 1990-1997: results of a follow-up national survey. JAMA 1998;280(18):1569–75.
5. Eisenberg DM, Kessler RC, Foster C, et al. Unconventional medicine in the United States. Prevalence, costs, and patterns of use. N Engl J Med 1993; 328(4):246–52.
6. Tindle HA, Davis RB, Phillips RS, et al. Trends in use of complementary and alternative medicine by US adults: 1997-2002. Altern Ther Health Med 2005; 11(1):42–9.
7. Barnes PM, Powell-Griner E. Complementary and alternative medicine use among adults: United States, 2002. Adv Data. Vital Health Stat 2004; 27(343):1–19.
8. Krouse JH, Krouse HJ. Patient use of traditional and complementary therapies in treating rhinosinusitis before consulting an otolaryngologist. Laryngoscope 1999;109(8):1223–7.
9. Asher BF, Seidman M, Snyderman C. Complementary and alternative medicine in otolaryngology. Laryngoscope 2001;111(8):1383–9.
10. Pletcher SD, Goldberg AN, Lee J, et al. Use of acupuncture in the treatment of sinus and nasal symptoms: results of a practitioner survey. Am J Rhinol 2006; 20(2):235–7.
11. Blanc PD, Trupin L, Earnest G, et al. Alternative therapies among adults with a reported diagnosis of asthma or rhinosinusitis: data from a population-based survey. Chest 2001;120(5):1461–7.
12. Rotenberg BW, Bertens KA. Use of complementary and alternative medical therapies for chronic rhinosinusitis: a Canadian perspective. J Otolaryngol Head Neck Surg 2010;39(5):586–93.
13. Newton JR, Santangeli L, Shakeel M, et al. Use of complementary and alternative medicine by patients attending a rhinology outpatient clinic. Am J Rhinol Allergy 2009;23(1):59–63.
14. Yakirevitch A, Bedrin L, Migirov L, et al. Use of alternative medicine in Israeli chronic rhinosinusitis patients. J Otolaryngol Head Neck Surg 2009;38(4): 517–20.
15. Taw MB, Nguyen CT, Wang MB. Complementary and integrative treatments: rhinosinusitis. Otolaryngol Clin North Am 2013;46(3):345–66.
16. Rosenfeld RM, Andes D, Bhattacharyya N, et al. Clinical practice guideline: adult sinusitis. Otolaryngol Head Neck Surg 2007;137(3 Suppl):S32–45. Review.
17. Report of the Rhinosinusitis Task Force Committee Meeting. Alexandria, Virginia, August 17, 1996. Otolaryngol Head Neck Surg 1997;117(3 Pt 2):S1–68.
18. Benninger MS, Ferguson BJ, Hadley JA, et al. Adult chronic rhinosinusitis: definitions, diagnosis, epidemiology and pathophysiology. Otolaryngol Head Neck Surg 2003;129(3 Suppl):S1–32.

19. Meltzer EO, Hamilos DL, Hadley JA, et al. Rhinosinusitis: establishing definitions for clinical research and patient care. Otolaryngol Head Neck Surg 2004;131(6 Suppl):S1–62.
20. Bladt S, Wagner H. From the Zulu medicine to the European phytomedicine Umckaloabo. Phytomedicine 2007;14(Suppl 6):2.
21. Kolodziej H. Fascinating metabolic pools of *Pelargonium sidoides* and *Pelargonium reniforme*, traditional and phytomedicinal sources of the herbal medicine Umckaloabo. Phytomedicine 2007;14(Suppl 6):9–17.
22. Janecki A, Kolodziej H. Anti-adhesive activities of flavan-3-ols and proanthocyanidins in the interaction of group A-streptococci and human epithelial cells. Molecules 2010;15(10):7139–52.
23. Kolodziej H, Kayser O, Radtke OA, et al. Pharmacological profile of extracts of *Pelargonium sidoides* and their constituents. Phytomedicine 2003;10(Suppl 4): 18–24.
24. Michaelis M, Doerr HW, Cinatl J Jr. Investigation of the influence of EPs® 7630, a herbal drug preparation from *Pelargonium sidoides*, on replication of a broad panel of respiratory viruses. Phytomedicine 2011;18(5):384–6.
25. Kayser O, Kolodziej H, Kiderlen AF. Immunomodulatory principles of *Pelargonium sidoides*. Phytother Res 2001;15(2):122–6.
26. Conrad A, Hansmann C, Engels I, et al. Extract of *Pelargonium sidoides* (EPs 7630) improves phagocytosis, oxidative burst, and intracellular killing of human peripheral blood phagocytes in vitro. Phytomedicine 2007;14(Suppl 6):46–51.
27. Janecki A, Conrad A, Engels I, et al. Evaluation of an aqueous-ethanolic extract from *Pelargonium sidoides* (EPs® 7630) for its activity against group A-streptococci adhesion to human HEp-2 epithelial cells. J Ethnopharmacol 2011;133(1): 147–52.
28. Bachert C, Schapowal A, Funk P, et al. Treatment of acute rhinosinusitis with the preparation from *Pelargonium sidoides* EPs 7630: a randomized, double-blind, placebo-controlled trial. Rhinology 2009;47(1):51–8.
29. Timmer A, Günther J, Motschall E, et al. *Pelargonium sidoides* extract for treating acute respiratory tract infections. Cochrane Database Syst Rev 2013;(10): CD006323.
30. Perić A, Gaćeša D, Barać A, et al. Herbal drug EPs 7630 versus amoxicillin in patients with uncomplicated acute bacterial rhinosinusitis: a randomized, open-label study. Ann Otol Rhinol Laryngol 2020;129(10):969–76.
31. Maurer HR. Bromelain: biochemistry, pharmacology and medical use. Cell Mol Life Sci 2001;58(9):1234–45.
32. Seltzer AP. Adjunctive use of bromelains in sinusitis: a controlled study. Eye Ear Nose Throat Mon 1967;46(10):1281–8.
33. Ryan RE. A double-blind clinical evaluation of bromelains in the treatment of acute sinusitis. Headache 1967;7(1):13–7.
34. Taub SJ. The use of bromelains in sinusitis: a double-blind clinical evaluation. Eye Ear Nose Throat Mon 1967;46(3):361–2.
35. Guo R, Canter PH, Ernst E. Herbal medicines for the treatment of rhinosinusitis: a systematic review. Otolaryngol Head Neck Surg 2006;135(4):496–506.
36. Braun JM, Schneider B, Beuth HJ. Therapeutic use, efficiency and safety of the proteolytic pineapple enzyme Bromelain-POS in children with acute sinusitis in Germany. In Vivo. Mar-Apr 2005;19(2):417–21.
37. Passali D, Passali GC, Bellussi LM, et al. Bromelain's penetration into the blood and sinonasal mucosa in patients with chronic rhinosinusitis. Acta Otorhinolaryngol Ital 2018;38(3):225–8.

38. Hidaka M, Nagata M, Kawano Y, et al. Inhibitory effects of fruit juices on cytochrome P450 2C9 activity in vitro. Biosci Biotechnol Biochem 2008;72(2): 406–11.

39. Kelly GS. Bromelain: a literature review and discussion of its therapeutic applications. Alt Med Rev 1996;1(4):243–57.

40. Sudhoff H, Klenke C, Greiner JF, et al. 1,8-Cineol reduces mucus-production in a novel human ex vivo model of late rhinosinusitis. PLoS One 2015;10(7): e0133040.

41. Juergens UR, Engelen T, Racké K, et al. Inhibitory activity of 1,8-cineol (eucalyptol) on cytokine production in cultured human lymphocytes and monocytes. Pulm Pharmacol Ther 2004;17(5):281–7.

42. Santos FA, Rao VS. Antiinflammatory and antinociceptive effects of 1,8-cineole a terpenoid oxide present in many plant essential oils. Phytother Res 2000;14(4): 240–4.

43. Kehrl W, Sonnemann U, Dethlefsen U. Therapy for acute nonpurulent rhinosinusitis with cineole: results of a double-blind, randomized, placebo-controlled trial. Laryngoscope 2004;114(4):738–42.

44. Tesche S, Metternich F, Sonnemann U, et al. The value of herbal medicines in the treatment of acute non-purulent rhinosinusitis. Results of a double-blind, randomised, controlled trial. Eur Arch Otorhinolaryngol 2008;265(11):1355–9.

45. Rajakumar K. Vitamin D, cod-liver oil, sunlight, and rickets: a historical perspective. Pediatrics 2003;112(2):e132–5.

46. Karkos PD, Leong SC, Arya AK, et al. Complementary ENT': a systematic review of commonly used supplements. J Laryngol Otol 2007;121(8):779–82.

47. Linday LA, Dolitsky JN, Shindledecker RD. Nutritional supplements as adjunctive therapy for children with chronic/recurrent sinusitis: pilot research. Int J Pediatr Otorhinolaryngol 2004;68(6):785–93.

48. Manji J, Thamboo A, Sunkaraneni V, et al. The association of Leptospermum honey with cytokine expression in the sinonasal epithelium of chronic rhinosinusitis patients. World J Otorhinolaryngol Head Neck Surg 2018;5(1):19–25.

49. Alandejani T, Marsan J, Ferris W, et al. Effectiveness of honey on *Staphylococcus aureus* and *Pseudomonas aeruginosa* biofilms. Otolaryngol Head Neck Surg 2009;141(1):114–8.

50. Jervis-Bardy J, Foreman A, Bray S, et al. Methylglyoxal-infused honey mimics the anti-*Staphylococcus aureus* biofilm activity of manuka honey: potential implication in chronic rhinosinusitis. Laryngoscope 2011;121(5):1104–7.

51. Paramasivan S, Drilling AJ, Jardeleza C, et al. Methylglyoxal-augmented manuka honey as a topical anti-*Staphylococcus aureus* biofilm agent: safety and efficacy in an in vivo model. Int Forum Allergy Rhinol 2014;4(3):187–95.

52. Yang C, Mavelli GV, Nacharaju P, et al. Novel nitric oxide-generating platform using manuka honey as an anti-biofilm strategy in chronic rhinosinusitis. Int Forum Allergy Rhinol 2020;10(2):223–32.

53. Thamboo A, Thamboo A, Philpott C, et al. Single-blind study of manuka honey in allergic fungal rhinosinusitis. J Otolaryngol Head Neck Surg 2011;40(3):238–43.

54. Lee VS, Humphreys IM, Purcell PL, et al. Manuka honey sinus irrigation for the treatment of chronic rhinosinusitis: a randomized controlled trial. Int Forum Allergy Rhinol 2017;7(4):365–72.

55. Ooi ML, Jothin A, Bennett C, et al. Manuka honey sinus irrigations in recalcitrant chronic rhinosinusitis: phase 1 randomized, single-blinded, placebo-controlled trial. Int Forum Allergy Rhinol 2019;9(12):1470–7.

56. Lee VS, Humphreys IM, Purcell PL, et al. Manuka honey versus saline sinus irrigation in the treatment of cystic fibrosis-associated chronic rhinosinusitis: a randomised pilot trial. Clin Otolaryngol 2021;46(1):168–74.

57. Schulz V, Hänsel R, Blumenthal M, et al. Rational phytotherapy: a physicians' guide to herbal medicine. 5th edition. Heidelberg, Germany: Springer; 2004.

58. Glatthaar-Saalmüller B, Rauchhaus U, Rode S, et al. Antiviral activity in vitro of two preparations of the herbal medicinal product Sinupret against viruses causing respiratory infections. Phytomedicine 2011;19(1):1–7.

59. Virgin F, Zhang S, Schuster D, et al. The bioflavonoid compound, Sinupret, stimulates transepithelial chloride transport in vitro and in vivo. Laryngoscope 2010; 120(5):1051–6.

60. Richstein A, Mann W. [Treatment of chronic sinusitis with Sinupret]. Therapie der Gegenwart 1980;119(9):1055–60 [in German].

61. Berghorn LW, März RW. Placebo-controlled, randomized double-blind clinical trial with Sinupret solution (SE) in addition to a basic therapy with antibiotics and decongestant nasal drops in acute sinusitis [unpublished clinical and biometrical report]. Neumarkt: Bionorica GmbH; 1991.

62. Neubauer N, März RW. Placebo-controlled, randomized double-blind clinical trial with Sinupret sugar coated tablets on the basis of a therapy with antibiotics and decongestant nasal drops in acute sinusitis. Phytomedicine 1994;1:177–81.

63. Zimmer M. Gezielte konservative Therapie der akuten Sinusitis in der HNO-Praxis. Therapiewoche 1985;35:4042–408.

64. Passali D, Loglisci M, Passali GC, et al. A prospective open-label study to assess the efficacy and safety of a herbal medicinal product (Sinupret) in patients with acute rhinosinusitis. ORL J Otorhinolaryngol Relat Spec 2015;77(1): 27–32.

65. Palm J, Steiner I, Abramov-Sommariva D, et al. Assessment of efficacy and safety of the herbal medicinal product BNO 1016 in chronic rhinosinusitis. Rhinology 2017;55(2):142–51.

66. Reden J, El-Hifnawi DJ, Zahnert T, et al. The effect of a herbal combination of primrose, gentian root, vervain, elder flowers, and sorrel on olfactory function in patients with a sinonasal olfactory dysfunction. Rhinology 2011;49(3):342–6.

67. Popovych VI, Beketova HV, Koshel IV, et al. An open-label, multicentre, randomized comparative study of efficacy, safety and tolerability of the 5 plant - extract BNO 1012 in the delayed antibiotic prescription method in children, aged 6 to 11 years with acute viral and post-viral rhinosinusitis. Am J Otolaryngol 2020; 41(5):102564.

68. Wüstenberg P, Henneicke-von Zepelin HH, Köhler G, et al. Efficacy and mode of action of an immunomodulator herbal preparation containing Echinacea, wild indigo, and white cedar. Adv Ther 1999;16(1):51–70.

69. Naser B, Lund B, Henneicke-von Zepelin HH, et al. A randomized, double-blind, placebo-controlled, clinical dose-response trial of an extract of Baptisia, Echinacea and Thuja for the treatment of patients with common cold. Phytomedicine 2005;12(10):715–22.

70. Beuscher N, Kietzmann M, Bien E, et al. Interference of Myrtol standardized with inflammatory and allergic mediators. Arzneimittelforschung 1998;48(10):985–9.

71. Federspil P, Wulkow R, Zimmermann T. [Effects of standardized Myrtol in therapy of acute sinusitis: results of a double-blind, randomized multicenter study compared with placebo]. Laryngorhinootologie 1997;76(1):23–7 [in German].

72. Gottschlich S, Röschmann K, Candler H. Phytomedicines in acute rhinosinusitis: a prospective, non-interventional parallel-group trial. Adv Ther 2018;35(7): 1023–34.

73. Zalmanovici Trestioreanu A, Barua A, Pertzov B. Cyclamen europaeum extract for acute sinusitis. Cochrane Database Syst Rev 2018;5(5):CD011341.

74. Ponikau JU, Hamilos DL, Barreto A, et al. An exploratory trial of Cyclamen europaeum extract for acute rhinosinusitis. Laryngoscope 2012;122(9):1887–92.

75. Pfaar O, Mullol J, Anders C, et al. Cyclamen europaeum nasal spray, a novel phytotherapeutic product for the management of acute rhinosinusitis: a randomized double-blind, placebo-controlled trial. Rhinology 2012;50(1):37–44.

76. Conrad A, Kolberg T, Engels I, et al. [In vitro study to evaluate the antibacterial activity of a combination of the haulm of nasturtium (Tropaeoli majoris herba) and of the roots of horseradish (Armoraciae rusticanae radix)]. Arzneimittelforschung 2006;56(12):842–9 [in German].

77. Goos KH, Albrecht U, Schneider B. [On-going investigations on efficacy and safety profile of a herbal drug containing nasturtium herb and horseradish root in acute sinusitis, acute bronchitis and acute urinary tract infection in children in comparison with other antibiotic treatments]. Arzneimittelforschung 2007;57(4):238–46 [in German].

78. Dugasani S, Pichika MR, Nadarajah VD, et al. Comparative antioxidant and anti-inflammatory effects of [6]-gingerol, [8]-gingerol, [10]-gingerol and [6]-shogaol. J Ethnopharmacol 2010;127(2):515–20.

79. Chirumbolo S. The role of quercetin, flavonols and flavones in modulating inflammatory cell function. Inflamm Allergy Drug Targets 2010;9(4):263–85.

80. Xiao X, Shi D, Liu L, et al. Quercetin suppresses cyclooxygenase-2 expression and angiogenesis through inactivation of P300 signaling. PLoS One 2011;6(8): e22934.

81. Park HH, Lee S, Son HY, et al. Flavonoids inhibit histamine release and expression of proinflammatory cytokines in mast cells. Arch Pharm Res 2008;31(10): 1303–11.

82. Zhang S, Smith N, Schuster D, et al. Quercetin increases cystic fibrosis transmembrane conductance regulator-mediated chloride transport and ciliary beat frequency: therapeutic implications for chronic rhinosinusitis. Am J Rhinol Allergy 2011;25(5):307–12.

83. Maeda-Yamamoto M, Ema K, Shibuichi I. In vitro and in vivo anti-allergic effects of 'benifuuki' green tea containing O-methylated catechin and ginger extract enhancement. Cytotechnology 2007;55(2–3):135–42.

84. Chang JH, Song KJ, Kim H-J, et al. Dietary polyphenols affect MUC5AC expression and ciliary movement in respiratory cells and nasal mucosa. Am J Rhinol Allergy 2010;24(2):e59–62.

85. Jonas WB, Kaptchuk TJ, Linde K. A critical overview of homeopathy. Ann Intern Med 2003;138(5):393–9.

86. Witt CM, Lüdtke R, Willich SN. Homeopathic treatment of patients with chronic sinusitis: a prospective observational study with 8 years follow-up. BMC Ear Nose Throat Disord 2009;9:7.

87. Zabolotnyi DI, Kneis KC, Richardson A, et al. Efficacy of a complex homeopathic medication (Sinfrontal) in patients with acute maxillary sinusitis: a prospective, randomized, double-blind, placebo-controlled, multicenter clinical trial. Explore 2007;3(2):98–109.

88. Kneis KC, Gandjour A. Economic evaluation of Sinfrontal in the treatment of acute maxillary sinusitis in adults. Appl Health Econ Health Policy 2009;7(3): 181–91.

89. Yap L, Pothula VB, Warner J, et al. The root and development of otorhinolaryngology in traditional Chinese medicine. Eur Arch Otorhinolaryngol 2009;266(9): 1353–9.

90. Cabioğlu MT, Cetin BE. Acupuncture and immunomodulation. Am J Chin Med 2008;36(1):25–36.

91. Zijlstra FJ, van den Berg-de Lange I, Huygen FJ, et al. Anti-inflammatory actions of acupuncture. Mediators Inflamm 2003;12(2):59–69.

92. Carpenter RJ, Dillard J, Zion AS, et al. The acute effects of acupuncture upon autonomic balance in healthy subjects. Am J Chin Med 2010;38(5):839–47.

93. Zhou W, Longhurst JC. Neuroendocrine mechanisms of acupuncture in the treatment of hypertension. Evid Based Complement Alternat Med 2012;2012: 878673.

94. Hui KK, Marina O, Liu J, et al. Acupuncture, the limbic system, and the anticorrelated networks of the brain. Auton Neurosci 2010;157(1–2):81–90.

95. Zhao ZQ. Neural mechanism underlying acupuncture analgesia. Prog Neurobiol 2008;85(4):355–7.

96. Tai S, Wang J, Sun F, et al. Effect of needle puncture and electro-acupuncture on mucociliary clearance in anesthetized quails. BMC Complement Altern Med 2006;6:4.

97. Sertel S, Bergmann Z, Ratzlaff K, et al. Acupuncture for nasal congestion: a prospective, randomized, double-blind, placebo-controlled clinical pilot study. Am J Rhinol Allergy 2009;23(6):e23–8.

98. Lundeberg T, Laurell G, Thomas M. Effect of acupuncture on sinus pain and experimentally induced pain. Ear Nose Throat J 1988;67(8):565–6, 571–2, 574-566.

99. Pothman R, Yeh HL. The effects of treatment with antibiotics, laser and acupuncture upon chronic maxillary sinusitis in children. Am J Chin Med 1982; 10(1–4):55–8.

100. Stavem K, Røssberg E, Larsson PG. Health-related quality of life in a trial of acupuncture, sham acupuncture and conventional treatment for chronic sinusitis. BMC Res Notes 2008;1:37.

101. Røssberg E, Larsson PG, Birkeflet O, et al. Comparison of traditional Chinese acupuncture, minimal acupuncture at non-acupoints and conventional treatment for chronic sinusitis. Complement Ther Med 2005;13(1):4–10.

102. Wu AW, Gettelfinger JD, Ting JY, et al. Alternative therapies for sinusitis and rhinitis: a systematic review utilizing a modified Delphi method. Int Forum Allergy Rhinol 2020;10(4):496–504.

103. Bensky D, Gamble A. Chinese herbal medicine: materia medica. Revised Edition. Seattle: Eastland Press; 1993.

104. Bensky D, Barolet R. Chinese herbal medicine: formulas & strategies. Seattle: Eastland Press; 1990.

105. Haller CA, Benowitz NL. Adverse cardiovascular and central nervous system events associated with dietary supplements containing ephedra alkaloids. N Engl J Med 2000;343(25):1833–8.

106. An HJ, Jeong HJ, Lee EH, et al. Xanthii fructus inhibits inflammatory responses in LPS-stimulated mouse peritoneal macrophages. Inflammation 2004;28(5): 263–70.

107. Hong SH, Jeong HJ, Kim HM. Inhibitory effects of Xanthii fructus extract on mast cell-mediated allergic reaction in murine model. J Ethnopharmacol 2003; 88(2–3):229–34.

108. Huang MH, Wang BS, Chiu CS, et al. Antioxidant, antinociceptive, and anti-inflammatory activities of Xanthii Fructus extract. J Ethnopharmacol 2011; 135(2). 545-5.

109. Fan W, Fan L, Peng C, et al. Traditional uses, botany, phytochemistry, pharmacology, pharmacokinetics and toxicology of xanthium strumarium L.: a review. Molecules 2019;24(2):359.

110. Zhao Y, Woo KS, Ma KH, et al. Treatment of perennial allergic rhinitis using Shi-Bi-Lin, a Chinese herbal formula. J Ethnopharmacol 2009;122(1):100–5.

111. West PL, Mckeown NJ, Hendrickson RG. Muscle spasm associated with therapeutic use of Cang Er Zi Wan. Clin Toxicol (Phila) 2010;48(4):380–4.

112. Zhang XM, Zhang ZH. [The study of intoxication and toxicity of Fructus Xanthii]. Zhong Xi Yi Jie He Xue Bao 2003;1(1):71–3 [in Chinese].

113. Shen Y, Li CG, Zhou SF, et al. Chemistry and bioactivity of Flos Magnoliae, a Chinese herb for rhinitis and sinusitis. Curr Med Chem 2008;15(16):1616–27.

114. Kimura M, Suzuki J, Yamada T, et al. Anti-Inflammatory effect of Neolignans Newly Isolated from the Crude Drug "Shin-i" (Flos Magnoliae). Planta Med 1985;51(4):291–3.

115. Baek JA, Lee YD, Lee CB, et al. Extracts of Magnoliae flos inhibit inducible nitric oxide synthase via ERK in human respiratory epithelial cells. Nitric Oxide 2009; 20(2):122–8.

116. Kim HM, Yi JM, Lim KS. Magnoliae flos inhibits mast cell-dependent immediate-type allergic reactions. Pharmacol Res 1999;39(2):107–11.

117. Yen HR, Sun MF, Lin CL, et al. Adjunctive traditional Chinese medicine therapy for patients with chronic rhinosinusitis: a population-based study. Int Forum Allergy Rhinol 2015;5(3):240–6.

118. Liang C-Y, Wen P, Zhen Y, et al. Multi-centre randomized controlled trial of bi yuan shu liquid on patients with chronic nasal sinusitis or nasal polyp after endoscopic sinus surgery [in Chinese]. Chin J Evid Based Med 2004;4:377–81.

119. Liang KL, Su YC, Tsai CC, et al. Postoperative care with Chinese herbal medicine or amoxicillin after functional endoscopic sinus surgery: a randomized, double-blind, placebo-controlled study. Am J Rhinol Allergy 2011;25(3):170–5.

120. Jiang RS, Wu SH, Tsai CC, et al. Efficacy of Chinese herbal medicine compared with a macrolide in the treatment of chronic rhinosinusitis without nasal polyps. Am J Rhinol Allergy 2012;26(4):293–7.

121. Weber U, Luedtke R, Friese KH, et al. A non-randomised pilot study to compare complementary and conventional treatments of acute sinusitis. Forsch Komplementarmed Klass Naturheilkd 2002;9(2):99–104.

122. Suh JD, Wu AW, Taw MB, et al. Treatment of recalcitrant chronic rhinosinusitis with integrative east-west medicine: a pilot study. Arch Otolaryngol Head Neck Surg 2012;138(3):294–300.

123. Helms S, Miller A. Natural treatment of chronic rhinosinusitis. Altern Med Rev 2006;11(3):196–207.

124. Ivker RS. Chronic sinusitis. In: Rakel: Integrative Medicine. 4th Edition. Philadelphia: Saunders (Elsevier); 2018.

125. Federoff HJ, Gostin LO. Evolving from reductionism to holism: is there a future for systems medicine? JAMA 2009;302(9):994–6.

126. Weston AD, Hood L. Systems biology, proteomics, and the future of health care: toward predictive, preventative, and personalized medicine. J Proteome Res 2004;3(2):179–96.
127. Goldberger AL, Peng CK, Lipsitz LA. What is physiologic complexity and how does it change with aging and disease? Neurobiol Aging 2002;23(1):23–6.
128. Ferguson BJ, Seiden A. Chronic rhinosinusitis: preface. Otolaryngol Clin North Am 2005;38(6). xiii-xv.

Allergies and Natural Alternatives

Walter M. Jongbloed, MD, Seth M. Brown, MD, MBA*

KEYWORDS

- Allergic rhinitis • Allergy treatment • Integrative medicine • Complementary medicine

KEY POINTS

- Allergic rhinitis (AR) is a treatable disease with the typical otolaryngologist often using many conventional approaches including antihistamines, corticosteroids, decongestants, and immunotherapy.
- Complementary and integrative therapies have been investigated to varying degrees, and nutritional supplements, herbal medications, traditional medicines, and other techniques have shown varying efficacy in treating AR.
- Certain risks are associated with the use of complementary and integrative medicine and include risks of bleeding and drug interactions.
- Obtaining a thorough history of the use of complementary and integrative therapies is the responsibility of the otolaryngologist treating this condition.

INTRODUCTION

Complementary and integrative medicine (CIM) is defined as "diagnosis, treatment, and/or prevention which complements mainstream medicine by contributing to a common whole, by satisfying a demand not met by orthodoxy or by diversifying the conceptual frameworks of medicine."[1] It is a broad category of practices and treatments that is outside the realm of conventional medicine, including nutritional supplements, herbal treatments, acupuncture, traditional or cultural practices, homeopathy, naturopathy, mind–body medicine, and chiropractic or osteopathic manipulations. This discussion explores the role of CIM in the treatment of allergic rhinitis (AR).

The pathophysiology of AR centers on defining this condition as a systemic inflammatory process associated with inflammatory disorders of the mucous membranes including asthma, rhinosinusitis, and allergic conjunctivitis. It is a state of hypersensitivity that occurs when the body reacts to an allergen. Modern treatment of AR began with the emergence of antihistamine therapy in the 1930s. Topical corticosteroids were developed in the 1950s which, when added to antihistamines, became the

Division of Otolaryngology, Department of Surgery, University of Connecticut, School of Medicine, 263 Farmington Avenue, Farmington, CT 06030, USA
* Corresponding author.
E-mail address: sbrown1@prohealthmd.com

Otolaryngol Clin N Am 55 (2022) 965–982
https://doi.org/10.1016/j.otc.2022.06.005
0030-6665/22/© 2022 Elsevier Inc. All rights reserved.

mainstay of therapy. Since this time, decongestants, mast cell stabilizers, and leukotriene receptor antagonists have offered additional options for treatment. Throughout this time, the use of complementary and integrative therapies has paralleled during this surge of therapies. CIM therapies that target atopic conditions, such as AR, are second only to therapies for back pain.[2] CIM therapies are not unpopular as approximately 40% of adults in the United States[3] have used at least one type of CIM therapy.

The prevalence of AR in the United States has been estimated to be as high as 36%, and before the age of 6 years, 40% of children are affected by AR.[4,5] Subsequently, AR is a major cause of school and work absences, therefore, creating a high cost to the health care system.[6] As a result, it is not surprising that most patients and parents who adopt CIM therapies use it as a complement to conventional care.[7,8] The reasons why patients use natural alternatives are complicated; they include a distrust in conventional medicine and the belief that CIM is more natural and safer.[9] Even with natural alternatives and conventional care, many patients do not believe that their symptoms are well controlled.[10] The negative motivation for using CIM emphasizes the important role of the physician in advising patients on these methods. However, a significant portion (40%–70%) of patients does not disclose the use of CIM therapies to their physicians.[11–13]

Physicians play an integral role in advising patients on the use of natural alternatives. Maintaining an awareness of the efficacy and contraindications of these alternatives is a critical responsibility. However, physicians face a challenge; there is a void of randomized controlled trials and experimental data to support the routine use of these alternatives. It is therefore, the responsibility of the physician to diligently review the data that are available, and then offer advice and recommendations to his or her patients. Many physicians are intimated by CIM because they are unaware of the clinical evidence and feel uncomfortable advising their patients on its efficacy.[9] An obstacle that cannot be understated is that herbal remedies are usually not standardized and most, to varying degrees, contain a mixture of substances. This lack of standardization potentiates the possibility of toxicity, drug-to-drug interactions, and a discrepancy even within what may be marketed as the same supplement. Knowledge of CIM therapies that impact the bleeding time is vital for the perioperative period.[14] Compared with proprietary marketing drugs, herbal remedies carry the risk of impurities, incorrect collection of plants, wrong preparation, and inappropriate/incorrect dosing.[15] Regardless of the obstacles that may limit a physician's knowledge of these alternatives, many patients are using or have used these therapies. Consequently, there is a need for physicians to inquire and discuss these alternatives with their patients while maintaining an understanding of the available data on these natural alternatives. This discussion addresses each natural alternative that has played a role in the treatment of AR, discusses the evidence behind the remedy, and offers recommendations for the physician.

DISCUSSION

The use of CIM therapies in allergy can be split into the broad categories of nutritional supplements, herbal supplements, Ayurvedic medicine, and Chinese traditional medicine.

NUTRITIONAL SUPPLEMENTS

Various nutritional supplements have been reported to improve the symptoms of allergy and AR or hasten recovery of upper respiratory infections. **Table 1** details the active ingredients, intended use, and mechanism of action of each of these

Table 1
Nutritional supplements used in the treatment of allergy and allergic rhinitis

Supplement	Active Ingredient	Uses and Mechanism of Action	Adverse Effects	Drug–Drug Interactions
Vitamin C	Ascorbic acid	Acute viral or bacterial rhinitis Inhibit histamine secretion by lymphocytes[16] Decrease nasal secretions, congestion. and edema[16]	Kidney stones Diarrhea Delayed wound healing Increase iron absorption in blood-iron disorders (thalassemia, hemochromatosis) Worsen sickle cell disease	Decrease effectiveness of HIV/AIDS medications Decrease effectiveness of warfarin (Coumadin) Delay metabolism of aspirin
Capsaicin	8-methyl-N-vanillyl-6-nonenamide	Allergic rhinitis Inhibit release of substance P from nasal mucosal cells, decreasing IL-6 production[17]	Localized irritation at application site	Unknown
Fish Oil	Eicosapentaenoic acid and docosahexaenoic acids, ω-3 fatty acids	Allergic rhinitis Anti-inflammatory properties Reduce production and effectiveness of prostaglandins[17]	Dose-related increase in bleeding time Hypotension by increasing the effects of antihypertensive medications	Unknown
Spirulina	Filamentous cyanobacteria, blue-green algae *Arthrospira platensis*, *Aporosa fusiformis, and Aristolochia maxima*	Allergic rhinitis Anti-inflammatory Inhibition of histamine release from mast cells Reduce IL-4, enhances IgA production[18,19]	Hepatotoxicity Heavy metal contamination	Unknown

(continued on next page)

Table 1
(continued)

Supplement	Active Ingredient	Uses and Mechanism of Action	Adverse Effects	Drug–Drug Interactions
Manuka/Tualang honey	Methylglyoxal	Allergic rhinitis Anti-inflammatory Modulates mast cell response[20] Suppresses antigen-specific IgE levels[21]	Unknown	Unknown

HIV/AIDS, Human immunodeficiency virus/acquired immunodeficiency syndrome; IgA, Immunoglobulin A; IgE, Immunoglobulin E; IL, interleukin; MIC, minimum inhibitory concentration; OTC, over-the-counter.

supplements, as well as the adverse effects and known drug–drug interactions. Unfortunately, much is still unknown about the side effects and interactions of these supplements.

Vitamin C, also known as ascorbic acid, has been used for the treatment of acute bacterial and viral rhinitis by inhibition of histamine secretion by lymphocytes.[16] It has been shown to decrease nasal secretions, congestion, and edema.[16] The most common adverse effects include kidney stones, diarrhea, delayed wound healing, increased iron absorption in diseases like thalassemia and hemochromatosis, and it may worsen sickle cell disease. Vitamin C also decreases the effectiveness of HIV/AIDS medications including amprenavir, nelfinavir, ritonavir, and saquinavir. It also decreases the effectiveness of warfarin and delays the metabolism of aspirin.

Capsaicin contains the active ingredient 8-methyl-N-vanillyl-6-nonenamide and is used as a topical treatment of AR by blocking neuropeptide substance P, thereby reducing IL-6 production.[16] However, one study has shown no therapeutic effect in the treatment of AR.[17] Side effects are relatively benign, mainly limited to localized irritation at application site.

Fish oil contains eicosapentaenoic acid and docosahexaenoic acids (omega-3 fatty acids), which are used in the treatment of AR via anti-inflammatory properties of reducing the production and effectiveness of prostaglandins. However, the efficacy of fish oil has not been overly positive, with some studies showing no benefit, and another showing an increase in the prevalence of AR in those with reduced intake of fish oil.[17] Fish oil has a dose-related increase in bleeding time and has been shown to decrease blood pressure by increasing the effect of antihypertensive medications, thereby causing hypotension.

Spirulina is a filamentous cyanobacteria or blue-green algae of the genus *Arthrospira*. It has been used in the management of AR by inhibiting the release of histamine from mast cells and reducing IL-4 in the IgE-mediated allergy pathway, thereby enhancing IgA production.[19] Spirulina has been shown to decrease IL-4 and improve nasal symptoms in patients with AR after 6 months of spirulina dosing.[18,19] In addition, spirulina has been cited as inhibiting histamine release from mast cells and increased interferon (INF)-gamma levels.[19] On the negative side, spirulina has been shown to cause hepatotoxicity and reaction from heavy metal contamination.

Manuka honey and Tualang honey contain the active ingredient of methylglyoxal and are used in the treatment of AR. They have been shown to modulate mast cell response and suppress IgE levels.[20,21] Clinically, they have been shown in clinical trials to improve the symptoms of AR, and the findings state that ingestion of honey along with standard antihistamines is beneficial in relieving the AR symptoms without any reported adverse effect.[22] However, another study showed no decrease in allergy symptoms when compared with placebo.[23]

HERBAL SUPPLEMENTS

Various herbal supplements have been used in the treatment of allergy and AR. **Table 2** details the active ingredients, intended use, and mechanism of action, as well as adverse effects and drug–drug interactions.

Angelica, also known as Danggui, is from the *Angelica archangelica* plant. It is an expectorant used for bronchial illnesses, allergies, colds, and coughs, as well as for treatment of mild spasms of the gastrointestinal tract, loss of appetite (anorexia nervosa), flatulence, and satiety. Isolated forms of the various furanocoumarins have shown to have an inhibitory effect on the lipopolysaccharide-induced prostaglandin E2 production with decreased expressions of cyclooxygenase-2 and microsomal

Table 2
Herbal supplements used in the treatment of allergy and allergic rhinitis

Supplement	Active Ingredient	Uses and Mechanism of Action	Adverse Effects	Drug–Drug Interactions
Angelia (*A archangelica*) Danngui	Furanocoumarins	Allergic rhinitis, upper respiratory infections Inhibitory effect on prostaglandin E2[24]	Photodermatitis and phototoxicity[25,26]	Inhibition of cytochrome P450
Bromelain (*A comosus*)	Proteolytic enzyme of the pineapple plant	Allergic rhinitis, sinusitis, anti-inflammatory Mucolytic; thins nasal mucus secretion Inhibits production of prostaglandin E1[16]	Gastrointestinal upset Allergic reactions overlap with allergies to pineapple, wheat, celery, papain, carrot, fennel, and cypress pollen or grass pollen	Unknown
Butterbur (*Petasites hydridus*)	Petasin	Allergic rhinitis Inhibits leukotrienes, mast cell degranulation, and nasal levels of histamine[27–29]	Removal of pyrrolizidine alkaloids is essential Pyrrolizidine alkaloids are hepatotoxic and carcinogenic Petasin is a processed butterbur extract with alkaloids removed[30–32] Gastrointestinal upset	Unknown
Cineole	Eucalyptol, 1,8-cineole, an extract from eucalyptus oil	Acute rhinosinusitis, anti-inflammatory Increased beat frequency of cilia[33]	Reflux, headache, and nausea Undiluted eucalyptus oil is toxic (3.5 mL of undiluted oil can be fatal) Symptoms of poisoning include dizziness, weakness, mydriasis, shortness of breath and abdominal pain/burning	Unknown

Herb	Active constituents	Indications/actions	Adverse effects	Drug interactions
Echinacea (E angustifolia, E pallida, and E purpurea)	Alkamides, chicoric acid, and polysaccharides	Acute infectious rhinitis; Activates T and B lymphocytes in vitro[35]	Gastrointestinal upset, tongue numbness, headache, muscular aches, and dizziness; Associated with hepatotoxicity, especially after 8 wk of use	May delay metabolism of caffeine, causing tachycardia and nervousness
Ephedra (E sinica) Ma huang	Ephedrine	Nasal congestion, asthma, bronchitis, and nasal congestion, weight loss aid and stimulant; Central nervous system stimulant via noradrenaline on adrenergic receptors[36,37]	Tachycardia, palpitations, hallucinations, hypertension, paranoia, and potentially death[38-42]; Banned for OTC use as a dietary supplement[45]	Interactions with glycosides and halothane, may cause arrhythmias and potentiation of monoamine oxidase inhibitors (MAOIs)[43-45]
Esberitox (T occidentalis, E purpurea, and B tinctoria)	Alkamides, chicoric acid, and polysaccharides	Acute sinusitis; Immune stimulant	Rashes, retching, facial swelling, vertigo, and hypotension	Unknown
Garlic (A sativum)	Allicin (diallyl-thiosulfinate)	Acute infectious rhinitis, cough; Inhibition of prostaglandins, thromboxanes	Rare allergic reactions, hypoglycemia, prolonged bleeding time; Decreased platelet aggregation within 5 d of oral dosing via inhibition of epinephrine-induced platelet aggregation[12]; Recommend discontinuation 1 wk before surgery	Inhibits cytochrome P450[2]; May interfere with paracetamol and chlorpropamide; Hypoglycemia; Increase MIC of ampicillin
Ginkgo (Ginkgo biloba)	Ginkgolides; Terpene lactones and ginkgo flavone glycosides	Inhibits development of bronchial hyperreactivity; Inhibits eosinophil influx into animal airways induced by platelet activating factor or antigen exposure[46,47]	Unknown	Inhibition of cytochrome P450; Increase in blood pressure when combined with thiazide diuretics[48] and coma with trazodone[49,50]

(continued on next page)

Table 2
(continued)

Supplement	Active Ingredient	Uses and Mechanism of Action	Adverse Effects	Drug–Drug Interactions
Grape seed extract	Proanthocyanidins	Chemoprevention of cellular damage[51]	Unknown	Unknown
Licorice root (*G glabra*)	Glycoside glycyrrhizin	Allergic rhinitis, conjunctivitis, and bronchitis Anti-inflammatory and antiviral Inhibit 11-beta-hydroxysteroid dehydrogenase and the classic complement pathway	Hypokalemia, muscle pain, extremity numbness, pseudo-aldosteronism which may lead to hypertension, headaches, and cardiac events[12]	Interferes with ACE inhibitors, diuretics, corticosteroids, insulin and other diabetic drugs, MAOIs, oral contraceptives, and digoxin, and can dangerously increase the toxicity of digoxin[43]
Myrtol (*Pinus spp* (pine), *C aurantifolia* (lime) and *Eucalyptus globulus*)	Monoterpenes, D-limonene, 1,8-cineole, alpha-pinene	Acute rhinosinusitis, chronic rhinosinusitis, anti-inflammatory Secretolytic and secretomotoric effects, increase upper and lower airway patency[52]	Gastrointestinal disturbance, facial swelling, allergic reactions, and taste disturbances	Unknown
N-acetylcysteine	N-acetylcysteine	Sinusitis Mucolytic Cleavage of disulfide bonds in mucoproteins by its sulfhydryl group resulting in less viscous mucus[16]	Gastrointestinal upset	Unknown
P frutescens	Phenolic acids, flavonoids, anthocyanins	Upper respiratory infections, asthma, allergic rhinitis Antioxidant, anti-	Pulmonary toxicity in animal studies, no evidence to support toxicity in humans[53,54]	Unknown

		inflammatory, antibacterial		
Quercetin (3,3',4'5-7-pentahydroxyflavone)	Bioflavonoid	Anti-inflammatory Inhibition of inflammatory enzymes (cyclooxygenase and lipoxygenase, regulators of leukotrienes and prostaglandins) Mast cell stabilizer, inhibits release of histamine	Unknown	May lessen the effects of quinolone antibiotics Not recommended in those with hypertension, immunosuppression, or kidney stones[34]
Sinupret Elder flower (Sambucus nigra), cowslip flowers (Primula veris), common sorrel (Rumex acetosa) European vervain (Verbena officinalis), and gentian (Gentiana lutea) root	Unknown	Allergic rhinosinusitis Mucolytic, antiviral, anti-inflammatory[33]	Kidney stones, allergic reactions, gastrointestinal symptoms, numbness, and mild dermatitis	Interacts with therapeutic monoclonal antibodies, hypertensive medications, and immunosuppressants (tacrolimus, methotrexate, corticosteroids, mycophenolate, etanercept, and cyclosporine)
Stinging nettle (U dioica)	Unknown	Allergic rhinitis[55]	Application to mucosal surfaces causes burning and itching, contact dermatitis, GI disturbances[2]	Unknown

prostaglandin E synthetase.[24] It also has inhibitory effects on cytochrome P450. Adverse effects include skin sensitization to sunlight due to the furanocoumarins causing photodermatitis and phototoxicity.[25,26]

Bromelain is an extract from the pineapple plant *Ananas comosus*. It contains a proteolytic enzyme used in the treatment of AR, sinusitis, and for anti-inflammatory properties. It is a mucolytic, which thereby thins nasal mucus and inhibits the production of prostaglandin E1.[26] It has been shown to aid in a faster symptomatic recovery from sinusitis.[16] An adverse side effect is gastrointestinal upset. It should not be used in those with allergies to pineapple, wheat, celery, papain, carrot, fennel, cypress pollen, or grass pollen because of an allergic reaction overlap with the pineapple plant.

Butterbur (*Petasites hybridus*) is a perennial shrub found in Europe and parts of Asia and North America which contains petasin, a compound believed to have anti-inflammatory and leukotriene inhibitory properties.[32,56,57] Petasin inhibits the biosynthesis of cysteinyl leukotrienes in vitro[27-29] and decreases nasal levels of histamine and cysteinyl leukotrienes in vivo.[56] In a randomized clinical trial, butterbur was shown to relieve symptoms, attenuate peak nasal inspiratory flow recovery, and reduce maximum percentage of peak nasal inspiratory flow decrease from baseline.[58,59] When compared against fexofenadine, it has been shown to be non-inferior in relieving symptoms of AR.[60] Trials suggest that *P hybridus* is superior to placebo or similarly effective when compared with nonsedative antihistamines.[60,61] Butterbur contains pyrrolizidine alkaloids which have been shown to cause acute hepatotoxicity, DNA damage, and neurologic damage.[30-32] Only butterbur with pyrrolizidine alkaloids removed should thus be considered for use.

Cineole is an herbal supplement containing eucalyptol (1,8-cineole), which is an extract from the eucalyptus plant. It has been used for the treatment of acute rhinosinusitis by increasing cilia beat frequency.[33] Clinical trials have shown efficacy when used with decongestants; it improves the effectiveness of nasal decongestants for the treatment of acute rhinosinusitis compared with placebo when dosed early in the course of an infection.[34] The known side effects include reflux, headache, and nausea. Importantly, undiluted eucalyptus oil is toxic, with a fatal dose of 3.5 mL. The symptoms of eucalyptus poisoning include dizziness, weakness, mydriasis, shortness of breath, and abdominal pain/abdominal burning.

Echinacea has been used for the treatment of the common cold and upper respiratory tract allergies. It reportedly has antiviral and immunomodulating properties.[35] Three species of *Echinacea* commonly used are *Echinacea angustifolia*, *Echinacea pallida,* and *Echinacea purpurea*. Studies to date have shown no benefit in the prevention of acute otitis media in children.[62] In treatment of the common cold, most recent randomized clinical trials have shown that *Echinacea* provides no detectable benefit or harm.[63] Older studies reported a reduction in severity and duration of upper respiratory tract disorders such as a cold, but more recent literature has not supported these claims.[64-66] Regardless, there are no clinical trials to support the use of *Echinacea* in the management of AR.

Ephedra (*Ephedra sinica*), also known as ma huang, is commonly used to treat asthma, bronchitis, and nasal congestion. It is also used as a diet aid for weight loss, enhancement of athletic performance, and as a central nervous system stimulant.[36,37] It has been used for nasal congestion, asthma, bronchitis, and nasal congestion, as well as a weight loss aid and stimulant. It works by simulating adrenergic receptors via norepinephrine. Therefore, common adverse side effects include hypertension, insomnia, tremor, heart palpitations, stroke, and even fatalities[38-42] There are also known drug interactions, including arrhythmias with cardiac glycosides and halothane, enhanced sympathomimetic effect with guanethidine, and monoamine oxidase inhibitors.[42–45] Ephedra was banned in 2004 for its over-the-counter use as a dietary supplement by the US federal government due to increasing reports of adverse effects.[45]

Esberitox is an herbal supplement derived from three species of plants, *Thuja occidentalis, E purpurea,* and *Baptisia tinctoria.* The active ingredients include alkamides, chicoric acid, and polysaccharides which are reported to be immune stimulants used to treat acute sinusitis. It has been shown to have a positive effect as an adjunct to doxycycline for treatment of acute sinusitis.[34] Significant side effects include rashes, retching, facial swelling, vertigo, and hypotension.

Garlic (Allium sativum) contains allicin (diallyl-thiosulfinate). It is used in the treatment of acute infectious rhinitis and cough via the inhibition of prostaglandins and thromboxanes. There are rare side effects including hypoglycemia, prolonged bleeding time due to decreased platelet aggregation prompting the recommendation for discontinuation 1 week before surgery.[12] Garlic inhibits cytochrome P450, thereby potentiating warfarin.[2] It may also interfere with paracetamol and chlorpropamide and may increase the minimum inhibitory concentration of ampicillin.

Ginkgo (Ginkgo biloba) and ginkgo derivatives containing ginkgolides are commonly used for decreased vascular perfusion type syndromes, such as peripheral arterial insufficiency, cerebral insufficiency associated with memory loss, difficulties in concentration, fatigue, anxiety, headaches, and depressed mood. In asthmatic patients, it has been shown to inhibit the development of bronchial hyperreactivity.[46,47] However, drug interactions include increased bleeding when combined with warfarin and spontaneous hemorrhage, which has led to its cautious use in patients receiving aspirin, nonsteroidal anti-inflammatory drugs, anticoagulants, or other platelet inhibitors. An increase in blood pressure when combined with thiazide diuretics[48] and coma when combined with trazodone have also been reported.[49,50]

Grape seed extract contains proanthocyanidins, which have been reported to prevent cellular damage.[67] In vivo studies have showed that grape seed extract may generate possible beneficial effects in the chemoprevention of cellular damage, chemotherapy-induced toxic effects of anthracycline, tissue damage in acute and chronic pancreatitis, acetaminophen-induced hepatotoxicity, and b-cell lymphoma (bcl) and cellular myelocytomatosis (c-myc) oncogene expression and had some cardioprotective effect with red wine consumption.[51,68–70] In the treatment of AR, clinical trials have shown no improvement.[67]

Licorice root (Glycyrrhiza glabra) contains glycoside and glycyrrhizin which are used in the treatment of AR, conjunctivitis, and bronchitis. It inhibits 11-beta-hydroxysteroid dehydrogenase and the classic complement pathway. Owing to the mechanism of action, side effects are primarily hypokalemia and pseudo-aldosteronism, which leads to hypertension, headaches, and cardiac events.[12] It is known to interfere with angiotensin-converting enzyme (ACE) inhibitors, diuretics, corticosteroids, insulin, monoamine oxidase inhibitors , and oral contraceptives and may dangerously increase the toxicity of digoxin.[45]

Myrtol is a combination of extracts from pine *(Pinus spp),* lime *(Citrus aurantifolia),* and eucalyptus. It contains monoterpenes, D-limonene, 1,8-cineole, and alpha-pinene. It is used for its secretolytic and secretomotoric properties in the treatment of AR and chronic rhinosinusitis (CRS).[52] Research has only shown a modest benefit in one study, but the data were insufficient to draw any significant conclusions.[35] Primary side effects include gastrointestinal disturbance, facial swelling, allergic reactions, and disturbance of taste.

N-acetylcysteine is a mucolytic used in the treatment of sinusitis via cleavage of di-sulfide bonds in mucoproteins, thereby reducing the viscosity of mucus.[16] There have been no trials assessing the efficacy of this compound. The only described side effect is gastrointestinal disturbance.

Perilla frutescens is an annual herb native to eastern Asia. It contains phenolic acids, flavonoids, and anthocyanins which are used in the treatment of upper respiratory in-fections, asthma, and AR. Clinical trials to date have not shown any significant improvement in symptoms of AR.[71] In animal studies, it has been shown to cause pul-monary toxicity, although it has not been studied sufficiency in humans to assess for this side effect.[53,54]

Quercetin contains 3,3′,4′5-7-pentahydroxyflavone, a bioflavonoid, which is used for anti-inflammatory properties via inhibition of cyclooxygenase and lipoxygenase which regulate leukotrienes and prostaglandins. It is reportedly a mast cell stabilizer which inhibits the release of histamine. However, no definitive evidence of its effect has been shown in clinical trials. It may lessen the effects of quinolone antibiotics and is not recommended for use in those with hypertension, immunosuppression, or kidney stones.[34]

Sinupret is a proprietary combination of elder flower, cowslip flowers, common sor-rel, European vervain, and gentian root. It is used in the treatment of AR as a mucolytic with antiviral and anti-inflammatory properties. Its efficacy has been tested in three large studies which have shown positive efficacy.[33] Side effects include kidney stones, allergic reactions, gastrointestinal symptoms, numbness, and mild dermatitis. It interacts with therapeutic monoclonal antibodies, hypertensive medications, and immunosuppressants.

Stinging nettle (*Urtica dioica*) is a perennial plant found in Africa, Europe, and North America. Its application to mucosal surfaces causes burning and itching and at times contact dermatitis, whereas its ingestion is known to cause mild gastrointestinal dis-turbances such as diarrhea.[55] Double-blind randomized studies in the treatment of AR have shown no, or only subjective benefit. [2,55]

AYURVEDIC MEDICINE

The goal of Ayurvedic medicine is to balance body, mind, and spirit through herbal medications, massage, and diet. In Sanskrit, *ayur* means life and *veda* means science. Of the multitude of Ayurvedic herbs and formulas, Aller-7 and Tinofend are both used for the treatment of AR.

Aller-7/NR-A2 is a formulation of herbal extracts including quercetin, stinging nettle, methylsulfonylmethane, turmeric, feverfew, ginger, and vitamin C. Randomized clin-ical trials testing Aller-7 against placebo in relieving symptoms of AR have shown potentially some benefit in relieving symptoms.[72,73] In animal models, Aller-7 has shown anti-inflammatory effects.[74] Overall, it has shown some improvement in AR symptoms by reducing inflammation.[17]

Tinofend (Tinospora cordifolia) or guduchi in Sanskrit has historically *been* used in the treatment of fever, jaundice, chronic diarrhea, cancer, dysentery, bone fracture, pain, asthma, skin disease, poisonous insect, snake bite, and eye disorders.[75] It has been reported to boost the phagocytic activity of macrophages and increase the production of reactive oxygen species in neutrophil cells.[76] It may influence cyto-kine production, mitogenicity, and stimulation and activation of immune effector cells.[77] In animal models, it has been shown to upregulate IL-6, activate cytotoxic T cells, and affect B cell differentiation.[78] It has been shown to also enhance immune response in mice by inducing secretion of IL-1 and activating macrophages. The(1,4)-

alpha-d-glucan, derived *T cordifolia* has been shown to activate human lymphocytes with downstream synthesis of the pro- and anti-inflammatory cytokines.[79] There has, however, only been one randomized clinical trial in patients with AR, which showed the reduction of symptoms in the test group.[80]

CHINESE TRADITIONAL MEDICINE

Shi-bi-lin is a Chinese herbal medication used in the treatment of AR by inhibiting release of IL-4 and TNF-alpha.[17] Animal trials have shown a decrease in eosinophil infiltration; however, human safety trials have not emerged.

Xiao-qing-long-tang, Sho-seiryu-to in Japanese or *TJ-19,* is a granule made from 8 Chinese herbs: *Paeonia lactiflora, E sinica, Cinnamomum cassia,* calcium sulfate, *Prunus armeniaca, Glycyrrhiza uralensis, Zingiber officinale,* and *Ziziphus jujube.* It is used for infectious rhinitis, asthma, and AR and shows the inhibition of histamine signaling and IL-4 and IL-5 expression in rat models.[17] One study has shown improvement in symptoms of sneezing, stuffy nose, and running nose, but not for nasal membrane edema.[81]

Biminne (11-herb CHM) is a capsule composed of 11 Chinese herbs (*Rehmannia glutinosa, Scutellaria baicalensis, Polygonatum sibiricum, Ginkgo biloba, Epimedium sagittatum, Psoralea corylifolia, Schisandra chinensis,* pulp of *Prunus mume, Ledebouriella divaricata, Angelica dahurica,* and *Astragalus membranaceus*). In one clinical trial, only one symptom (sneezing) was significantly reduced compared with placebo and there was no improvement in nasal obstruction.[82]

An extract of *18 Chinese herbs* (*Angelica sinensis*; Asari, herba; Astragali, radix; *Atractylodis macrocephalae,* rhizome; Bupleuri, radix; Cimicifugae, rhizome; *Codonopsis pilosulae,* radix; Glycyrrhizae, radix; Chuanxiong, rhizome; Magnoliae, flos; Menthae, herba; *Citri reticulatae,* pericarpium; Plantaginis, semen; Schisandrae, fructus; Schizonepetae, herba; Saposhnikoviae, radix; Chebulae, fructus; and Xanthii, fructus) has been studied in one small (*n* = 55) trial in the treatment of AR, which showed improvement in symptoms after 5 to 6 weeks of treatment.[83]

Acupuncture. Please refer to the chapter on acupuncture for further discussion.

ADDITIONAL THERAPIES

Homeopathy uses stimulating active ingredients dosed in ultra-dilution based on an individual's symptomatic response.[17] Homeopathic treatments have varied efficacy but have been shown to worsen symptoms.

Phototherapy uses light wavelengths to stimulate an immunosuppressive response. Phototherapy reduces antigen presentation by dendritic cells and inhibits proinflammatory factors, thereby decreasing levels of IL-5 and eosinophils.[17] Further studies have demonstrated efficacy, especially for patients for who use of other drugs are contraindicated.[84–86]

SUMMARY

CIM therapies in the treatment of allergy and AR are divided broadly into the categories of nutritional supplements, herbal supplements, Ayurvedic, and Chinese traditional medicine. The efficacy of these therapies is varied and under-researched. The therapies with the strongest evidence in the treatment of allergy and AR are Manuka honey, Butterbur, and Sinupret. It is at the discretion of the physician to balance efficacy against risks when advising patients of these treatment options.

CLINICS CARE POINTS

- Maintaining knowledge of complementary and integrative medicine (CIM) therapies is essential in the treatment of allergic rhinitis (AR).
- The otolaryngologist must ask patients about the use of CIM therapies and monitor for adverse effects and drug interactions.
- In the perioperative period, a thorough understanding of CIM therapy's impact on bleeding and interaction with conventional medications is critical.
- American Society of Anesthesiologists recommends the discontinuation all herbal medications 2 to 4 weeks before surgery.
- Research on the efficacy of CIM therapies is lacking for many supplements and herbs; therefore, randomized clinical trials are needed to improve standardization of CIM therapies.

DISCLOSURE

The authors have no relevant disclosures related to this topic.

REFERENCES

1. Ernst E, Resch KL, Mills S, et al. Complementary medicine—a definition. Br J Gen Pract 1995;45:506.
2. Bielory L. Complementary and alternative interventions in asthma, allergy, and immunology. Ann Allergy Asthma Immunol 2004;93(2 Suppl 1):S45–54.
3. Neiberg RH, Aickin M, Grzywacz JG, et al. Occurrence and co-occurrence of types of complementary and alternative medicine use by age, gender, ethnicity, and education among adults in the United States: the 2002 National Health Interview Survey (NHIS). J Altern Complement Med 2011;17(4):363–70.
4. Blaiss MS. Cognitive, social and economic costs of allergic rhinitis. Allergy Asthma Proc 2000;21:7–13.
5. Schoenwetter WF. Allergic rhinitis: epidemiology and natural history. Allergy Asthma Proc 2000;21:1–6.
6. Malone DC, Lawson KA, Smith DH, et al. A cost of illness study of allergic rhinitis in the United States. J Allergy Clin Immunol 1997;99:22–7.
7. Astin JA. Why patients use alternative medicine: results of a national study. JAMA 1998;279:1548–53.
8. Eisenberg DM, Kessler RC, Foster C, et al. Unconventional medicine in the United States: prevalence, costs and patterns of use. N Engl J Med 1993;328:246–52.
9. Passalacqua G, Compalati E, Schiappoli M, et al. Complementary and alternative medicine for the treatment and diagnosis of asthma and allergic diseases. Monaldi Arch Chest Dis 2005;63:47–54.
10. Storms W, Meltzer EO, Nathan RA. Allergic rhinitis: the patient's perspective. J Allergy Clin Immunol 1997;99:S825–9.
11. Shakeel M, Trinidade A, Ah-See KW. Complementary and alternative medicine use by otolaryngology patients: a paradigm for practitioners in all surgical specialties. Eur Arch Otorhinolaryngol 2010;267(6):961–71.
12. Miller LG. Herbal medicinals: selected clinical considerations focusing on known or potential drug-herb interactions. Arch Intern Med 1998;158(20):2200–11.

13. Shakeel M, Newton JR, Ah-See KW. Complementary and alternative medicine use among patients under-going otolaryngologic surgery. J Otolaryngol Head Neck Surg 2009;38(3):355–61.
14. Roehm CE, Tessema B, Brown SM. The role of alternative medicine in rhinology. Facial Plast Surg Clin North Am 2012;20(1):73–81.
15. Ernst E. Adulteration of Chinese herbal medicines with synthetic drugs: a systematic review. J Intern Med 2002;252:107–13.
16. Helms S, Miller A. Natural treatment of chronic rhinosinusitis. Altern Med Rev 2006;11(3):196–207.
17. Man LX. Complementary and alternative medicine for allergic rhinitis. Curr Opin Otolaryngol Head Neck Surg 2009;17(3):226–31.
18. Karkos PD, Leong SC, Arya AK, et al. "Complementary ENT": a systematic review of commonly used supplements. J Laryngol Otol 2007;121(8):779–82.
19. Mao TK, Van de Water J, Gershwin ME. Effects of a *Spirulina*- based dietary supplement on cytokine production from allergic rhinitis patients. J Med Food 2005;8: 27–30.
20. Alangari AA, Morris K, Lwaleed BA, et al. Honey is potentially effective in the treatment of atopic dermatitis: clinical and mechanistic studies. Immun Inflamm Dis 2017;5:190–9.
21. Duddukuri GR, Kumar PS, Kumar VB, et al. Immunosuppressive effect of honey on the induction of allergen-specific humoral antibody response in mice. Int Arch Allergy Immunol 1997;114:385–8.
22. Asha'Ari ZA, Ahmad MZ, Wan Din WSJ, et al. Ingestion of honey improves the symptoms of allergic rhinitis: evidence from a randomized placebo-controlled trial in the East Coast of Peninsular Malaysia. Ann Saudi Med 2013;33:469–75.
23. Rajan TV, Tennen H, Lindquist RL, et al. Effect of ingestion of honey on symptoms of rhinoconjunctivitis. Ann Allergy Asthma Immunol 2002;88(2):198–203. Honey is generally very well tolerated with no known side effects or drug interactions.
24. Ban HS, Lim SS, Suzuki K, et al. Inhibitory effects of furanocoumarins isolated from the roots of *Anglelica dahurica* on prostaglandin E2 production. Planta Med 2003;69:408–12.
25. Hann SK, Park YK, Im S, et al. Angelica-induced phytophotodermatitis. Photodermatol Photoimmunol Photomed 1991;8:84–5.
26. Baek NI, Ahn EM, Kim HY, et al. Furanocoumarins from the root of. Angelia Dahurica Arch Pharm Res 2000;23:467–70.
27. Thomet OA, Wiesmann UN, Blaser K, et al. Differential inhibition of inflammatory effector functions by petasin, isopetasin and neopetasin in human eosinophils. Clin Exp Allergy 2001;31:1310–20.
28. Thomet OA, Wiesmann UN, Schapowal A, et al. Role of petasin in the potential anti-inflammatory activity of a plant extract of. Petasites Hybridus Biochem Pharmacol 2001;61:1041–7.
29. Bickel D, Roder T, Bestmann HJ, et al. Identification and characterization of inhibitors of peptido-leukotriene-synthesis from. Petasites Hybridus Planta Med 1994; 60:318–22.
30. Chen T, Mei N, Fu PP. Genotoxicity of pyrrolizidine alkaloids. J Appl Toxicol 2010; 30:183–96. https://doi.org/10.1002/jat.1504.
31. Glück J, Ebmeyer J, Waizenegger J, et al. Hepatotoxicity of pyrrolizidine alkaloids in human hepatocytes and endothelial cells. Toxicol Lett 2018;295:S142. https://doi.org/10.1016/j.toxlet.2018.06.72.
32. Jank B, Rath J. The risk of pyrrolizidine alkaloids in human food and animal feed. Trends Plant Sci 2017;22:191–3. https://doi.org/10.1016/j.tplants.2017.01.002.

33. Tesche S, Metternich F, Sonnemann U, et al. The value of herbal medicines in the treatment of acute non-purulent rhinosinusitis. Results of a double-blind, randomised, controlled trial. Eur Arch Otorhinolaryngol 2008;265(11):1355–9.

34. Guo R, Canter PH, Ernst E. Herbal medicines for the treatment of rhinosinusitis: a systematic review. Otolaryngol Head Neck Surg 2006;135(4):496–506.

35. David S, Cunningham R. Echinacea for the prevention and treatment of upper respiratory tract infections: A systematic review and meta-analysis. Complement Ther Med 2019;44:18–26.

36. Shekelle P, Morton S, Maglione M, et al. Ephedra and ephedrine for weight loss and athletic performance enhancement: clinical efficacy and side effects. In: Database of abstracts of reviews of effects (DARE): quality-assessed reviews [Internet]. York (UK): Centre for Reviews and Dissemination (UK); 2003.

37. Hutchins GM. Dietary supplements containing ephedra alkaloids. N Engl J Med 2001;344:1095–6 [author reply: 1096-1097].

38. Morgenstern LB, Viscoli CM, Kernan WN, et al. Use of Ephedra-containing products and risk for hemorrhagic stroke. Neurology 2003;60:132–5.

39. Charatan F. Ephedra supplement may have contributed to sportman's death. BMJ 2003;326:464.

40. Bent S, Tiedt TN, Odden MC, et al. The relative safety of ephedra compared with other herbal products. Ann Intern Med 2003;138:468–71.

41. Fontanarosa PB, Rennies D, DeAngelia CD. The need for regulation of dietary supplements: lessons from ephedra. JAMA 2003;289:1568–70.

42. Kalman DS, Antonio J, Kreider RB. The relative safety of ephedra compared with other herbal products. Ann Intern Med 2003;138:1006 [author reply 1006-1007].

43. Ernst E. Cardiovascular adverse effects of herbal medicines: a systematic review of the recent literature. Can J Cardiol 2003;19:818–27.

44. Samenuk D, Link MS, Homoud MK, et al. Adverse cardiovascular events temporally associated with ma huang, an herbal source of ephedrine. Mayo Clin Proc 2002;77:12–6.

45. Meadows M. Public health officials caution against ephedra use: health officials caution consumers against using dietary supplements containing ephedra: the stimulant can have dangerous effects on the nervous system and heart. FDA Consum 2003;37:8–9.

46. Guinot P, Brambilla C, Duchier J, et al. Effect on BN 52063, a specific PAF-acether antagonist, on bronchial provocation test to allergens in asthmatic patients: a preliminary study. Prostaglandins 1987;34:723–31.

47. Coyle AJ, Urwin SC, Page CP, et al. The effect of the selective PAF antagonist DB 52021 on PAF- and antigen-induced bronchial hyper-reactivity and eosinophil accumulation. Eur J Pharmacol 1988;148:51–8.

48. Aggarwal A, Ades PA. Interactions of herbal remedies with prescription cardiovascular medications. Coron Artery Dis 2001;12:581–4.

49. Isso AA, Ernst E. Interactions between herbal medicines and prescribed drugs: a systematic review. Drugs 2001;61:2163–75.

50. Deral JM, Gold JL, Laxer DA, et al. Potential interactions between herbal medicines and conventional drug therapies used by older adults attending a memory clinic. Drugs Aging 2002;19:879–86.

51. Joshi SS, Kuszynski CA, Bagchi D. The cellular and molecular bases of health benefits for grape seed proanthocyanidin extract. Curr Pharm Biotechnol 2001;2:187–200.

52. Paparoupa M, Gillissen A. Is Myrtol® Standardized a New Alternative toward Antibiotics? Pharmacogn Rev 2016;10(20):143–6.

53. Kerr LA, Johnson BJ, Burrows GE. Intoxication of cattle by Perilla frutescens (purple mint). Vet Hum Toxicol 1986;28:412–6.

54. Bassoli A, Borgonovo G, Morini G, et al. Analogues of perillaketone as highly potent agonists of TRPA1 channel. Food Chem 2013;141:2044–51.

55. Bossuyt L, Dooms-Goosens A. Contact sensitivity to nettles and chamomile in alternative remedies. Contact dermatitis 1994;31:131–2.

56. Thomet OA, Schapowal A, Heinisch IV, et al. Anti-inflammatory activity of an extract of *Petasites hybridus* in allergic rhinitis. Int Immunopharmacol 2002;2: 997–1006.

57. Thomet OAR, Simon HU. Petasins in the treatment of allergic diseases: results of preclinical and clinical studies. Int Arch Allergy Immunol 2002;129:108–12.

58. Lee DKC, Carstairs IJ, Haggart K, et al. Butterbur, a herbal remedy, attenuates adenosine monophosphate induced nasal responsiveness in seasonal allergic rhinitis. Clin Exp Allergy 2003;33:882–6.

59. Schapowal A. Butterbur Ze339 for the treatment of intermittent allergic rhinitis: dose-dependent efficacy in a prospective, randomized, double-blind, placebo-controlled study. Arch Otolaryngol Head Neck Surg 2004;130:1381–6.

60. Lee DKC, Gray RD, Robb FM, et al. A placebo-controlled evaluation of butterbur and fexofenadine on objective and subjective outcomes in perennial allergic rhinitis. Clin Exp Allergy 2004;34:646–9.

61. Gray RD, Haggart K, Lee DKC, et al. Effects of butterbur treatment in intermittent allergic rhinitis: a placebo- controlled evaluation. Ann Allergy 2004;93:56–60.

62. Aldous MB, Wahl R, Worden K, Grant KL. A randomized, controlled trial of cranial osteopathic manipulative treatment and Echinacae in children with recurrent otitis media. In: Program and abstracts of the 2003 Pediatric Academic Societies' Annual Meeting; May 3-6, 2003;Seattle, WA. Abstract 1062.

63. Barrett BP, Brown RL, Locken K, et al. Treatment of the common cold with unrefined Echinacae: a randomized, double-blind, placebo-controlled trial. Ann Intern Med 2002;137:939–46.

64. Melchart D, Linde K, Fischer P, et al. Echinacea for preventing and treating the common cold. Cochrane Database Syst Rev 2000;2:CD000530.

65. Melchart D, Walther E, Linde K, et al. Echinacea root extracts for the prevention of upper respiratory tract infections: a double-blind, placebo-controlled randomized trial. Arch Fam Med 1998;7:541–5.

66. Melchart D, Linde K, Worku F, et al. Results of five randomized studies on the immunomodulatory activity of preparations of Echinacea. J Altern Complement Med 1995;1:145–60.

67. Bernstein DI, Bernstein CK, Deng C, et al. Evaluation of the clinical efficacy and safety of grapeseed extract in the treatment of fall seasonal allergic rhinitis: a pilot study. Ann Allergy Immunol 2002;88:272–8.

68. Banergee B, Bagchi D. Beneficial effects of a novel ih636 grape seed proanthocyanidin extract in the treatment of chronic pancreatitis. Digestion 2001;63: 203–6.

69. Ray SD, Parikh H, Hickey E, et al. Differential effects of IH636 grapde seed proanthocyanidin extract and a DNA repair modulator 4-aminobenzamide on liver microsomal cytochrome 4502E1-dependent aniline hydroxylation. Mol Cell Biochem 2001;218:27–33.

70. Sato M, Bagchi D, Tosaki A, et al. Grape seed proanthocyanidin reduces cardiomyocyte apoptosis by inhibiting ischemia/reperfusion-induced activation of JNK-1 and C-JUN. Free Radic Biol Med 2001;31:729–37.

71. Takano H, Osakabe N, Sanbongi C, et al. Extract of *Perilla frutescens* enriched for rosmarinic acid, a polyphenolic phyto- chemical, inhibits seasonal allergic rhino-conjunctivitis in humans. Exp Biol Med (Maywood) 2004;229:247–54.

72. Saxena VS, Venkateshwarlu K, Nadig P, et al. Multicenter clinical trials on a novel polyherbal formulation in allergic rhinitis. Int J Clin Pharmacol Res 2004;24:79–94.

73. Vyjayanthi G, Shetty S, Saxena VS, et al. Randomized, double- blind, placebo-controlled trial of Aller-7 in patients with allergic rhinitis. Res Commun Pharmacol Toxicol 2003;8:15–24.

74. Pratibha N, Saxena VS, Amit A, et al. Anti-inflammatory activities of Aller-7, a novel polyherbal formulation for allergic rhinitis. Int J Tissue React 2004; 26(1–2):43–51.

75. Parthipan M, Aravindhan V, Rajendran A. Medico-botanical study of Yercaud hills in the eastern Ghats of Tamil Nadu, India. Anc Sci Life. 2011;30:104–109.The Ayurvedic Pharmacopoeia India . 1st ed. Vol. 1. New Delhi: Department Of AYUSH, Ministry of Health and FW; 2001. pp. 53–109.

76. More P, Pai K. In vitro NADH-oxidase, NADPH-oxidase and myeloperoxidase activity of macrophages after Tinospora cordifolia (guduchi) treatment. Immunopharmacol Immunotoxicol 2012;34:368–72.

77. Upadhyaya R, PR, Sharma V, et al. Assessment of the multifaceted immunomodulatory potential of the aqueous extract of Tinospora cordifolia. Res J Chem Sci 2011;1:71–9.

78. Sudhakaran DS, Srirekha P, Devasree LD, et al. Immunostimulatory effect of Tinospora cordifolia Miers leaf extract in Oreochromis mossambicus. Indian J Exp Biol 2006;44:726–32.

79. Koppada R, Norozian FM, Torbati D, et al. Physiological effects of a novel immune stimulator drug, (1,4)-α-D-glucan, in rats. Basic Clin Pharmacol Toxicol 2009;105: 217–21.

80. Badar VA, Thawani VR, Wakode PT, et al. Efficacy of *Tinos- pora cordifolia* in allergic rhinitis. J Ethnopharmacol 2005;96:445–9.

81. Baba S. Double-blind clinical trial of Sho-seiryu-to (TJ-19) for perennial nasal allergy. Pract Otol 1995;88:389–405.

82. Hu G, Walls RS, Bass D, et al. The Chinese herbal formulation Biminne in management of perennial allergic rhinitis: a randomized, double-blind, placebo-controlled, 12-week clinical trial. Ann Allergy 2002;88:478–87.

83. Xue CC, Thien FC, Zhang JJ, et al. Treatment for seasonal allergic rhinitis by Chinese herbal medicine: a randomized placebo controlled trial. Altern Ther Health Med 2003;9:80–7.

84. Cingi C, Cakli H, Yaz A, et al. Phototherapy for allergic rhinitis: a prospective, randomized, single-blind, placebo-controlled study. Ther Adv Respir Dis 2010;4(4): 209–13.

85. Ural A, Oktemer TK, Kizil Y, et al. Impact of isotonic and hypertonic saline solutions on mucociliary activity in various nasal pathologies: clinical study. J Laryngol Otol 2009;123:517–21.

86. Blanc PD, Trupin L, Earnest G, et al. Alternative therapies among adults with a reported diagnosis of asthma or rhinosinusitis: data from a population- based survey. Chest 2001;120(5):1461–7.

The Use of Antioxidants in the Prevention and Treatment of Noise-Induced Hearing Loss

Haley Hullfish, BS[a],*, Luis P. Roldan, MD[a], Michael E. Hoffer, MD[a,b]

KEYWORDS

- Noise-induced hearing loss • Antioxidants • Reactive oxygen species
- N-acetylcysteine • Acetyl-L-carnitine • D-methionine • Resveratrol

KEY POINTS

- Continuous or excessively loud noise exposure leads to an accumulation of intracellular free radicals, particularly reactive oxygen species (ROS) and reactive nitrogen species (RNS), for at least 7 to 10 days after injury.
- Experimental animal studies with systemic or local antioxidant use have been shown to protect hair cells and reduce hearing loss from acoustic trauma.
- Combination antioxidant therapy may better attenuate NIHL than single-agent therapy by targeting multiple pathways in ROS and RNS formation.

INTRODUCTION TO NOISE-INDUCED HEARING LOSS

Noise-induced hearing loss (NIHL), which occurs due to excessive noise exposure, is a preventable cause of sensorineural hearing loss. The CDC approximates that at least 40 million adults aged between 20 and 69 years in the United States have audiological evidence of NIHL in one or both ears,[1] affecting as much as 17% of the adolescent population.[2] The severity of hearing loss relies on several factors, including individual characteristics, sound intensity, and duration of sound exposure. Although sensitivities vary among individuals, sound intensity at or above 85 decibels (dB) can precipitate hearing loss, a sound level equivalent to that of a food blender or city traffic. Those exposed to sound exceeding 85 dB for only 5 hours per week can suffer permanent hearing loss.[3] There are several proposed theories to explain the pathogenesis of NIHL. Evidence demonstrates that inflammation, increased oxidative stress,

[a] Department of Otolaryngology, University of Miami Miller School of Medicine, 1120 Northwest 14th Street, Miami, FL 33136, USA; [b] Department of Neurological Surgery, University of Miami Miller School of Medicine, 1120 Northwest 14th Street, Miami, FL 33136, USA
* Corresponding author.
E-mail address: hmhullfish@med.miami.edu

Otolaryngol Clin N Am 55 (2022) 983–991
https://doi.org/10.1016/j.otc.2022.06.006
0030-6665/22/© 2022 Elsevier Inc. All rights reserved.
oto.theclinics.com

Abbreviations	
ABR	Auditory brainstem response
ALCAR	acetyl-l-carnitine
BBB	Blood-brain barrier
CDC	Centers for Disease Control and Prevention
COX-2	Cyclooxygenase-2
dB	Decibels
D-met	D-methionine
DPOAE	Distortion product otoacoustic emission
FDA	Food and Drug Administration
GSH	Glutathione
HC	Hair cell
NAC	N-acetyl cysteine
NIHL	Noise-induced hearing loss
OBN	Octave band noise
PTS	Permanent threshold shift
ROS	Reactive oxygen species
RNS	Reactive nitrogen species
TTS	Temporary threshold shift

elevated calcium, and reduced blood flow are all mechanisms underlying NIHL.[4] Importantly, no treatment has proven effective in reversing the damage inflicted by excessive noise exposure. Primary prevention by noise avoidance and regular use of personal protective hearing equipment is the standard of care at this time.

Impulse noise is defined as a quick burst of acoustic energy. Common examples are gunfire, explosions, fireworks, and heavy machinery. These acoustic bursts can elicit acute effects, including transient tinnitus, hyperacusis, and tympanic membrane perforations. High-intensity exposure can cause loss of cochlear sensory hair cells (HCs), leading to permanent threshold shift (PTS). In contrast, hearing loss associated with more mild acoustic exposure is typically reversible and recovers in days to weeks, referred to as temporary threshold shift (TTS). This is thought to be due to reversible swelling and damage to the stereocilia of HCs.[5] However, the impact of TTS may misrepresent the damage of noise-induced cochlear toxicity. Recent studies have demonstrated that even mild acoustic trauma associated with TTS can lead to the loss of more than 50% of the synapses between cochlear nerve fibers and inner HCs, without HC loss and without alteration of hearing thresholds.[6] The resulting synaptopathy is sometimes referred to as "hidden hearing loss." Although seemingly plausible, there is no current data to support this synaptopathy in humans; thus, the concept of hidden hearing loss remains controversial.

Hearing loss may also result from continuous moderate noise exposure. In contrast to impulse noise, continuous noise has been shown to be more damaging because there is less recovery time between acoustic insults.[7] Initial hearing loss patterns for both acute and chronic noise exposure seem similar. Nerve fiber degeneration and HC damage occur bilaterally at the cochlear region corresponding to a 4-kHz notch on audiograms.[8] As noise exposure persists, the damage extends in the basilar direction toward the high-frequency portion of the cochlea, eventually resulting in mid-frequency to high-frequency hearing loss. There is a limit to the severity of hearing loss because NIHL rarely exceeds 70 to 90 dB threshold even after many years of continuous noise exposure.[8] Because both chronic and acute noise exposure can induce NIHL, it is important to obtain an adequate patient history of environmental risk factors, including occupational and recreational noise exposures.

INTRODUCTION TO ANTIOXIDANTS

Continuous or excessively loud noise exposure leads to an accumulation of intracellular free radicals, particularly reactive oxygen species (ROS) and reactive nitrogen species (RNS), for at least 7 to 10 days after injury.[9] At high levels, these agents overwhelm the cells' antioxidant systems, which maintain redox homeostasis. Glutathione (GSH), GSH peroxidase, GSH reductase, methionine sulfoxide reductase, superoxide dismutase, catalase, and coenzyme Q_{10} are all redox enzymes found in the inner ear.[5] Once these natural defenses are depleted, toxic reactive species induce inflammation, permanent damage, and cell death of cochlear neurons and HCs. The cochlear distribution of these defensive proteins may correspond to the pattern of hearing loss observed in noise exposure. The antioxidant GSH is distributed in a high-to-low gradient from the apex to the base in the organ of Corti, suggesting a lower tolerance of basal HCs to acoustic insult.[10]

The pathophysiological mechanism underlying NIHL has translational potential for pharmacological intervention to prevent or rescue HC injury from free radical damage. Multiple antioxidants have been investigated for both the prophylaxis and treatment of NIHL. The various antioxidants work via different mechanisms involving scavenging free radical species, quenching singlet oxygen molecules, reducing concentrations of intracellular oxygen, chelating metals, interrupting free radical reactions, and preventing the oxidation of protein or DNA.[11] Given the variety of pathways by which ROS and RNS are generated, the use of multiple antioxidants that target different pathways of noise-induced ototoxicity may be most effective in preventing cochlear damage.

ANTIOXIDANT STUDIES

Experimental animal studies with systemic or local antioxidant use have been shown to protect HCs and reduce hearing loss from acoustic trauma. Among the most extensively studied are N-acetyl cysteine (NAC), methionine, acetyl-L-carnitine (ALCAR), and resveratrol.

N-Acetyl Cysteine

NAC is one of the few antioxidants that have been studied in both animal and human trials for the treatment of NIHL. It is an over-the-counter anti-inflammatory medication commonly used to treat acetaminophen-induced oxidative hepatic injury. NAC replenishes cysteine, the limiting substrate in GSH synthesis. GSH reduces and conjugates ROS and RNS formed during intracellular oxidative stress and is a major antioxidant enzyme in HCs.[12] Similar to GSH, NAC also acts as a scavenger of reactive oxygen species through the reduction of disulfide bonds.

In animal studies, NAC has shown promising otoprotectant results. Kopke and colleagues exposed chinchillas to 6 hours of 105 dB octave band noise (OBN) centered at 4 kHz. Animals received salicylate and NAC 1 hour before or 1 hour after the noise exposure. PTSs were significantly reduced to approximately 10 dB in the pretreatment groups compared with the 20 to 40 dB threshold shift in controls at 3 weeks postexposure. Those treated after noise exposure had no protection from HC loss.[13] Additionally, Kopke's laboratory investigated combining NAC with 2,4-disulfophenyl-N-tert-butylnitrone (HPN-07), a nitrone-based free radical trap. HPN-07 has been shown to be effective in treating acute acoustic trauma in chinchillas.[14] Rats exposed to 115 dB OBN (10–20 kHz) for 1 hour were treated with combined NAC and HPN-07 starting 1 hour after noise exposure for 2 consecutive days. Results demonstrated reduced auditory brainstem response (ABR) threshold shifts, decreased distortion product otoacoustic emission (DPOAE) shifts, and HC loss reduction by 85% to 64% in the outer and inner HC regions, respectively.[15]

In contrast, NAC administration in humans with extreme noise exposure has shown varying results. Kramer and colleagues[16] administered 900 mg of NAC or placebo to 31 participants 30 minutes before exposure to live music at a nightclub and no significant difference between treatment groups was found in distortion product otoacoustic emissions (DPOE) measurements before and 2 hours after exposure. However, the inconsistency of sound exposure and the wide variance of subject sensitivity could be confounders. Lin and colleagues performed a prospective, double-blind crossover study on 53 male industrial workers exposed to approximately 88 to 89 dB of noise daily. The intervention was 1,200 mg/day of NAC for 2 weeks followed by placebo for 2 weeks or vice versa. The data indicate reduced high-frequency TTS by NAC with such effects more prominent among men carrying GSH S-transferase M1 and T1 null genotypes. The TTS at low frequency was not significantly different between the postplacebo and post-NAC phases of the study.[11] In 2003, the US Department of the Navy conducted a large trial with 566 Marine Corps. The subjects received 900 mg of NAC or placebo with each meal for a total dose of 2700 mg during the first 16 days of weapon training. There was no statistical evidence that NAC reduced the rate of threshold shifts; however, post hoc analysis showed significant decreases in threshold shift rates when handedness was considered.[17] Due to the lack of significant differences in overall hearing loss between treatment and placebo, further studies are warranted to clarify dose–response and other factors, including differences in risks between ears. Trials in human subjects have been limited in scale and current evidence demonstrates varied support for NAC alone as a reliable otoprotectant in NIHL.

Methionine

Methionine is one of the most easily oxidized amino acids and can react readily with various reactive oxygen species to form methionine sulfoxide.[18] Its functional role as an otoprotectant has been elicited by studies that demonstrate HC apoptosis and deafness in subjects with mutations that reduce cochlear concentrations of methionine.[19,20] Methionine can also increase intracellular stores of GSH, and similar to NAC, can serve as a cysteine supplier for GSH synthesis.[21,22] The enantiomer D-methionine (D-met) is often used clinically because it has a more stable shelf life and better bioavailability than L-methionine.

D-met has been widely shown to protect against cisplatin-induced and carboplatin-induced ototoxicity in animals.[23–25] Kopke and colleagues[26] demonstrated that D-met delivered 48 hours before and 48 hours after noise exposure protected against permanent NIHL and HC loss in chinchillas. Campbell further demonstrated that D-met could rescue permanent NIHL when given 1 hour after noise exposure.[27] Claussen and colleagues[28] also illustrated that D-met preloading 2 to 3 days before noise exposure reduced ABR threshold shifts and outer HC loss in chinchillas. Clifford and colleagues investigated the effects of low-dose intraperitoneal D-met and NAC administered to chinchillas before and after continuous noise exposure. D-met and NAC together demonstrated significant improvement of ABR thresholds. D-met seemed to be the primary compound responsible for hearing restoration as D-met alone showed gradual improvement with statistically significant recovery in middle frequencies.[29] Furthermore, dose-dependent otoprotective effects of D-met have been reported in guinea pigs with NIHL. Animals were treated 1 hour after noise exposure with 200, 400, or 600 mg/kg of D-met by intraperitoneal injection. The level of rescue from noise-induced PTS was dose-dependent. Administration of D-met 200 mg/kg did not reduce the mean PTS but 600 mg/kg dosage achieved a complete rescue response.[30] In addition, dose-dependent decreases in ATPase activity, mean lipid peroxidation, and nitric oxide levels were also observed.[30] Clinical trials are necessary to evaluate the efficacy of D-met for preventing and treating NIHL in humans.

Acetyl-L-Carnitine

ALCAR is a naturally occurring amino acid stored in high quantities in muscle and heart tissue. It is a readily available over-the-counter supplement that has been administered in doses ranging from 20 to 50 mg/kg daily in both animal and human studies.[31] ALCAR stabilizes mitochondrial membranes during respiration and aids in cellular energy production by regulating acetyl-CoA, a key substrate in the citric acid cycle. Through several parallel reactions, ALCAR reduces oxidative stress by scavenging ROS and increases cellular stores of other antioxidants, including GSH and coenzyme Q_{10}.[31] Its effect on hearing restoration following acoustic trauma has been studied in animal models suggesting a positive effect.

In one such animal model, Coleman and colleagues investigated the combined efficacy of ALCAR and NAC administered 1, 4, and 12 hours after sustained noise exposure (105 dB for 6 hours). Both ALCAR and NAC demonstrated time-dependent effects on outer and inner HC counts and undamaged mitochondrial density. The most significant reduction in hearing loss for both ALCAR and NAC treated animals occurred in the 1-hour postexposure groups. Treatment groups with delayed administration of more than 4 hours failed to improve hearing suggesting a short window of therapeutic efficacy after noise exposure.[32] In addition to NIHL, Seidman's laboratory demonstrated that ALCAR could protect against age-related hearing loss in rats by preventing and repairing age-induced cochlear mitochondrial DNA damage.[33] The effects of ALCAR to reduce NIHL warrants further study before routine recommendation.

Resveratrol

Resveratrol (trans 3,5,4'-trihydroxystilbene) is a phytoalexin and nutritional supplement found in the skin and seed of red grapes. It is studied in cancer and heart disease due to its antioxidant and anti-inflammatory properties.[34,35] In a study published in 2003, resveratrol supplementation for 7 weeks was noted to reduce threshold shifts in rats exposed to significant acoustic trauma compared with controls.[36] Seidman and colleagues further elicited the protective mechanism of resveratrol by measuring its effect on cyclooxygenase-2 (COX-2) and ROS formation following noise exposure in rats. The data demonstrated that at a dose of 5 mg/kg for 3 days before 24 hour noise exposure, resveratrol reduced noise-induced COX-2 expression and ROS formation in the blood.[37] No trials exist that study the effects of resveratrol on NIHL in humans.

CHALLENGES IN ANTIOXIDANT USE

The animal studies previously mentioned advocate for the translation of these promising antioxidant studies to human trials. However, the route of administration, high experimental dosages, and ability to control noise exposure in animal studies are often not feasible in human subjects. In addition, the bioavailability of antioxidants is varied and needs to be fully elucidated before application in humans. To date, no antioxidant agent for NIHL is approved by the U.S. Food and Drug Administration (FDA).

The selection of an appropriate medication for NIHL should consider bioavailability at the cochlear target organ and its ability to permeate the blood–brain barrier (BBB). Various antioxidants possess potential therapeutic benefits for central nervous system diseases but have limited availability across the BBB. GSH, for instance, penetrates the BBB by <1% when given exogenously thereby diminishing its effect in reducing oxidative stress in the CNS.[38] Other antioxidants including derivatives of Vitamins A, D, and E have demonstrated similar shortcomings in crossing the BBB, even when given at high doses.[38] However, when the BBB is damaged, for example, in traumatic brain injury, increased brain permeability may facilitate selective drug delivery to affected sites.[39]

Numerous animal studies have validated the use of antioxidants for NIHL in preexposure and postexposure settings. However, experimental study in human populations is far more limited, with many studies relying on cross-sectional data to infer differences between populations and exposures. Both ethical and epidemiological factors restrict further development and research in the clinical setting. Although feasible, obvious ethical considerations exist that prohibit the deliberate exposure of damaging sound in human subjects. Enrollment of subjects with environmental exposure to extreme noise also poses a unique challenge because the therapeutic window for antioxidant therapy is limited and the wait period to obtain appropriate medical attention may be exceedingly long. Additional factors including poor public awareness of NIHL, subclinical symptoms, individual variations in noise susceptibility, and limitations in access to health care make it increasingly difficult to recruit participants in a timely manner immediately following acoustic trauma and before noise-induced cochlear damage becomes permanent.

Early-onset of antioxidant therapy confers the greatest protective benefit against NIHL. Similarly, there is a time-dependent response to therapy, with reduced responses to therapy with greater delay to initial administration. There is strong data that supports the protective effects of antioxidants when given before and immediately after extreme noise exposure. Coleman and colleagues[32] revealed a significant reduction in hearing loss when ALCAR and NAC therapy was given within 4 hours of noise exposure but not when given after 12 hours. D-met has been demonstrated to provide significant PTS rescue up to 7 hours after noise exposure.[40] Prophylactic administration of antioxidants also provides otoprotection from noise-induced trauma. NAC, D-met, and magnesium are among the antioxidants that have reduced HC loss and hearing loss in animal models when given days to hours before exposure.[13,28,41] However, prophylactic treatment in humans is not always feasible because patients usually present once permanent hearing loss has already occurred. Prophylactic administration could be considered especially in settings when occupational noise exposure is anticipated, for example, in military or construction settings. However, this raises further questions about the duration of treatment and long-term drug effects.

Less data exist regarding the efficacy of delayed treatment in NIHL. Yamashita and colleagues[9] found that ROS and RNS persist in HCs for up to 7 to 10 days after acoustic trauma. Consequently, they reported that the greatest window of opportunity was within 3 days of exposure achievable by using a combination of antioxidants with different mechanisms of action and prolonging the duration of treatment.[42] Altogether, there is a need for more conclusive evidence demonstrating the protective effects of antioxidant drug administration if given at least 1 week following exposure. Unfortunately, initial diagnosis and subsequent treatment may often be delayed, minimizing the therapeutic efficacy of antioxidants.

SUMMARY

Antioxidant compounds seem very promising in the prevention and treatment of noise-induced cochlear trauma. However, no single protective agent has proved fruitful at the bedside. It is likely that a combination antioxidant therapy may better attenuate NIHL than a single-agent therapy. The enhanced efficacy of combination therapy can be explained by the targeting of multiple pathways in ROS and RNS formation. Of course, the benefits of combination therapy should be weighed against the potential for cross-drug reactions and the variable side effects of polypharmacy. The success of these therapies depends on factors such as type of antioxidant, dosage, route of administration, bioavailability, the timing of therapy in relation to noise exposure, and duration of therapy.

In 2011, experts estimated that oral drug therapy to protect against NIHL would be available in the next decade.[43] Although this was not achieved, we can continue to move forward by developing a better understanding of the complex biochemical and molecular mechanisms of cell death in the cochlea and the biochemistry of antioxidants relevant to the cochlea in order to design more effective treatment strategies in hearing loss.[44] Large, randomized, double-blind, placebo-controlled clinical trials demonstrating the efficacy of antioxidant therapy are essential to attest to their value in treating NIHL. In addition, a statistically significant reduction in hearing loss is different than functionally significant. Therapies that can reliably reduce hearing loss by at least 15 dB are needed. Although we have made significant strides in combating acoustic injury, it is apparent we still have a long way to go until an oral drug therapy is available for NIHL. However, antioxidants are a promising option that require further exploration.

DISCLOSURES

There are no conflicts of interest with respect to the research, authorship, and publication of this article. The authors received no financial support for the research, authorship, and publication of this article.

REFERENCES

1. Center for Disease Control and Prevention. Too loud! For too long 2020. Available at: https://www.cdc.gov/vitalsigns/hearingloss/index.html. Accessed May 01, 2022.
2. Henderson E, Testa MA, Hartnick C. Prevalence of noise-induced hearing-threshold shifts and hearing loss among US youths. Pediatrics 2011;127(1): e39–46.
3. Imam L, Hannan SA. Noise-induced hearing loss: a modern epidemic? Br J Hosp Med 2017;78(5):286–90.
4. Le Prell CG, Yamashita D, Minami SB, et al. Mechanisms of noise-induced hearing loss indicate multiple methods of prevention. Hearing Res 2007;226(1–2): 22–43.
5. Kurabi A, Keithley EM, Housley GD, et al. Cellular mechanisms of noise-induced hearing loss. Hearing Res 2017;349:129–37.
6. Liberman MC. Noise-Induced hearing loss: permanent versus temporary threshold shifts and the effects of hair cell versus neuronal degeneration. Adv Exp Med Biol 2016;875:1–7.
7. Pourbakht A, Yamasoba T. Cochlear damage caused by continuous and intermittent noise exposure. Hearing Res 2003;178(1):70–8.
8. Le Prell C. Noise-induced hearing loss. In: Cummings Otolaryngol Head Neck Surg,. 7th edition.2020:154, 2342-2355.e2344.
9. Yamashita D, Jiang HY, Schacht J, et al. Delayed production of free radicals following noise exposure. Brain Res 2004;1019(1–2):201–9.

10. Sha SH, Taylor R, Forge A, et al. Differential vulnerability of basal and apical hair cells is based on intrinsic susceptibility to free radicals. Hear Res 2001; 155(1–2):1–8.

11. Lin CY, Wu JL, Shih TS, et al. N-Acetyl-cysteine against noise-induced temporary threshold shift in male workers. Hear Res 2010;269(1–2):42–7.

12. Pedre B, Barayeu U, Ezeriņa D, et al. The mechanism of action of N-acetylcysteine (NAC): The emerging role of H2S and sulfane sulfur species. Pharmacol Ther 2021;228:107916.

13. Kopke RD, Weisskopf PA, Boone JL, et al. Reduction of noise-induced hearing loss using L-NAC and salicylate in the chinchilla. Hear Res 2000;149(1–2): 138–46.

14. Ewert D, Hu N, Du X, et al. HPN-07, a free radical spin trapping agent, protects against functional, cellular and electrophysiological changes in the cochlea induced by acute acoustic trauma. PLoS One 2017;12(8):e0183089.

15. Lu J, Li W, Du X, et al. Antioxidants reduce cellular and functional changes induced by intense noise in the inner ear and cochlear nucleus. J Assoc Res Otolaryngol 2014;15(3):353–72.

16. Kramer S, Dreisbach L, Lockwood J, et al. Efficacy of the antioxidant N-acetylcysteine (NAC) in protecting ears exposed to loud music. J Am Acad Audiol 2006; 17(4):265–78.

17. Kopke R, Slade MD, Jackson R, et al. Efficacy and safety of N-acetylcysteine in prevention of noise induced hearing loss: a randomized clinical trial. Hear Res 2015;323:40–50.

18. Luo S, Levine RL. Methionine in proteins defends against oxidative stress. FASEB J 2009;23(2):464–72.

19. Kwon TJ, Cho HJ, Kim UK, et al. Methionine sulfoxide reductase B3 deficiency causes hearing loss due to stereocilia degeneration and apoptotic cell death in cochlear hair cells. Hum Mol Genet 2014;23(6):1591–601.

20. Ahmed ZM, Yousaf R, Lee BC, et al. Functional null mutations of MSRB3 encoding methionine sulfoxide reductase are associated with human deafness DFNB74. Am J Hum Genet 2011;88(1):19–29.

21. Lu SC. Regulation of hepatic glutathione synthesis: current concepts and controversies. FASEB J 1999;13(10):1169–83.

22. Ghibelli L, Fanelli C, Rotilio G, et al. Rescue of cells from apoptosis by inhibition of active GSH extrusion. FASEB J 1998;12(6):479–86.

23. Campbell KCM, Rybak LP, Meech RP, et al. d-Methionine provides excellent protection from cisplatin ototoxicity in the rat. Hearing Res 1996;102(1):90–8.

24. Lockwood DS, Ding DL, Wang J, et al. D-Methionine attenuates inner hair cell loss in carboplatin-treated chinchillas. Audiol Neurootol 2000;5(5):263–6.

25. Wimmer C, Mees K, Stumpf P, et al. Round window application of d-methionine, sodium thiosulfate, brain-derived neurotrophic factor, and fibroblast growth factor-2 in cisplatin-induced ototoxicity. Otology & Neurotology 2004;25(1):33–40.

26. Kopke RD, Coleman JK, Liu J, et al. Candidate's thesis: enhancing intrinsic cochlear stress defenses to reduce noise-induced hearing loss. Laryngoscope 2002;112(9):1515–32.

27. Campbell KC, Meech RP, Klemens JJ, et al. Prevention of noise- and drug-induced hearing loss with D-methionine. Hear Res 2007;226(1–2):92–103.

28. Claussen AD, Fox DJ, Yu XC, et al. D-methionine pre-loading reduces both noise-induced permanent threshold shift and outer hair cell loss in the chinchilla. Int J Audiol 2013;52(12):801–7.

29. Clifford RE, Coleman JK, Balough BJ, et al. Low-dose D-methionine and N-acetyl-L-cysteine for protection from permanent noise-induced hearing loss in chinchillas. Otolaryngol Head Neck Surg 2011;145(6):999–1006.

30. Lo WC, Liao LJ, Wang CT, et al. Dose-dependent effects of D-methionine for rescuing noise-induced permanent threshold shift in guinea-pigs. Neuroscience 2013;254:222–9.

31. Ferreira GC, McKenna MC. L-Carnitine and Acetyl-L-carnitine Roles and Neuroprotection in Developing Brain. Neurochem Res 2017;42(6):1661–75.

32. Coleman JK, Kopke RD, Liu J, et al. Pharmacological rescue of noise induced hearing loss using N-acetylcysteine and acetyl-L-carnitine. Hear Res 2007; 226(1–2):104–13.

33. Seidman MD, Khan MJ, Bai U, et al. Biologic activity of mitochondrial metabolites on aging and age-related hearing loss. Am J Otol 2000;21(2):161–7.

34. Bertelli AA, Ferrara F, Diana G, et al. Resveratrol, a natural stilbene in grapes and wine, enhances intraphagocytosis in human promonocytes: a co-factor in antiinflammatory and anticancer chemopreventive activity. Int J Tissue React 1999; 21(4):93–104.

35. Jiang H, Zhang L, Kuo J, et al. Resveratrol-induced apoptotic death in human U251 glioma cells. Mol Cancer Ther 2005;4(4):554–61.

36. Seidman M, Babu S, Tang W, et al. Effects of resveratrol on acoustic trauma. Otolaryngol Head Neck Surg 2003;129(5):463–70.

37. Seidman MD, Tang W, Bai VU, et al. Resveratrol decreases noise-induced cyclooxygenase-2 expression in the rat cochlea. Otolaryngology–Head Neck Surg 2013;148(5):827–33.

38. Gilgun-Sherki Y, Melamed E, Offen D. Oxidative stress induced-neurodegenerative diseases: the need for antioxidants that penetrate the blood brain barrier. Neuropharmacology 2001;40(8):959–75.

39. Hoffer ME, Balaban C, Slade MD, et al. Amelioration of acute sequelae of blast induced mild traumatic brain injury by N-acetyl cysteine: a double-blind, placebo controlled study. PLoS One 2013;8(1):e54163.

40. Campbell K, Claussen A, Meech R, et al. d-methionine (d-met) significantly rescues noise-induced hearing loss: Timing studies. Hearing Res 2011;282(1): 138–44.

41. Scheibe F, Haupt H, Ising H. Preventive effect of magnesium supplement on noise-induced hearing loss in the guinea pig. Eur Arch Otorhinolaryngol 2000; 257(1):10–6.

42. Yamashita D, Jiang HY, Le Prell CG, et al. Post-exposure treatment attenuates noise-induced hearing loss. Neuroscience 2005;134(2):633–42.

43. Oishi N, Schacht J. Emerging treatments for noise-induced hearing loss. Expert Opin Emerg Drugs 2011;16(2):235–45.

44. Shirwany NA, Seidman MD. Antioxidants and Their Effect on Stress-Induced Pathology in the Inner Ear. In: Miller J, Le Prell CG, Rybak L, editors. Free radicals in ENT pathology. Cham: Springer International Publishing; 2015. p. 57–89.

Complementary and Integrative Medicine in Head and Neck Cancer

Joseph F. Goodman, MD[a],*, Marilene B. Wang, MD[b]

KEYWORDS

- Complementary • Integrative • Alternative • Medicine • Oncology • CIM • CAM

KEY POINTS

- Physicians have an obligation to ask patients about their beliefs, preferences, and intended use of complementary and integrative medicine (CIM) during conventional cancer treatments.
- Referral to a trained integrative oncologist can help provide holistic care without undermining standard of care treatment of cancer.
- By encouraging communication between doctors, patients, family members, and other CIM providers, collaborative care can be established that is patient-centered and evidence-informed to optimize cancer treatments and maximize quality of life.

INTRODUCTION

Integrative oncology (IO) for head and neck cancer (HNC) refers to a holistic approach to cancer care that includes conventional approaches such as surgery and radiation, alongside a broad range of complementary and alternative medicine (CAM) approaches and treatments which may be regionally variable across the United States and in other countries.[1] Complementary and integrative medicine (CIM) is now the preferred term, to make a distinction from "alternative medicine," which by definition usually falls outside of conventional cancer treatment[2] (**Table 1**). Integrative oncology (IO) has become the preferred term for collaborative cancer care focused on whole-person health using complementary treatments which are patient-centered and evidence-informed alongside standard of care therapies.[3] Several key principles have emerged within IO: treatments seek to maximize quality of life while minimizing toxicities or potential interactions with standard therapy; "alternative" therapies

[a] Otolaryngology/Head & Neck Surgery, George Washington University, 2300 M Street, Northwest, 4th Floor (ENT), Washington, DC 20037, USA; [b] Department of Head & Neck Surgery, UCLA David Geffen School of Medicine, 200 Medical Plaza Ste. 550, Los Angeles, CA 90095, USA
* Corresponding author.
E-mail address: jfgoodman@mfa.gwu.edu

Otolaryngol Clin N Am 55 (2022) 993–1006
https://doi.org/10.1016/j.otc.2022.06.007
oto.theclinics.com

Abbreviations	
13-cRA	13-cis-retinoic acid
EGFR	estimated glomerular filtration rate
NF-κB	nuclear factor kappa beta
AKT	
MAPK	mitogen-activated protein kinase
COX-2	cyclooxygenase-2
iNOS	inducible nitric oxide synthase
IL	interleukinsinhibitor of NFKB
IKKβ	

outside of this integrative approach are not recommended; and the process of discovery and exploration allows patients and physicians to collaborate on complementary therapies which may be of real importance to patients from different traditions and value systems.

Historically, cancer has been feared more than any other diseases. This has been noted in up to 60% of patients in some surveys, particularly in an older population as prevalence of cancer increases.[4] The implication of this cancer worry has not been borne out well in preventive strategies or screening, but fears regarding treatment effects of cancer seem to be as significant as the fear of cancer itself.[5] Fear of cancer recurrence affects up to 73% percent of cancer survivors and can be associated with increased used of CIM approaches.[6] Behavioral modification such as tobacco cessation, exercise, and eating more fruits and vegetables have been shown to reduce cancer risk in the general population, and a significant number of cancers have been linked to modifiable lifestyle choices.[7] Nevertheless, when a diagnosis of cancer has been made, patients have diverse beliefs and strategies for seeking treatment and pursuing complementary approaches during treatment. It has been estimated that 50% of patients with cancer have used some form of CIM in addition to conventional cancer treatment.[8] Patients have been shown to use CIM for prevention of cancer, treatment of cancer, and mitigation of side effects of cancer and treatment.[9]

BACKGROUND

HNC encompasses a broad group of malignancies colocated in terms of anatomy, but quite distinct in terms of etiology, treatment strategies, morbidity/mortality, and survivorship. Most of the HNC are squamous cell carcinomas (SCCs) of the upper aerodigestive tract to include the sinonasal cavity, oral cavity, larynx, nasopharynx, oropharynx, and hypopharynx.[10] Other significant contributors include salivary gland malignancies, cutaneous malignancies, and rare lesions such as adnexal malignancies, sarcoma, and mucosal melanoma.[11] Either surgery or radiation could be considered as primary treatment of most head and neck SCCs (HNSCCs), with addition of cisplatin-based chemotherapy reserved for advanced disease.[12] Each treatment modality causes specific side effects that significantly affect quality of life; combined treatments often amplify these side effects with both acute and chronic disability associated.

A recent systematic review documents reasons for CIM use by patients with cancer, in order of frequency; to treat or help with treating their cancer, to mitigate the complications of their cancer or cancer treatments; to provide holistic health care and influence general health; to have a sense of taking control of their health; and on recommendation from others and/or personal beliefs.[13] Whereas patients have a

Table 1 Definitions	
Integrative oncology	A holistic approach to cancer care that includes conventional approaches such as surgery and radiation, alongside a broad range of CAM approaches, evidence-informed and patient-centered with an emphasis on safety
Complementary and alternative medicine (CAM)	Therapies and approaches for diagnosis, treatment, and/or prevention of disease outside of conventional allopathic medicine
Complementary and integrative medicine	Therapies and approaches for diagnosis, treatment, and/or prevention of disease outside of conventional allopathic medicine, which are overseen and integrated into standard treatment for the prevention and mitigation of symptoms and treatment side effects

variety of reasons for pursuing CIM, most clinical practice guidelines (CPG) focus on mitigation of symptoms and a way of integrating treatments.[14] Although many small studies with lower quality evidence have reported on prevention and treatment, oncologists are hesitant to recommend CIM that has not been shown to be safe or efficacious, especially outside of established guidelines. Specific CIM interventions for HNC have been primarily investigated as an adjunct for reducing the effects of treatment or improved tolerance of posttreatment sequelae, such as lymphedema, fibrosis, fatigue, pain, xerostomia, dysgeusia, and depression/anxiety.[15]

DISCUSSION
The Role of Government Regulation and Funding

The US Government has devoted significant resources to funding research in CIM therapies for a variety of diseases. In 1991, Congress established the Office of Alternative Medicine (OAM) within the National Institutes of Health (NIH). The OAM was elevated in status and funding in 1998 as the National Center for Complementary and Alternative Medicine (NCCAM). In 2014, NCCAM was rebranded the National Center for Complementary and Integrative Health (NCCIH) with an annual budget of $120 million reported in 2019. Altogether over $500 million dollars (of a total NIH budget of $39 billion) are spent annually to support research in CIM, a 40% increase in the past 5 years.[16] The Institute of Medicine has also advocated for research into CIM.[17]

NCCIH divides CAM into natural products, including dietary supplements and herbal supplements (botanicals); mind–body practices, including meditation, yoga, qigong/tai-chi, acupuncture, and manipulation practices (such as chiropractic and osteopathic medicine); and alternative systems, such as homeopathy, naturopathy, traditional Chinese medicine (TCM), and Ayurveda.[18]

The Office of Cancer Complementary and Alternative Medicine (OCCAM) was established in 1998 within the National Cancer Institute (NCI) in the Division of Cancer Treatment and Diagnosis. OCCAM supports various CIM-related research projects on cancer prevention, treatment, symptom/side effect management and epidemiology, with an annual budget of about $60 million reported in 2019. A joint US-China collaboration has been established for investigation of TCM in conventional cancer care.[19]

The Role of Professional Organizations and Patient Advocacy Groups

A definition for IO has been proposed by the Society for Integrative Oncology (SIO), established in 2003 "to encourage scientific evaluation, dissemination of evidence-based information, and appropriate clinical integration of complementary therapies."[20] The process of establishing consensus within the medical community regarding IO has been slow and deliberate. Several practice guidelines have been established in collaboration with other oncology organization such as American Society for Clinical Oncology (ASCO) for breast cancer[21,22] and the American College of Chest Physicians for lung cancer.[23] Not until 2017 was a comprehensive definition of IO published as such: IO is a patient-centered, evidence-informed field of cancer care that uses mind–body practices, natural products, and/or lifestyle modifications from different physicians alongside conventional cancer treatments. IO aims to optimize health, quality of life, and clinical outcomes across cancer care continuum and to empower people to prevent cancer and become active participants before, during, and beyond cancer treatment.[24]

Other collaborative guidelines between SIO and ASCO are in progress with regard to cancer-related pain management, cancer fatigue, and depression/anxiety in cancer.[25] A consensus for categorization of treatment modalities has started to emerge, with a recognition of considerable overlap. Generally, the categories can include nutritional approaches (herbal supplements or botanicals, vitamins and minerals, probiotics, and dietary regimens); and/or mind-body practices, which seek to integrate psychological/emotional health with physical health, often promoting mental calming strategies alongside gentle physical movement (yoga, tai chi, qi gong, mindfulness meditation, art/music therapy, and dance). There are a growing number of training and certification options available to allopathic physicians interested in IO.[3] Medical massage, acupuncture, chiropractic, and osteopathic manipulation all have deep roots with a significant body of literature and rigorous training/licensing requirements.

Complementary and Integrative Medicine for Palliation of Symptoms/Side Effects of Treatment in Head and Neck Cancer

Although many late effects of radiation therapy cause significant morbidity, the additive effects after surgery can be quite debilitating.[26] It is in the setting of posttreatment palliation and improvement of quality of life that most integrative approaches have been incorporated into HNC treatment. Randomized controlled trials have shown acupuncture to be effective in treating side effects of chemoradiation for HNC, including dysphagia[27] and xerostomia,[28,29] as well as side effects after neck dissection surgery, including shoulder pain and dysfunction.[30,31] Several systematic reviews have shown patient-reported outcomes document utility for dermatitis, mucositis, fatigue, xerostomia, anxiety, and nausea using a wide variety of CIM modalities.[32,33]

Organizations such as the American Head and Neck Society (AHNS) have become increasingly attentive to quality of life in the context of survivorship,[34] and working groups have been established to provide patient recommendations regarding CIM treatments. Acupuncture is now recommended as a CIM treatment for pain management in HNC with level 1A evidence (systematic review of randomized controlled trials). It has been shown that patients seeking alternative care to conventional cancer treatment often delay definitive treatment and have poor outcomes,[35,36] whereas complementary treatments that can be integrated into standard of care cancer treatment may provide benefit regarding treatment side effects and overall quality of life. Patients value being able to discuss these concerns with their oncologists, including HNC surgeons, and this engagement and communication has been increasingly advocated in the medical literature to improve outcomes.[37] The SIO definition of IO notes the importance of using evidence to inform collaborative treatment decisions. Although it is important for physicians to understand the values and experiences patients bring related to traditional whole health systems (such as Ayurveda, TCM and other agents systems, Native American wisdom, and other folk traditions from around the world), it is also paramount that physicians guide patients with evidence-based recommendations as to which treatments may or may not be helpful with the ultimate goal of curing cancer, preventing relapses, minimizing treatment-related toxicities, and maximizing quality of life outcomes.

Increasingly, NCI-designated Comprehensive Cancer Centers are offering integrative treatments for HNC patients to include yoga, massage, acupuncture, mindfulness meditation, music therapy, and other strategies for reducing anxiety, insomnia, and pain associated with treatment.[38] Numerous randomized controlled clinical trials (RCTs) have shown benefit–for instance in very specific treatments to include acupuncture for nausea and vomiting–and there is a suggestion of improvement for fibrosis, xerostomia, pain, and other sequelae of treatment of cancer.[39] Memorial Sloan-Kettering Cancer Center (MSKCC) operates an herbal dispensary overseen by physicians and pharmacists trained in IO, for mitigation of side effects during treatment of various cancers.[40] A smart phone app has been developed to help guide practitioners of IO discuss herbal supplements with patient in reference to potential side effects.[41] Current guidelines have been established for investigating mechanisms and safety behind TCM herbal medications for cancer treatment symptoms management.[42]

Complementary and Integrative Medicine for Prevention/Treatment of Cancer

Natural products have provided highly effective treatment of cancer to include such chemotherapy agents as the vinca alkaloids (periwinkle flower), taxanes (yew tree bark), and rapamycin (*Streptomyces* strain from Rapa Nui island). It is estimated that 60% of current anticancer drugs have been derived from natural sources.[43] Some products have some promise for chemoprevention, although many promising basic science and animal studies have not borne out similarly compelling results in human trials. Herbal products are the most commonly used category of CIM therapies by patients with cancer.[44] Whereas some botanicals have been investigated for mechanisms pertaining to prevention of cancer or premalignant lesions, none have been established within conventional cancer treatment. In fact, some natural products are known to be counterproductive or harmful during conventional cancer treatment.[45]

Juxtaposed against the fact that dietary supplements, herbal medications, and botanicals are the most frequently used CIM products by patients in cancer care, high-level recommendations from within the IO community do not support use of these products for cancer treatment, without clear evidence, because of potential side effects.[46] Direct discussions with patients and close monitoring are advised to ensure no adverse events.[47] A review of the NIH Clinical Trials database (www.clinicaltrials.gov/) for HNC and CIM therapies reveals over 2180 active trials for head and neck neoplasms, and over half investigating side effects of treatment, but only a handful examining herbal products or botanicals. Several recent publications have reported some benefit for certain natural products as treatment of oral mucositis during radiation therapy.[48–50]

As the diagnosis and treatment of HNSCC involve tremendous health burden, prevention of both primary and secondary tumors remains a worthwhile yet elusive goal.[51] The population at risk for HNSCC includes individuals with heavy tobacco and/or alcohol use, human papillomavirus infection, previous HNC, and radiation exposure. Such individuals would be the obvious targets for chemoprevention efforts. It is imperative to understand the molecular pathways involved in the development and progression of HNSCC to identify targets for chemopreventive agents.[44]

Retinoids

Early studies demonstrated that high-dose 13-cRA treatment for 1 year significantly reduced the incidence of second primary tumors in Stages I to IV HNSCC patients.[52,53] Unfortunately, a subsequent large-scale Phase III clinical trial of low-dose 13-cRA in randomized Stages I and II HNSCC patients failed to demonstrate a significant reduction in the development of second primary or recurrent tumors.[54] Although combinations of multiple compounds such as 13-cRA, a-interferon, and a-tocopherol appeared to be promising in delaying disease recurrence, it was difficult to enroll patients in clinical trials because of the refusal of subjects to be randomized.[55] Because of the challenges of these clinical trials, retinoids are no longer being used as chemopreventive agents for HNSCC, although a study of genetic variations from the Retinoid Second Primary Trial indicated that patients with certain genotypes had a more favorable response to 13-cRA and that the stratification of patients with HNSCC may lead to more effective chemoprevention measures.[56] Future trials targeting patients with specific genotypes who may exhibit a greater response to retinoids will support a pharmacogenetic approach to chemoprevention.

Curcumin

Curcumin (diferuloylmethane) is the chief component of the spice turmeric and is derived from the rhizome of the East Indian plant Curcuma longa. Turmeric contains a class of compounds known as the curcuminoids, which includes curcumin, demethoxycurcumin, and bisdemethoxycurcumin.[57] Curcumin is the principal curcuminoid and constitutes approximately 2% to 5% of turmeric; it is responsible for the yellow color of the spice as well as the majority of therapeutic effects of turmeric.[58] Apart from being used as a flavoring and coloring agent in food, turmeric has also been widely used in Ayurvedic medicine for its antioxidant, antiseptic, analgesic, antimalarial, and anti-inflammatory properties.[59] Curcumin has been consumed as a dietary supplement for centuries and is considered pharmacologically safe.

Curcumin's inhibitory effect on the NF-κB pathway is central to providing the compound with its anti-inflammatory properties. NF-κB regulates a variety of pro-inflammatory gene products such as COX-2, tumor necrosis factor (TNF)-a, iNOS, and various IL and inflammatory cytokines. Studies involving the suppression of NF-κB activation show a subsequent downregulation of COX-2 and iNOS and decreased production of inflammatory markers.[60–66] Curcumin has been shown to inhibit the production of inflammatory cytokines by activated monocytes and macrophages; in addition, the free-radical scavenging activity of curcumin also contributes to its anti-inflammatory properties by decreasing the amount of oxidative stress that can trigger the inflammatory cascade.

Curcumin has been studied in multiple human carcinomas including melanoma, head and neck, breast, colon, pancreatic, prostate, and ovarian cancers.[67–75] Epidemiologic studies attribute the low incidence of colon cancer in India to the chemopreventive and antioxidant properties of diets rich in curcumin.[76] The mechanisms by which curcumin exerts its anticancer effects are comprehensive and diverse, targeting many levels of regulation in the processes of cellular growth and apoptosis. Besides the vertical effects of curcumin on various transcription factors, oncogenes, and signaling proteins, it also acts at various temporal stages of carcinogenesis—from the initial insults leading to DNA mutations through the process of tumorigenesis, growth, and metastasis. Because of the far-reaching effects and multiple targets of curcumin on the cell growth regulatory processes, it holds much promise as a potential chemotherapeutic agent for many human cancers.

Recent trials in HNC patients have shown promise. A pilot study of oral curcumin patients with oral cancer demonstrated reduction in inflammatory cytokines, including IKKβ kinase, in the saliva following administration of a single dose of 1000 mg of curcumin.[77] A recent Phase I clinical trial of an oral turmeric pastille in subjects with oral cancer demonstrated systemic absorption, with circulating levels of curcumin in the blood as well as reduction in inflammatory cytokines in the saliva and T-cell recruitment to the tumor microenvironment.[78] This suggests potential for use of curcumin as an adjunctive or chemopreventive treatment of HNC. Further trials are necessary in HNC to establish the value and feasibility of curcumin as a chemopreventive agent.

Green tea

Green tea contains four major polyphenols: epigallocatechin-3-gallate (EGCG), epicatenin-3-gallate, epigallocatechin, and epicatechin. EGCG seems to be the most active agent and has been shown to function as an antioxidant and mediate signaling transduction pathways involving EGFR, NF-κB, TNF-a, AKT, MAPK, and p53. Through these pathways, it inhibits cell proliferation, angiogenesis, and invasion.[79,80] Because of the low bioavailability of the catechins in green tea, several cups a day must be consumed to achieve active levels of the phenols.[81] A Japanese cohort study of data collected prospectively over 10 years demonstrated that consumption of more than 10 cups of green tea a day resulted in a decreased incidence of cancer, with a hazard ratio of 0.59.[82] A Phase I trial of oral green tea extracts in patients with advanced solid tumors found that doses of 1000 mg/m^2 three times a day were well tolerated.[83] A pilot study using green tea extracts in doses of 2000 to 2500 mg/d demonstrated reduced smoking-induced DNA damage and aneuploidy, as well as increased apoptosis, in oral cells of smokers.[84] In vivo studies of the combination of EGCG and the EGFR tyrosine kinase inhibitor erlotinib demonstrated a synergistic inhibition of head and neck tumor growth in an animal model.[85] This combination treatment regimen may have promise as a chemopreventive protocol for HNSCC.

Dietary and Lifestyle Factors in Chemoprevention

Epidemiologic studies have documented the risk factors for development of HNSCC, including smoking, consuming alcohol, and chewing betel nut. Other factors such as poor dietary practices and nutritional deficiencies have also been linked to the development of oral cancer. A meta-analysis examined 16 studies describing the association between consumption of fruits and vegetables and oral cancer. A multivariate meta-regression analysis was performed and found that each portion of fruit consumed per day reduced the risk of oral cancer by 49% and vegetable consumption reduced the overall risk of oral cancer by 50%. There was no significantly different effect for green vegetable consumption compared with overall vegetable consumption, although greater protection against oral cancer was associated with citrus fruit consumption compared with overall fruit consumption.[86] The American Cancer Society has recommendations regarding nutrition and physical activity for prevention of cancer recurrence.[87]

Controversies in Evidence-Based Complementary and Integrative Medicine Practice

Many complementary therapies take their origin from non-Western healing systems such as Ayurveda, TCM and folk-healing traditions, which are quite comprehensive and have been relied on for thousands of years. Evidence-based medicine has increasingly become the standard-bearer in Western medicine; however, a critical component of this paradigm is continual reassessment of outcomes and incorporation of new information as it becomes understood and studied. The RCT has been elevated as the gold standard of evidence but for many reasons, including cost, it has been impractical or impossible to base all treatment decisions on RCT-level evidence.[88] In some cases, specifically with CIM therapies for cancer care, meta-analyses have found differing conclusions within similarly designed RCTs, thereby concluding a lack of evidence exists.[89]

On the other hand, there are many therapies which have been investigated in the medical literature with lower levels of evidence—not just case reports or anecdotes, but significant case series and even prospective trials that physicians can use to help patients guide treatment decision. Increasingly, practitioners with advanced training in IO have begun to compile recommendations and collaborate on clinical practice guidelines (CPG). Given that very little of our current medical knowledge has come from randomized controlled clinical studies, we must acknowledge our own "sliding scale" of evidence-informed decision-making. A graded response to incorporating lower levels of evidence[90] using Strength of Recommendation Taxonomy with additional grading of possible adverse effects has been advocated.[91]

SUMMARY

CIM in HNC is an evolving area of collaboration between conventional oncology, patient values and beliefs, and practitioners of complementary medicine. Evidence-informed decision-making is necessary to advise patients on which treatments may be incorporated into standard of care treatment of cancer. Patients use CIM for a variety of reasons and often have unrealistic expectations of cure or disease modifications.[92] On the other hand, there is increasing evidence that symptoms, side effects, and dysfunction related to cancer and its treatment can be ameliorated by CIM approaches to improve patient satisfaction and quality of life. Open communication between patients and providers is paramount.[93]

CLINICS CARE POINTS

- Most patients use some sort of complementary and integrative medicine (CIM) during conventional treatments of cancer.
- Patients consider using CIM for prevention and treatment of cancer as well as for mitigation of side effects of conventional cancer treatment.
- It is up to physicians and other members of the oncology team to advocate for CIM as opposed to "alternative" treatments which may be harmful or counter-productive.
- Physicians have an obligation to ask patients about their beliefs, preference, and intended use of CIM during conventional cancer treatments.
- Referral to a certified Integrative Oncologist can help provide holistic care without undermining standard of care treatment of cancer.
- As communication between doctors, patients, family members, and other CIM providers improves, collaborative care can be established that is patient-centered and evidence-informed to optimize cancer treatments and maximize quality of life.

DISCLOSURES

None. The authors do not have any commercial or financial conflicts of interest or any funding sources to disclose.

REFERENCES

1. Abrams DI, Weil A. Integrative oncology. 2nd edition. New York, (NY): Oxford University Press; 2014.
2. Miller MC. Complementary and integrative treatments: expanding the continuum of care. Otolaryngol Clin North Am 2013;46(3):261–76.
3. Latte-Naor S, Mao JJ. Putting Integrative Oncology Into Practice: Concepts and Approaches. J Oncol Pract 2019;15(1):7–14.
4. Vrinten C, van Jaarsveld CH, Waller J, et al. The structure and demographic correlates of cancer fear. BMC Cancer 2014;14:597.
5. Vrinten C, McGregor LM, Heinrich M, et al. What do people fear about cancer? A systematic review and meta-synthesis of cancer fears in the general population. Psychooncology 2017;26(8):1070–9.
6. Simard S, Thewes B, Humphris G, et al. Fear of cancer recurrence in adult cancer survivors: a systematic review of quantitative studies. J Cancer Surviv 2013;7(3): 300–22.
7. Niederdeppe J, Levy AG. Fatalistic beliefs about cancer prevention and three prevention behaviors. Cancer Epidemiol Biomarkers Prev 2007;16(5):998–1003.
8. Horneber M, Bueschel G, Dennert G, et al. How many cancer patients use complementary and alternative medicine: a systematic review and metaanalysis. Integr Cancer Ther 2012;11(3):187–203.
9. Matovina C, Birkeland AC, Zick S, et al. Integrative Medicine in Head and Neck Cancer. Otolaryngol Head Neck Surg 2017;156(2):228–37.
10. Chow LQM. Head and Neck Cancer. N Engl J Med 2020;382(1):60–72.
11. Huang SH, O'Sullivan B. Overview of the 8th Edition TNM Classification for Head and Neck Cancer. Curr Treat Options Oncol 2017;18(7):40.
12. Pfister DG, Spencer S, Adelstein D, et al. Head and Neck Cancers, Version 2.2020, NCCN Clinical Practice Guidelines in Oncology. J Natl Compr Canc Netw 2020;18(7):873–98.
13. Keene MR, Heslop IM, Sabesan SS, et al. Complementary and alternative medicine use in cancer: A systematic review. Complement Ther Clin Pract 2019;35: 33–47.
14. Ng JY, Dogadova E. The Presence of Complementary and Alternative Medicine Recommendations in Head and Neck Cancer Guidelines: Systematic Review and Quality Assessment. Curr Oncol Rep 2021;23(3):32.
15. Hendershot KA, Dixon M, Kono SA, et al. Patients' perceptions of complementary and alternative medicine in head and neck cancer: a qualitative, pilot study with clinical implications. Complement Ther Clin Pract 2014;20(4):213–8.
16. Available at: https://www.nccih.nih.gov/about/budget/complementary-and-alternative-medicine-funding-by-nih-institutecenter. Accessed date March 12 2022.
17. Complementary and Alternative Medicine in the United States. Washington, DC: National Academies Press (US); 2005. Institute of Medicine (US) Committee on the Use of Complementary and Alternative Medicine by the American Public. http://www.ncbi.nlm.nih.gov/books/NBK83799/(Accessed date March 12 2022)
18. Available at: https://www.nih.gov/about-nih/what-we-do/nih-almanac/national-center-complementary-integrative-health-nccih. Accessed date March 12 2022.
19. Jia L, Lin H, Oppenheim J, et al. US National Cancer Institute-China Collaborative Studies on Chinese Medicine and Cancer. J Natl Cancer Inst Monogr 2017; 2017(52).

20. Deng GE, Cassileth BR, Cohen L, et al. Integrative Oncology Practice Guidelines. J Soc Integr Oncol 2007;5(2):65–84.
21. Greenlee H, Balneaves LG, Carlson LE, et al. Clinical practice guidelines on the use of integrative therapies as supportive care in patients treated for breast cancer. J Natl Cancer Inst Monogr 2014;2014(50):346–58.
22. Lyman GH, Bohlke K, Cohen L. Integrative Therapies During and After Breast Cancer Treatment: ASCO Endorsement of the SIO Clinical Practice Guideline Summary. J Oncol Pract 2018;14(8):495–9.
23. Deng GE, Rausch SM, Jones LW, et al. Complementary therapies and integrative medicine in lung cancer: Diagnosis and management of lung cancer, 3rd ed: American College of Chest Physicians evidence-based clinical practice guidelines. Chest 2013;143(5 Suppl):e420S–36S.
24. Witt CM, Balneaves LG, Cardoso MJ, et al. A Comprehensive Definition for Integrative Oncology. J Natl Cancer Inst Monogr 2017;2017(52):10.
25. Available at: https://integrativeonc.org/latest-news/216-sio-asco-collaboration-on-guidelines. Accessed March 12 2022.
26. Mowery YM, Salama JK. Interpreting ORATOR: Lessons Learned From a Randomized Comparison of Primary Surgical and Radiation Approaches for Early-Stage Oropharyngeal Cancer. J Clin Oncol 2022;JCO2102813.
27. Lu W, Wayne PM, Davis RB, et al. Acupuncture for Chemoradiation Therapy-Related Dysphagia in Head and Neck Cancer: A Pilot Randomized Sham-Controlled Trial. Oncologist 2016;21(12):1522–9.
28. Garcia MK, Meng Z, Rosenthal DI, et al. Effect of True and Sham Acupuncture on Radiation-Induced Xerostomia Among Patients With Head and Neck Cancer: A Randomized Clinical Trial. JAMA Netw Open 2019;2(12):e1916910.
29. Meng Z, Garcia MK, Hu C, et al. Randomized controlled trial of acupuncture for prevention of radiation-induced xerostomia among patients with nasopharyngeal carcinoma. Cancer 2012;118(13):3337–44.
30. Pfister DG, Cassileth BR, Deng GE, et al. Acupuncture for pain and dysfunction after neck dissection: results of a randomized controlled trial. J Clin Oncol 2010;28(15):2565–70.
31. Deganello A, Battat N, Muratori E, et al. Acupuncture in shoulder pain and functional impairment after neck dissection: A prospective randomized pilot study. Laryngoscope 2016;126(8):1790–5.
32.. Bonomo P, Stocchi G, Caini S, et al. Acupuncture for radiation-induced toxicity in head and neck squamous cell carcinoma: a systematic review based on PICO criteria [published online ahead of print, 2021 Jul 31]. Eur Arch Otorhinolaryngol 2022;279(4):2083–97.
33. Lapen K, Cha E, Huang CC, et al. The use of complementary and integrative therapies as adjunct interventions during radiotherapy: a systematic review. Support Care Cancer 2021;29(11):6201–9.
34. Goyal N, Day A, Epstein J, et al. Head and neck cancer survivorship consensus statement from the American Head and Neck Society. Laryngoscope Investig Otolaryngol 2021;7(1):70–92.
35. Sahovaler A, Gualtieri T, Palma D, et al. Head and neck cancer patients declining curative treatment: a case series and literature review. Acta Otorhinolaryngol Ital 2021;41(1):18–23.
36. Balogh LC, Matthews TW, Schrag C, et al. Clinical outcomes of head and neck cancer patients who refuse curative therapy in pursuit of alternative medicine. Laryngoscope Investig Otolaryngol 2021;6(5):991–8.

37. Witt CM, Helmer SM, Schofield P, et al. Training oncology physicians to advise their patients on complementary and integrative medicine: An implementation study for a manual-guided consultation. Cancer 2020;126(13):3031–41.

38. Desai K, Liou K, Liang K, et al. Availability of Integrative Medicine Therapies at National Cancer Institute-Designated Comprehensive Cancer Centers and Community Hospitals. J Altern Complement Med 2021;27(11):1011–3.

39. Lin WF, Zhong MF, Zhou QH, et al. Efficacy of complementary and integrative medicine on health-related quality of life in cancer patients: a systematic review and meta-analysis. Cancer Manag Res 2019;11:6663–80.

40. Hou YN, Deng G, Mao JJ. [abstract online] Herbal medicine as a critical element of integrative cancer care: a retrospective analysis of the herbal dispensary program at Memorial Sloan-Kettering cancer center. J Altern Complement Med 2021;A1–3027. Available at: https://www.liebertpub.com/doi/abs/10.1089/acm. 2021.29097.abstracts. Accessed March 12 2022.

41. Hou YN, Deng G, Mao JJ. Practical Application of "About Herbs" Website: Herbs and Dietary Supplement Use in Oncology Settings. Cancer J 2019;25(5):357–66.

42. Liu J, Mao JJ, Wang XS, et al. Evaluation of Traditional Chinese Medicine Herbs in Oncology Clinical Trials. Cancer J 2019;25(5):367–71.

43. Cragg GM, Pezzuto JM. Natural Products as a Vital Source for the Discovery of Cancer Chemotherapeutic and Chemopreventive Agents. Med Princ Pract 2016;25(Suppl 2):41–59.

44. Lan XY, Chung TT, Huang CL, et al. Traditional Herbal Medicine Mediated Regulations during Head and Neck Carcinogenesis. Biomolecules 2020;10(9):1321.

45. Seidman MD, van Grinsven G. Complementary and integrative treatments: integrative care centers and hospitals: one center's perspective. Otolaryngol Clin North Am 2013;46(3):485–97.

46. Deng GE, Frenkel M, Cohen L, et al. Evidence-based clinical practice guidelines for integrative oncology: complementary therapies and botanicals. J Soc Integr Oncol 2009;7(3):85–120.

47. Truant TL, Porcino AJ, Ross BC, et al. Complementary and alternative medicine (CAM) use in advanced cancer: a systematic review. J Support Oncol 2013; 11(3):105–13.

48. Marucci L, Farneti A, Di Ridolfi P, et al. Double-blind randomized phase III study comparing a mixture of natural agents versus placebo in the prevention of acute mucositis during chemoradiotherapy for head and neck cancer. Head Neck 2017;39(9):1761–9.

49. Soltani GM, Hemati S, Sarvizadeh M, et al. Efficacy of the plantago major L. syrup on radiation induced oral mucositis in head and neck cancer patients: A randomized, double blind, placebo-controlled clinical trial. Complement Ther Med 2020; 51:102397.

50. Aghamohammadi A, Moslemi D, Akbari J, et al. The effectiveness of Zataria extract mouthwash for the management of radiation-induced oral mucositis in patients: a randomized placebo-controlled double-blind study. Clin Oral Investig 2018;22(6):2263–72.

51. Nguyen CT, Taw MB, Wang MB. Integrative care of the patient with head and neck cancer. Laryngoscope Investig Otolaryngol 2018;3(5):364–71.

52. Hong WK, Lippman SM, Itri LM, et al. Prevention of second primary tumors with isotretinoin in squamous-cell carcinoma of the head and neck. N Engl J Med 1990;323(12):795–801.

53. Benner SE, Pajak TF, Lippman SM, et al. Prevention of second primary tumors with isotretinoin in patients with squamous cell carcinoma of the head and neck: long-term follow-up. J Natl Cancer Inst 1994;86(2):140–1.

54. Khuri FR, Lee JJ, Lippman SM, et al. Randomized phase III trial of low-dose isotretinoin for prevention of second primary tumors in stage I and II head and neck cancer patients. J Natl Cancer Inst 2006;98(7):441–50.

55. Shin DM, Khuri FR, Murphy B, et al. Combined interferon-alfa, 13-cis-retinoic acid, and alpha-tocopherol in locally advanced head and neck squamous cell carcinoma: novel bioadjuvant phase II trial. J Clin Oncol 2001;19(12):3010–7.

56. Lee JJ, Wu X, Hildebrandt MAT, et al. Global assessment of genetic variation influencing response to retinoid chemoprevention in head and neck cancer patients. Cancer Prev Res (Phila) 2011;4(2):185–93.

57. Jurenka JS. Anti-inflammatory properties of curcumin, a major constituent of Curcuma longa: a review of preclinical and clinical research. Altern Med Rev 2009; 14(2):141–53.

58. Aggarwal BB, Sundaram C, Malani N, et al. Curcumin: the Indian solid gold. Adv Exp Med Biol 2007;595:1–75.

59. Ammon HP, Wahl MA. Pharmacology of Curcuma longa. Planta Med 1991; 57(1):1–7.

60. Brennan P, O'Neill LA. Inhibition of nuclear factor kappaB by direct modification in whole cells—mechanism of action of nordihydroguaiaritic acid, curcumin and thiol modifiers. Biochem Pharmacol 1998;55(7):965–73.

61. Jobin C, Bradham CA, Russo MP, et al. Curcumin blocks cytokine-mediated NF-kappa B activation and proinflammatory gene expression by inhibiting inhibitory factor I-kappa B kinase activity. J Immunol 1999;163(6):3474–83.

62. Plummer SM, Holloway KA, Manson MM, et al. Inhibition of cyclo-oxygenase 2 expression in colon cells by the chemopreventive agent curcumin involves inhibition of NF-kappaB activation via the NIK/IKK signaling complex. Oncogene 1999; 18(44):6013–20.

63. Barnes PJ, Karin M. Nuclear factor-kappaB: a pivotal transcription factor in chronic inflammatory diseases. N Engl J Med 1997;336(15):1066–71.

64. Wertz IE, O'Rourke KM, Zhou H, et al. De-ubiquitination and ubiquitin ligase domains of A20 downregulate NF-kappaB signalling. Nature 2004;430(7000):694–9.

65. Gilmore TD. Introduction to NF-kappaB: players, pathways, perspectives. Oncogene 2006;25(51):6680–4.

66. Brasier AR. The NF-kappaB regulatory network. Cardiovasc Toxicol 2006;6(2): 111–30.

67. Aggarwal S, Takada Y, Singh S, et al. Inhibition of growth and survival of human head and neck squamous cell carcinoma cells by curcumin via modulation of nuclear factor-kappaB signaling. Int J Cancer 2004;111(5):679–92.

68. LoTempio MM, Veena MS, Steele HL, et al. Curcumin suppresses growth of head and neck squamous cell carcinoma. Clin Cancer Res 2005;11(19 Pt 1): 6994–7002.

69. Wang D, Veena MS, Stevenson K, et al. Liposome-encapsulated curcumin suppresses growth of head and neck squamous cell carcinoma in vitro and in xenografts through the inhibition of nuclear factor kappaB by an AKT-independent pathway. Clin Cancer Res 2008;14(19):6228–36.

70. Mukhopadhyay A, Bueso-Ramos C, Chatterjee D, et al. Curcumin downregulates cell survival mechanisms in human prostate cancer cell lines. Oncogene 2001; 20(52):7597–609.

71. Mehta K, Pantazis P, McQueen T, et al. Antiproliferative effect of curcumin (diferuloylmethane) against human breast tumor cell lines. Anticancer Drugs 1997; 8(5):470–81.

72. Hanif R, Qiao L, Shiff SJ, et al. Curcumin, a natural plant phenolic food additive, inhibits cell proliferation and induces cell cycle changes in colon adenocarcinoma cell lines by a prostaglandin-independent pathway. J Lab Clin Med 1997;130(6):576–84.

73. Elattar TM, Virji AS. The inhibitory effect of curcumin, genistein, quercetin and cisplatin on the growth of oral cancer cells in vitro. Anticancer Res 2000; 20(3A):1733–8.

74. Lin YG, Kunnumakkara AB, Nair A, et al. Curcumin inhibits tumor growth and angiogenesis in ovarian carcinoma by targeting the nuclear factor-kappaB pathway. Clin Cancer Res 2007;13(11):3423–30.

75. Siwak DR, Shishodia S, Aggarwal BB, et al. Curcumin-induced antiproliferative and proapoptotic effects in melanoma cells are associated with suppression of IkappaB kinase and nuclear factor kappaB activity and are independent of the B-Raf/mitogen-activated/extracellular signal-regulated protein kinase pathway and the Akt pathway. Cancer 2005;104(4):879–90.

76. Mohandas KM, Desai DC. Epidemiology of digestive tract cancers in India. V. Large and small bowel. Indian J Gastroenterol 1999;18(3):118–21.

77. Kim SG, Veena MS, Basak SK, et al. Curcumin treatment suppresses IKKβ kinase activity of salivary cells of patients with head and neck cancer: a pilot study. Clin Cancer Res 2011;17(18):5953–61.

78. Basak SK, Bera A, Yoon AJ, et al. A randomized, phase 1, placebo-controlled trial of APG-157 in oral cancer demonstrates systemic absorption and an inhibitory effect on cytokines and tumor-associated microbes. Cancer 2020;126(8):1668–82.

79. Mukhtar H, Ahmad N. Tea polyphenols: prevention of cancer and optimizing health. Am J Clin Nutr 2000;71(Suppl 6):1698S–702S.

80. Yang CS, Maliakal P, Meng X. Inhibition of carcinogenesis by tea. Annu Rev Pharmacol Toxicol 2002;42:25–54.

81. Clinical development plan: tea extracts. Green tea polyphenols. Epigallocatechin gallate. J Cell Biochem Suppl 1996;26:236–57.

82. Suganuma M, Sueoka E, Sueoka N, et al. Mechanisms of cancer prevention by tea polyphenols based on inhibition of TNF-alpha expression. Biofactors 2000; 13(1–4):67–72.

83. Pisters KM, Newman RA, Coldman B, et al. Phase I trial of oral green tea extract in adult patients with solid tumors. J Clin Oncol 2001;19(6):1830–8.

84. Schwartz JL, Baker V, Larios E, et al. Molecular and cellular effects of green tea on oral cells of smokers: a pilot study. Mol Nutr Food Res 2005;49(1):43–51.

85. Zhang X, Zhang H, Tighiouart M, et al. Synergistic inhibition of head and neck tumor growth by green tea (-)-epigallocatechin-3-gallate and EGFR tyrosine kinase inhibitor. Int J Cancer 2008;123(5):1005–14.

86. Pavia M, Pileggi C, Nobile CGA, et al. Association between fruit and vegetable consumption and oral cancer: a meta-analysis of observational studies. Am J Clin Nutr 2006;83(5):1126–34.

87. Kushi LH, Doyle C, McCullough M, et al. American Cancer Society Guidelines on nutrition and physical activity for cancer prevention: reducing the risk of cancer with healthy food choices and physical activity. CA Cancer J Clin 2012;62(1): 30–67.

88. Devisch I, Murray SJ. 'We hold these truths to be self-evident': deconstructing 'evidence-based' medical practice. J Eval Clin Pract 2009;15(6):950–4.

89. Chung VC, Wu X, Hui EP, et al. Effectiveness of Chinese herbal medicine for cancer palliative care: overview of systematic reviews with meta-analyses. Sci Rep 2015;5:18111.

90. Ebell MH, Siwek J, Weiss BD, et al. Strength of recommendation taxonomy (SORT): a patient-centered approach to grading evidence in the medical literature. Am Fam Physician 2004;69(3):548–56.

91. Rakel D, editor. Integrative medicine. 4th editiom. Philadelphia, (PA): Elsevier; 2018.

92. Gansler T, Strollo S, Fallon E, et al. Use of complementary/integrative methods: cancer survivors' misconceptions about recurrence prevention. J Cancer Surviv 2019;13(3):418–28.

93. Latte-Naor S. Managing Patient Expectations: Integrative, Not Alternative. Cancer J 2019;25(5):307–10.

Complementary and Integrative Medicine and the Voice

Karuna Dewan, MD[a], Vanessa Lopez, BA[b], Nausheen Jamal, MD[c],*

KEYWORDS

- Dysphonia • Muscle tension dysphonia • Massage therapy • Acupuncture

KEY POINTS

- There are four broad categories in the realm of complementary medicine: nutritional, psychological, physical, and combined. Each of these has something to offer the dysphonic patient.
- A variety of herbal supplements can be used to decrease inflammation and edema within the vocal folds.
- Acupuncture, laryngeal manual therapy, and neuromuscular therapy are the primary means of releasing tension within the larynx.
- Hypnotherapy and neurolinguistic programming are the primary psychological methods of treating dysphonia.
- Treatment of dysphonia is a complex process that should use both traditional and complementary approaches.

INTRODUCTION

Voice disorders, including dysphonia, impact 7.6% of American adults yearly[1] . Dysphonia can be indicative of an underlying pathology, including laryngitis, functional or muscle tension dysphonia, lesions, or neurologic conditions.[2] Conventional treatment options include medications with limiting side effects, such as antibiotics, steroids, or acid-reducing medications.[3] Often, concerns about conventional treatment options lead patients with dysphonia to seek alternative options within complementary and integrative medicine (CIM).

[a] Department of Otolaryngology- Head and Neck Surgery, Louisiana State University Health Shreveport, Edinburg, TX 78541, USA; [b] The University of Texas Rio Grande Valley School of Medicine, 1210 West Schunior Street, EMEBL 3.145, Edinburg, TX 78541, USA; [c] Department of Otolaryngology–Head and Neck Surgery, The University of Texas Rio Grande Valley School of Medicine, 1210 West Schunior Street, EMEBL 3.145, Edinburg, TX 78541, USA
* Corresponding author.
E-mail address: Nausheen.Jamal@utrgv.edu

Otolaryngol Clin N Am 55 (2022) 1007–1016
https://doi.org/10.1016/j.otc.2022.06.008
0030-6665/22/© 2022 Elsevier Inc. All rights reserved.

The use of medicine, herbs, and practices or therapies that focus on the wellness of the entire individual has made CIM increasingly popular over recent years. In a survey of singers and voice students, Surow and Lovetri found that 71% of participants endorsed frequent use of alternative therapies. Of those users, 53% reported daily use.[4]

The National Center for Complementary and Integrative Health classifies complementary health approaches into four broad categories: nutritional, physical, psychological, and a combination of the previous three categories.

Nutritional

The most used complementary health approach is the use of natural products, defined as dietary supplements other than vitamins or minerals. Among professional voice users surveyed, the most common modalities of complementary medicine used to treat voice disorders fall into the category of natural products: hot teas and drinks that include lemon and honey, lozenges, and other herbal remedies.[5]

Herbal medicine is the culmination of many generations of knowledge used in conjunction with the practice of medicine as performed by ancient physicians. Herbal remedies are a complementary and alternative treatment option for voice disorders, especially those with minor symptoms. Traditional Chinese medicine supports performers and professional voice users by protecting the voice during times of increased vulnerability. Herbal therapy is helpful in reducing recovery time for the common cold and assisting during times of high vocal demand.

Calcinoni and colleagues have created a database of herbal medicines used in the treatment of voice disorders that includes forty-four plants, one fungus, and one lichen. The Herbs for Voice Database includes household names in the herbal treatment of voice disorders, such as tea, ginger, and peppermint, as well as some less popular species such as bitter kola and oroxylum.[6] Anti-inflammatory, analgesic, and antimicrobial effects are the three most important biological activities associated with these herbs, followed by antitussive and immunomodulatory effects. The major clinical uses of these herbs in the treatment of voice disorders are divided into four symptom categories: irritation, infection effects, respiratory impairments, and voice quality alteration. The most commonly represented biological target of the herbs included in this database is the transient receptor potential Ankyrin 1 (TRPA1) receptor ion channel, an anti-inflammatory and neurogenic pain mediator (**Table 1**).[6]

The aromatic herbs in the database are widely popular. These include ginger, mint, oregano, sage, cinnamon, eucalyptus, and thyme. *Sisymbrium officinale* (SO), known for its effects on the vocal tract, is the most common herb used in the treatment of voice disorders. It is often referred to as "the singer's plant." SO desensitizes TRPA1, making it a potent anti-inflammatory and analgesic agent.[6]

White willow bark extract, a natural source of salicylic acid, also demonstrates anti-inflammatory activities. These anti-inflammatory benefits are conferred without the irritating gastrointestinal effects seen with aspirin, and with less thrombocyte inhibition. *Astragalus membranaceus* is known for its energy enhancement as well as its anti-inflammatory and immunomodulating actions that increase resistance to disease.[7–9] It stimulates proliferation of stem cells, macrophages, and lymphocytes while increasing interferon production.[7–11]

Butterbur (*Petasites hybridus*), a member of the daisy family, is used to treat asthma and allergic rhinitis.[12] Randomized controlled trials have shown butterbur to be as effective for allergic rhinitis as fexofenadine and cetirizine, with fewer sedative side effects.[13] Its leaves and roots contain the active ingredient that is thought to inhibit leukotriene production.

Table 1
Most common herbal substances used in complementary treatment of voice disorders, adapted from the Herbs for Voice Database

Herbs	Activity	Clinical Use
S officinale	Analgesic, anti-inflammatory, antitussive, antimicrobial, acts on TRPA1	Vocal tract diseases, sore throat, cough, throat dryness or irritation, hoarseness
Ginger	Analgesic, anti-inflammatory, antibacterial, acts on TRPA1	Cough, fever, throat pain, asthma, cold, chest pain, bronchitis
Peppermint	Analgesic, anti-inflammatory, antimicrobial, acts on TRPA1, TRPM8	Sore throat, hoarseness, cough
Eucalyptus	Analgesic, anti-inflammatory, antimicrobial, antioxidant, acts on TRPA1	Sore throat, hoarseness, cough
Sage	Analgesic, anti-inflammatory, antimicrobial, acts on TRPA1	Acute sore throat, oral infection, or inflammation
A montana	Anti-inflammatory, acts on NF-kB through lactone helenalin	Postoperative sore throat with hoarseness, dysphonia or aphonia

Arnica montana, an herb with anti-inflammatory effects, is helpful in the setting of injury from a blunt instrument. Blunt instrument insertion may cause hematoma of the vocal folds and laryngeal swelling. *A montana* exerts its anti-inflammatory effects through the lactone helenalin, which inhibits nuclear factor kappa-beta (NF-kB) to effectively treat postoperative voice disorders. These positive effects of *A montana* on the postoperative sore throat with hoarseness has only been described in case studies, warranting further research into this plant's effect on voice disorders.[14]

Cordyceps sinensis, a fungus filled with polysaccharides, nucleosides, and fatty acids, has a variety of uses and is thought to enhance immunity and reduce coughing. It increases the activity of natural killer cells and demonstrates anti-inflammatory effects. Goldenseal (*Hydrastis canadensis*) has been used for the treatment of cold and flu.[15] It is noted to have antibacterial, antisecretory, and antitussive effects.[16,17] It is also noted to induce tracheal muscle relaxation.

Irritation of the larynx in laryngopharyngeal reflux (LPR) can lead to voice disorders. The first-line treatment for LPR is proton-pump inhibitor administration to suppress acid secretion. In patients with LPR refractory to acid-suppressing medication, an anti-reflux diet may provide symptom relief. An intensive dietary change is recommended, consisting of a low-acid diet with alkaline water (pH > 8.8) that can inactivate pepsin (**Tables 2** and **3**). Other possible dietary additions mentioned in the literature

Table 2
Low-acid food options from the induction reflux diet (nothing less than pH 5)[20]

Fruits	Vegetables	Grains	Meats	Others
Banana	Celery	Bagels	Chicken, skinless	Beans
Melons	Potatoes	Low-fat, non-fruit muffins	Turkey breast, skinless	Egg whites
	Turnip	Whole grain bread, pasta, and rice	Fish	Skim milk
	Broccoli	Rye bread		Tofu
		Oatmeal		Chamomile tea

Table 3
Acidic foods to avoid in laryngopharyngeal reflux treatment[20]

Fruits	Vegetables	Grains	Meats	Others
Almost all fruits, except for bananas and melons	Onions Peppers Tomatoes	Breads with fruit in them	Skin-on meats Red meat	Fried foods Coffee Garlic Cheese Chocolate Mints Most herbal teas Carbonated beverages Butter Eggs Beer Hard Liquor Wine

include chamomile tea, honey, vinegar, ginger, and turmeric; however, these foods have not been studied for efficacy in the treatment of voice disorders.[18] Pediatric voice disorders may also be caused by LPR because of the high rates of consumption of foods and beverages that are high in acid and sugar content, otherwise known as junk food.[19] A study comparing the dietary habits of children with vocal fold nodules to a control group of children without voice disorders showed higher rates of junk food consumption in the children with vocal fold nodules, suggesting that a poor diet may correlate with LPR symptoms and pediatric voice disorders.[19]

It is essential for health care providers to ask patients about herbal and supplement use. Alternative therapies do exist and should be considered. Patients should be counseled that although beneficial effects of natural treatments have been shown, safety is not guaranteed often due to a lack of sufficient research. However, the relative risk with natural therapies is generally quite low.

Physical

Speech and singing involve complex coordination of muscular activities in the larynx and throughout the body. Movement of the diaphragm, intercostal muscles, and abdominal muscles is necessary to generate adequate breath support for sustained phonation. This sound resonates within the pharynx, sinuses, and oral cavity. Resonance and transmission of sound can be hindered by excessive muscle tension in the neck, shoulders, mouth, and tongue. Mood disorders, anxiety, and increased muscle tension at inappropriate times have been implicated in conditions such as muscle tension dysphonia, laryngeal dystonia, tremor, and development of some phonotraumatic lesions.[20–22] Aronson noted that "the extrinsic and intrinsic laryngeal muscles are exquisitely sensitive to emotional stress, and their hyperconstriction is the common denominator behind the dysphonia and aphonia in virtually all psychogenic voice disorders."[23] Acupuncture releases muscle tension, reduces emotional disorders, relieves stress, and improves problems of digestion, breathing, and blood flow, potentially alleviating dysphonia.

There have been several studies evaluating the use of acupuncture to improve vocal pathology. These studies describe the treatment of vocal fold thickening, nodules, edema, polyps, and incomplete closure.[24] There are also case studies reporting improvements with acupuncture while treating dysphonia following radiation therapy for nasopharyngeal carcinoma, unilateral vocal fold paralysis, and acute laryngitis.[24]

Psychogenic voice disorders have also been treated with modest success.[25] Unfortunately, these studies are reported as small case series, and none of them have control groups. Acupuncture use in the treatment of laryngeal dystonia has been reported in two studies.[26] In both studies, patients showed some improvements in fundamental frequency and voice breaks, but once again, a placebo effect cannot be ruled out.[27] The utility of acupuncture in the treatment of muscle tension dysphonia remains to be seen. Using acupuncture to help with overall relaxation may allow a patient to center their emotions and help to improve skeletal alignment, breathing, and muscle performance, thereby promoting healthy voice use.

Addressing pathologies within the respiratory system plays a role in the treatment of voice disorders, because the respiratory and laryngeal systems work in tandem to produce voice. Engagement of respiratory muscles in professional voice users leads to easier voice production and projection, known as the "supported voice." In patients who are not professional voice users, there is an opportunity to engage respiratory muscles with voice exercises to functionally improve voice disorders. A survey of voice therapists reported that respiratory exercises were one of the most common strategies used in treating voice patients. Respiratory exercises are indicated when respiratory function is impaired and can lead to functional improvement that overcomes the patient's specific voice deficits.[28]

The most common respiratory exercises to treat voice disorders can be broken up into two categories: those that use a resistance device and those that do not. The most common intervention used is expiratory muscle strength training (EMST), a technique in which patients perform forceful expiration against a breathing device that offers resistance. EMST is thought to enhance airflow and control of laryngeal and respiratory muscles, leading to better stability of phonation, and reduced vocal fatigue. In patients with weaker expiratory muscles, laryngeal tension can overcompensate during phonation; by strengthening the expiratory muscles, this laryngeal overcompensation can be reduced. Although no improvements in respiratory function parameters are seen with EMST, improvements have been shown in phonation time, vocal fatigue, and voicing efficiency.[29]

The posture and muscle tone in cervical and perilaryngeal muscles have a role to play in voice production and quality. Patients may experience increased muscle tension and pain in the area surrounding the larynx, indicative of muscle tension dysphonia. In a survey of professional and amateur voice users, the most common alternative medicine practitioner sought for treatment of vocal symptoms was a massage therapist.[30] Massage techniques, including laryngeal manual therapy (LMT), massage of the neck or shoulder girdle, and passive stretching, are an effective way to reduce muscle tension in cervical and perilaryngeal muscles to improve voice quality.[31] LMT, also referred to as manual circumlaryngeal therapy or voice massage, is a technique that consists of massaging the sternocleidomastoid, suprahyoid, and other extrinsic laryngeal muscles while the patient is silent.[32] LMT has been shown to lead to decreased pain, increased positive self-perception of voice, and partial improvement in voice quality in dysphonic patients, particularly in vocal stability.[31] In the long-term, manual circumlaryngeal therapy was shown to be effective for treatment of muscle tension dysphonia for at least 6 months after treatment.[33] Another complementary relaxation technique is transcutaneous electrical nerve stimulation (TENS), in which a low-frequency analgesic current is applied to the perilaryngeal region, improving blood flow and leading to muscle relaxation.[32] In comparison to LMT, TENS showed similar improvements in pain and self-perception signs but with more immediate improvement among dysphonic patients in voice quality and stability.[32] However, there are no long-term studies of TENS as a complementary treatment of voice disorders. Both LMT and TENS have been shown to have similar effectiveness on vocal symptoms as other voice therapy options, and both can be used as complementary treatments of voice disorders.[34]

Another method to manipulate muscle tension and function is through neuromuscular therapy (NMT) that is used to manipulate the soft tissues of the body to restore homeostasis and balance between the muscular and nervous system. Dysphonia can be related to the improper use of various muscles of the body. The tone of facial muscles, oral cavity, pharynx, larynx, and even of chest and abdominal muscles impacts the quality, range, texture, resonance, and articulation of the voice produced. The source of excessive muscle activity can be attributed to the underlying personality of the person, learned adaptations during times of sickness or disease, and technical factors during voice production.[35–38] Excessive vocal tension leads to complaints of neck tightness, vocal effort, and vocal fatigue that worsen as the day progresses. The voice produced by these individuals can have variable quality, ranging from breathy to pressed. In NMT, muscular hypertonicity is thought to occur in areas of hypoperfusion or ischemia. These regions have decreased range of motion and may become trigger points. Sometimes the trigger point sites refer elsewhere in the body and manifest as pain, paresthesia, numbness, tingling, and diminished range of motion.[39] Treatment strategies using NMT and other massage techniques are applied after the muscular tone is assessed in the shoulders, anterior and lateral neck, and the tongue base. Therapy applied to areas of excess tension improves circulation and allows the muscles to relax and lengthen. NMT uses techniques of friction, static pressure, and trigger point therapy to treat the origin and insertion of the involved muscles. Circumlaryngeal massage closely relates to NMT through its role of manual repositioning of the larynx. Roy and colleagues describe pressure that is placed via palpation over the tips of the hyoid, along the thyrohyoid space and the lateral edges of the thyroid cartilage.[23,38] Any regions of muscular tension are addressed while pulling the larynx down. The identification of taut muscular bands, narrowed or absent thyrohyoid space, or trigger points is highly suggestive of excessive muscle tension.[35] These laryngeal manipulations will induce periods of improved voice during which therapeutic vocal maneuvers can be reinforced.[40] NMT and other massage techniques are low-cost, noninvasive methods to correct vocal dysfunction secondary to the inappropriate excessive muscular tension impacting the neck and throat. In conjunction with traditional voice therapy techniques, massage therapy should be considered before more invasive solutions are attempted. In addition to treating soft tissue pathology, this therapy encourages good vocal health. Massage therapy provides a strong beneficial physiologic effect, including the ability to enhance immune function and provide a sense of relaxation and well-being. Many professional performers find benefit with the healing properties of massage.

Psychological

Human beliefs and perceptions strongly influence behavior. Beliefs are so powerful that they can affect our neuroimmunopsychology, and they are an invaluable asset to assist a person in achieving their goals. Mind–body therapies include hypnotherapy and neurolinguistic programming. Hypnotherapy has been used for many years to facilitate relaxation and envision a perfect performance for the professional voice user. Many professional singers use this form of therapy. Initially, singers might practice with several sessions with a professional hypnotherapist, and then they can learn to do this on their own.

Neurolinguistic therapy is essentially the science of how to run one's brain in an optimal way to produce the result one wants. Neurolinguistic therapy addresses the mind and allows the individual to form positive images that are the foothold for success. These powerful techniques can also be used to assist patients with overcoming fears, phobias, anxiety, depression, and limiting beliefs. A hypnotherapist can also use the above strategies by incorporating them into a hypnosis script and using the techniques with the client during hypnosis.

Pediatric voice disorders arise from multiple factors and have a prevalence of 5% to 7% in most populations. The most common pediatric voice disorder is a functional voice disorder that can progress to vocal fold nodules. Although pediatric voice disorders are commonly treated with acid-suppressing medication, voice therapy, or vocal hygiene education, psychodynamic and family therapy is a complementary treatment option that can target the psychosomatic aspects of functional voice disorders. The Bernese Brief Dynamic Intervention (BBDI) was developed for children with functional voice disorders and involves alternating sessions of play therapy and family dynamic counseling to target the psychosomatic aspects of their voice issue(s). The play therapy allows children to better vocalize their emotions and feelings, soothing the child's uneasiness in their voice and reducing muscle tension. Following two sessions of play therapy, parents in Kollbrunner and Seifert's study were counseled on family dynamics, encouraging parent–parent and child–parent dialogue and the cycle was repeated. In that study, BBDI was shown to be as effective as traditional voice therapy for children with voice disorders, suggesting that it may be a complementary treatment option for pediatric voice disorders.[41]

SUMMARY

Complementary integrative therapies have been present since the advent of ancient medical practices. Despite the wealth of scientific knowledge that we have accumulated, especially over the past few hundred years, conventional "modern" medicine does not have all the answers. Many vocalists seek complementary and integrative treatments because of their appreciation that their body is their instrument. When the body is functioning optimally, the voice reflects that state. Nutritional, physical, and psychological treatments are helpful in prevention and management of dysphonia. As clinicians, we must guide patients regarding the integration of these alternative methods with traditional medical treatments.

CLINICS CARE POINTS

- Patients should be counseled that although beneficial effects of natural treatments have been shown, safety is not guaranteed often due to a lack of sufficient research. However, the relative risk with natural therapies is generally quite low.

- Muscular issues contributing to voice problems can be addressed in many different ways, including acupuncture, neuromuscular therapy, and a number of traditional voice therapy approaches, including laryngeal manual therapy and expiratory muscle strength training.

- The mind-body connection must be considered in voice pathologies. Therapies such as hypnotherapy and neurolinguistic programming are useful in addressing this connection when treating the impact of beliefs and perceptions on voice.

DISCLOSURE

The authors do not have any commercial or financial conflicts of interest. Dr N. Jamal receives partial salary support through a federal grant from the Department of Health and Human Services. The other authors have no funding sources to declare.

REFERENCES

1. Bhattacharyya N. The prevalence of voice problems among adults in the United States. Laryngoscope 2014;124(10):2359–62.
2. Neighbors C, Song SA. Dysphonia. In: StatPearls. FL: Treasure Island; 2022.
3. Asher BF. Complementary and integrative treatments: the voice. Otolaryngol Clin North Am 2013;46(3):437–45.
4. Surow JB, Lovetri J. Alternative medical therapy" use among singers: prevalence and implications for the medical care of the singer. J Voice 2000;14(3):398–409.
5. MacDonald AJ, You P, Fung K. Prevalence of complementary and alternative medicine use in professional voice users. J Voice 2021;S0892-1997(21):00240-X.
6. Calcinoni O, Borgonovo G, Cassanelli A, et al. Herbs for Voice Database: Developing a Rational Approach to the Study of Herbal Remedies Used in Voice Care. J Voice 2021;35(5):807 e833–41.
7. Cho WC, Leung KN. In vitro and in vivo immunomodulating and immunorestorative effects of Astragalus membranaceus. J Ethnopharmacol 2007;113(1):132–41.
8. Matkovic Z, Zivkovic V, Korica M, et al. Efficacy and safety of Astragalus membranaceus in the treatment of patients with seasonal allergic rhinitis. Phytother Res 2010;24(2):175–81.
9. Yang X, Huang S, Chen J, et al. Evaluation of the adjuvant properties of Astragalus membranaceus and Scutellaria baicalensis GEORGI in the immune protection induced by UV-attenuated Toxoplasma gondii in mouse models. Vaccine 2010;28(3):737–43.
10. Du X, Chen X, Zhao B, et al. Astragalus polysaccharides enhance the humoral and cellular immune responses of hepatitis B surface antigen vaccination through inhibiting the expression of transforming growth factor beta and the frequency of regulatory T cells. FEMS Immunol Med Microbiol 2011;63(2):228–35.
11. Shen B, Chen L, Zhou K, et al. [Effects of astragalus and angelica on bone marrow stem cells proliferation and VEGF protein expression in vitro]. Zhongguo Gu Shang 2011;24(8):652–5.
12. Schapowal A, Study G. Treating intermittent allergic rhinitis: a prospective, randomized, placebo and antihistamine-controlled study of Butterbur extract Ze 339. Phytother Res 2005;19(6):530–7.
13. Schapowal A, Petasites Study G. Randomised controlled trial of butterbur and cetirizine for treating seasonal allergic rhinitis. BMJ 2002;324(7330):144–6.
14. Tsintzas D, Vithoulkas G. Treatment of Postoperative Sore Throat With the Aid of the Homeopathic Remedy Arnica montana: A Report of Two Cases. J Evid Based Complement Altern Med 2017;22(4):926–8.
15. Hwang BY, Roberts SK, Chadwick LR, et al. Antimicrobial constituents from goldenseal (the Rhizomes of Hydrastis canadensis) against selected oral pathogens. Planta Med 2003;69(7):623–7.
16. Ettefagh KA, Burns JT, Junio HA, et al. Goldenseal (Hydrastis canadensis L.) extracts synergistically enhance the antibacterial activity of berberine via efflux pump inhibition. Planta Med 2011;77(8):835–40.
17. Cech NB, Junio HA, Ackermann LW, et al. Quorum quenching and antimicrobial activity of goldenseal (Hydrastis canadensis) against methicillin-resistant Staphylococcus aureus (MRSA). Planta Med 2012;78(14):1556–61.
18. Huestis MJ, Keefe KR, Kahn CI, et al. Alternatives to Acid Suppression Treatment for Laryngopharyngeal Reflux. Ann Otol Rhinol Laryngol 2020;129(10):1030–9.

19. Ozcelik Korkmaz M, Tuzuner A. The Role of Nutritional and Dietary Habits in Etiology in Pediatric Vocal Fold Nodule. J Voice 2020;S0892-1997(20):30358–61.

20. House A, Andrews HB. The psychiatric and social characteristics of patients with functional dysphonia. J Psychosom Res 1987;31(4):483–90.

21. Altman KW, Atkinson C, Lazarus C. Current and emerging concepts in muscle tension dysphonia: a 30-month review. J Voice 2005;19(2):261–7.

22. Andrade DF, Heuer R, Hockstein NE, et al. The frequency of hard glottal attacks in patients with muscle tension dysphonia, unilateral benign masses and bilateral benign masses. J Voice 2000;14(2):240–6.

23. Aronson AE, Bless DM. Clinical voice disorders. 4th edition. New York: Thieme; 2009.

24. Yang S. Clinical observations on 109 cases of vocal nodules treated with acupuncture and Chinese drugs. J Tradit Chin Med 2000;20(3):202–5.

25. Yao W. Prof. Sheng Canruo's experience in acupuncture treatment of throat diseases with yan si xue. J Tradit Chin Med 2000;20(2):122–5.

26. Crevier-Buchman L, Laccourreye O, Papon JF, et al. Adductor spasmodic dysphonia: case reports with acoustic analysis following botulinum toxin injection and acupuncture. J Voice 1997;11(2):232–7.

27. Lee L, Daughton S, Scheer S, et al. Use of acupuncture for the treatment of adductor spasmodic dysphonia: a preliminary investigation. J Voice 2003; 17(3):411–24.

28. Desjardins M, Bonilha HS. The impact of respiratory exercises on voice outcomes: a systematic review of the literature. J Voice 2020;34(4):648.e1–9.

29. Tsai YC, Huang S, Che WC, et al. The effects of expiratory muscle strength training on voice and associated factors in medical professionals with voice disorders. J Voice 2016;30(6):759 e721–7.

30. Weekly EM, Carroll LM, Korovin GS, et al. A vocal health survey among amateur and professional voice users. J Voice 2018;32(4):474–8.

31. Cardoso R, Meneses RF, Lumini-Oliveira J. The effectiveness of physiotherapy and complementary therapies on voice disorders: a systematic review of randomized controlled trials. Front Med (Lausanne) 2017;4:45.

32. Conde MCM, Siqueira LTD, Vendramini JE, et al. Transcutaneous electrical nerve stimulation (TENS) and laryngeal manual therapy (LMT): immediate effects in women with dysphonia. J Voice 2018;32(3):385 e317–25.

33. Dehqan A, Scherer RC. Positive effects of manual circumlaryngeal therapy in the treatment of muscle tension dysphonia (mtd): long term treatment outcomes. J Voice 2019;33(6):866–71.

34. Ribeiro VV, Vitor JDS, Honorio HM, et al. Surface electromyographic biofeedback for behavioral dysphonia in adult people: a systematic review. Codas 2018;30(6): e20180031.

35. Roy N, Ford CN, Bless DM. Muscle tension dysphonia and spasmodic dysphonia: the role of manual laryngeal tension reduction in diagnosis and management. Ann Otol Rhinol Laryngol 1996;105(11):851–6.

36. Morrison MD, Rammage LA. Muscle misuse voice disorders: description and classification. Acta Otolaryngol 1993;113(3):428–34.

37. Morrison MD, Nichol H, Rammage LA. Diagnostic criteria in functional dysphonia. Laryngoscope 1986;96(1):1–8.

38. Roy N, Bless DM, Heisey D. Personality and voice disorders: a multitrait-multidisorder analysis. J Voice 2000;14(4):521–48.

39. Simons DG, Travell JG, Simons LS, et al. Travell & Simons' myofascial pain and dysfunction : the trigger point manual. 2nd edition. Baltimore: Williams & Wilkins; 1999.

40. Roy N, Bless DM, Heisey D. Personality and voice disorders: a superfactor trait analysis. J Speech Lang Hear Res 2000;43(3):749–68.

41. Kollbrunner J, Seifert E. Functional hoarseness in children: short-term play therapy with family dynamic counseling as therapy of choice. J Voice 2013;27(5): 579–88.

Migrainous Vertigo, Tinnitus, and Ear Symptoms and Alternatives

Mehdi Abouzari, MD, PhD[a,1], Karen Tawk, MD[a,1], Darlene Lee, ND[b],
Hamid R. Djalilian, MD[a,c],*

KEYWORDS

- Tinnitus • Vertigo • Dizziness • Hearing loss • Alternative medicine

KEY POINTS

- Migraine is a chronic disorder that frequently coexists with vestibular and neuro-otological symptoms leading to significant physical and psychological disabilities including tinnitus and hearing loss.
- The evidence currently encourages the use of cognitive behavioral therapy and supplements for the treatment of tinnitus and vestibular rehabilitation for vertigo.
- Based on the review results, complementary and integrative medicine should undergo further high-quality clinical trials to obtain more definitive data to translate these therapies into routine recommendations for patients.

INTRODUCTION

Migraine headaches frequently coexist with vestibular symptoms such as vertigo, motion sickness, and gait instability. Migraine-related vasospasm can also damage the inner ear, which results in symptoms such as sudden sensorineural hearing loss (SSNHL) and tinnitus.[1] The pathophysiology of these symptoms is not yet fully understood, and despite their prevalence, there is no universally approved management.

Financial disclosure: M. Abouzari is supported by the National Center for Research Resources and the National Center for Advancing Translational Sciences, National Institutes of Health, through Grant TL1TR001415.
Conflicts of Interest: H.R. Djalilian. holds equity in MindSet Technologies, Elinava Technologies, and Cactus Medical LLC. He is a consultant to NXT Biomedical.
[a] Division of Neurotology and Skull Base Surgery, Department of Otolaryngology–Head and Neck Surgery, University of California Irvine, 19182 Jamboree Road, Otolaryngology-5386, Irvine, CA 92697, USA; [b] Susan Samueli Integrative Health Institute, University of California, 5141 California Avenue, Suite 200B, Irvine, CA 92617, USA; [c] Department of Biomedical Engineering, University of California, Irvine, USA
[1] These authors contributed equally to this article.
* Corresponding author.
E-mail address: hdjalili@hs.uci.edu

Otolaryngol Clin N Am 55 (2022) 1017–1033
https://doi.org/10.1016/j.otc.2022.06.017
0030-6665/22/© 2022 Elsevier Inc. All rights reserved.

Owing to patient belief, nonuniversal effectiveness, cost, and fear of the side effects of conventional treatments, many patients with migraine-related symptoms seek complementary and integrative medicine (CIM) alternatives. Traditional medicine (acupuncture, herbal supplements, and manual therapies) originated in China about 3000 years ago and then spread to Korea and Japan with Buddhism.[2] However, some in the United States still regard CIM therapies with skepticism mainly because of the lack of randomized clinical trials.[3,4] A cross-sectional study conducted between 2002 and 2012 reported that 33.2% of adults in the United States use complementary health approaches (dietary supplements, deep breathing exercises, and yoga),[5] with 75% of patients not informing their physician about this practice.[3] This review summarizes the data on CIM in treating patients with migrainous ear disorders (**Tables 1–3**).

COGNITIVE BEHAVIORAL THERAPY

Cognitive behavioral therapy (CBT) is an active approach that includes a wide array of strategic interventions such as cognitive restructuring, behavioral activation, exposure, and problem solving. CBT helps reduce emotional distress and increase adaptative behaviors, thus adopting a problem-solving strategy.[6] Several studies evaluating CBT for tinnitus have demonstrated its effectiveness as an alternative approach.[7–9]

In a randomized double-blind controlled study,[10] patients with tinnitus were allocated in 2 groups: the first one receiving CBT with sound-focused tinnitus retraining therapy and the second group was provided standard audiological intervention. Patients assigned to CBT showed a decrease in tinnitus severity and improvement in their quality of life (QOL). In another study, Beukes and colleagues[11] concluded that Internet-delivered CBT (iCBT) helped reduce tinnitus distress and associated difficulties (anxiety, depression, and insomnia), hence improving the QOL. Andersson[12] reported that iCBT is as effective as face-to-face CBT. Furthermore, a smartphone-based iCBT and customized sound therapy were found to be effective in treating tinnitus.[7] Although in this study no significant improvement was reported in the Generalized Anxiety Disorder 7-item and Perceived Stress Scale, a significant reduction of Tinnitus Handicap Index (THI), which measures tinnitus-related stress, anxiety, and QOL, was observed in the treatment group.[7] In addition, in a Cochrane systematic review, including 28 studies comparing CBT versus no intervention, audiological care, tinnitus retraining therapy, or any other active control, the investigators concluded that CBT may be effective in reducing tinnitus negative impact on QOL and associated depression.[13] In line with the previous results, Nolan and colleagues[14] showed a highly significant reduction in tinnitus, hyperacusis, and concomitant psychological symptoms posttreatment with CBT. Based on the data, CBT is a valuable treatment option for the treatment of tinnitus.

YOGA

There are several studies demonstrating the benefits of yoga in patients with tinnitus.[15–17] The first study by Köksoy and colleagues[15] showed that yoga practices reduce tinnitus severity and tinnitus stress score. Thus, practicing yoga improves the symptoms of tinnitus and QOL, and reduces stress and anxiety.[15] Another study in 25 patients with chronic tinnitus assessed 12 weeks of yoga training compared with a control group of 13 patients. The yoga group improved on the tinnitus functional index (TFI) global score.[16] Both studies were limited by the lack of longer-term follow-up and small sample sizes. Gazbare and colleagues[17] performed a randomized controlled trial comparing the effect of yogasanas (yoga postures) with gaze stabilization and

Table 1
Summary of alternative treatments of tinnitus

Symptom	Alternative Medicine Interventions	Study	Study Nature	Sample Size	Key Findings
Tinnitus	CBT	Abouzari et al,[7] 2021	Randomized controlled trial	30 Patients	Treatment group: significant higher improvement in THI scores after smartphone-based iCBT and sound therapy
		McKenna et al,[9] 2020	Meta-analysis		CBT is an effective treatment of tinnitus distress
		Cima et al,[10] 2012	Randomized controlled trial	492 Patients	CBT group: a significant improvement in QOL, decrease in tinnitus severity, and tinnitus impairment
		Beukes et al,[11] 2019	Meta-analysis	15 Studies	Tinnitus: significant favor of tinnitus iCBT over inactive and active controls. Hearing loss: no significant favor for either intervention. Study quality affected the outcome
		Andersson,[12] 2015	Systemic review	9 Controlled studies	iCBT is more effective than no-treatment condition. iCBT is as effective as face-to-face CBT
		Fuller et al,[13] 2020	Meta-analysis	28 Controlled studies	In all CBT groups, primary outcome: significant reduction of the impact of tinnitus on QOL. CBT vs no intervention: 14 studies. CBT vs audiological care: 3 studies. Secondary outcome: reduction is depression. CBT vs TRT: 1 study. No secondary outcome. CBT vs active control (relaxation, information, Internet-based discussion forums): 16 studies. Secondary outcome: reduction in depression and anxiety
		Nolan et al,[14] 2020	Cross-sectional	268 Patients	Reduction of TQ, QHS, BSI, and BDI-II
	Yoga	Köksoy et al,[15] 2018	Clinical trial	12 Patients	Yoga practices reduce stress, handicap, and severity of tinnitus
		Niedziatek et al,[16] 2019	Randomized controlled trial	38 Patients	Significant decrease in 5 of 8 subscales of TFI global score (intrusiveness, sense of control, sleep, auditory, and quality of life)
	Neurofeedback	Peter et al,[18] 2019	Review		TMS: to be used for tinnitus localization rather than tinnitus suppression. tDCS, transcranial random noise stimulation: qualify as a promising method in tinnitus treatment. Neurofeedback: should be further investigated as a treatment modality for tinnitus. Vagus nerve stimulation: promising treatment option for tinnitus. Invasive brain stimulation: more research is needed. It will always be limited to a very select group because it is invasive
		Guillard et al,[19] 2021	Clinical trial	33 Patients	Significant decrease of the THI score. Significant increase of the alpha-band power within sessions
		Güntensperger et al,[22] 2020	Randomized controlled trial	26 Patients	Significance reduction of tinnitus loudness and related distress (THI, TQ). An increase in the trained alpha/delta ratio

(continued on next page)

Table 1
(continued)

Symptom	Alternative Medicine Interventions	Study	Study Nature	Sample Size	Key Findings
		Güntensperger et al,[21] 2019	Randomized controlled trial	48 Patients	Significant reduction of tinnitus loudness and related distress in both groups. Significant increase in trained alpha/delta ratio over the course of training and follow-up period
		Emmert et al,[23] 2017	Randomized controlled trial	14 Patients	Significant deactivation of the secondary auditory cortex until the last session for the continuous group vs intermittent feedback showed the strongest downregulation in the first session. Decrease of the TFI scores that was not statistically significant
	Hypnosis	Ross et al,[26] 2007	Controlled clinical trial	393 Patients	Significant improvement of the TQ and SF-36 scores when compared with the waiting-list controls
		Maudoux et al,[27] 2007	Clinical trial	49 Patients	Significant improvement of the THI score in all patients (60.23 before EH therapy to 16.9 at discharge)
		Yazıcı et al,[28] 2012	Controlled clinical trial	39 Patients	Significant improvement of the THI and SF-36 scores
		Brüggemann et al,[36] 2021	Meta-analysis	3 Placebo-controlled clinical trials	Significant reduction in tinnitus severity. Significant improvement of anxiety, depression, and cognition
		Spiegel et al,[37] 2018	Review	5 Placebo-controlled clinical trials	EGb761 significantly superior to placebo in alleviating tinnitus and dizziness
		Radunz et al,[38] 2020	Randomized controlled trial	33 Patients	Significant improvement of the THI score with the individual HA and/or GB EGb71 HA were more effective in patients with shorter time to onset of tinnitus GB alone or in association with HA was effective regardless of tinnitus duration
	Zinc	Jun et al,[47] 2015	Case-control	2225 Patients	After adjustment of sex, age and hearing loss, no significant difference in zinc levels between a tinnitus population and a control population. Significant lower zinc levels in the most severe tinnitus group compared with the control group
		Berkiten et al,[48] 2015	Cross-sectional	100 Patients	Patients in group III (between 61 and 78 years old) have significantly lower serum zinc levels. Significantly higher hearing thresholds of air conduction in zinc-deficient patients. Significantly higher Tinnitus Severity Index Questionnaire and loudness scores in zinc-deficient patients
		Coelho et al,[49] 2013	Randomized controlled trial	116 patients	No significant improvement in THQ scores after zinc treatment or placebo
	Vitamin B and antioxidants	Person et al,[50] 2016	Systemic review	3 Randomized controlled trials 1435 Patients	Overall, no significant improvement in tinnitus severity and loudness. No significant improvement in any secondary outcome (QOL, anxiety, and depression)
		Lee and Kim,[58] 2018	Cross-sectional		Less intake of vitamin B_2 is associated with tinnitus in middle-aged patients. Less intake of water, protein, and vitamin B_3 is associated with tinnitus-related annoyance in elderly. It is recommended to use vitamin B_2 and B_3 in combination with pharmacologic or behavioral therapy
		Singh et al,[59] 2016	Randomized Controlled Trial	40 Patients	Significant improvement in mean TSI score and VAS after vitamin B_{12} treatment in patients with tinnitus and cobalamin deficiency

	Study	Study Type	Sample Size	Findings
	Hameed et al,[60] 2018	Observational Cohort	75 Patients	Supplementation with vitamin B complex improves the tinnitus severity, specifically in patients with tinnitus and without hearing loss. DPOAE changing amplitude can be used as a tool to assess the effect of vitamin B complex used in patient with tinnitus with or without hearing loss
	Dawes et al,[61] 2020	Cross-sectional	34,576 Patients	Higher intake of vitamin B_{12} and protein is associated with reduced odds of tinnitus. Meanwhile, a high intake of calcium, iron, and fat were associated with increased odds of tinnitus. High intake of vitamin D, fruits and vegetables, and protein is associated with reduced likelihood of hearing difficulties. High fat intake was associated with hearing difficulties
	Ekinci et al,[62] 2020	Randomized Controlled Trial	50 patients	Serum prolidase enzyme and oxidative stress might participate to the etiopathogenesis of tinnitus
	Khan et al,[63] 2007	Clinical Trial	20 patients	CoQ10 supply in patients with low CoQ10 levels may decrease tinnitus
Melatonin	Albu and Chirtes,[66] 2014	Randomized Controlled Trial	60 Patients	In the intratympanic dexamethasone plus melatonin (compared with melatonin alone): significant improvement in all of the following outcome measures: tinnitus loudness score, tinnitus awareness score, THI, PSQI, and BDI
	Rosenberg et al,[68] 1998	Randomized Controlled Trial	30 Patients	Statistically significant overall improvement among patients with high THI scores and/or difficulty sleeping taking melatonin when compared with placebo
	Abtahi et al,[69] 2017	Randomized Controlled Trial	70 Patients	THI scores were significantly reduced in the melatonin and sertraline groups, but the use of melatonin is more effective
	Miroddi et al,[70] 2015	Review	5 Clinical Studies	The authors were not able to confirm the effectiveness of melatonin in treating tinnitus; however, melatonin improved sleep disturbances associated with tinnitus
	Merrick et al,[71] 2014	Review		Patient with tinnitus can benefit from melatonin through its antioxidant and sleep enhancement properties
Acupuncture	Tu et al,[72] 2019	Randomized Controlled Trial	30 Patients	Significant reduction in THI in DA group greater than that in SA group. DA can modulate the autonomic nervous system by activating the sympathetic and parasympathetic nervous system balance
	Cai et al,[73] 2019	Clinical Trial	54 Patients	Significant reduction in temperature differentials of both sides after acupuncture implying an even distribution of blood in both cochlea
	Naderinabi et al,[74] 2018	Randomized Controlled Trial	88 Patients	TSI and VAS significantly improved in all groups; however, the differences by both measures were better with acupuncture compared with placebo at the end of the late sessions
	Pang et al,[75] 2019	Review	40 Randomized Controlled Trials	The 8 different methods of acupuncture are effective in treating tinnitus. The clinical effect from high to low is as follows: moxibustion acupuncture, moxibustion acupuncture combined with electroacupuncture, moxibustion acupuncture combined with supplementary medication, traditional acupuncture combined with supplementary medication, electroacupuncture combined with supplementary medication, electroacupuncture, traditional acupuncture, and medication-only treatment

Abbreviations: BDI-II, Beck Depression Inventory; BSI, Brief Symptom Inventory; CBT, cognitive behavioral therapy; DA, deep acupuncture; DPOAE, distortion product otoacoustic emissions; EH, Ericksonian hypnosis; GB, *Ginkgo biloba*; HA, hearing aid; iCBT, Internet-based CBT; PSQI, Pittsburgh Sleep Quality Index; SA, shallow acupuncture; SF-36, 36-Item Short Form Health Survey; tDCS, transcranial direct current stimulation; TFI, Tinnitus Functional Index; THI, Tinnitus Handicap Inventory; THQ, Tinnitus Handicap Questionnaire; TMS, transcranial magnetic stimulation; TQ, Tinnitus Questionnaire; TRT, tinnitus retraining therapy; TSI, Tinnitus Severity Index; QHS, Questionnaire on Hypersensitivity to Sound; QOL, Quality Of Life; VAS, visual analog scale.

Table 2
Summary of alternative treatments of vertigo/dizziness

Symptom	Alternative Medicine Interventions	Study	Study Nature	Sample Size	Key Findings
Vertigo	Yoga	Gazbare et al,[17] 2021	Randomized controlled trial	32 Patients	Both groups reduced symptoms of dizziness Yogasanas: better improvement in MSQ Gaze stabilization and habituation exercises: better improvement in DHI
	Physical therapy	Brown et al,[29] 2006	Case-series	48 Patients	Statistically significant improvement after physical therapy on the ABC, DHI, DGI, the timed up & go test, and the FTSTS test
		Whitney et al,[30] 2000	Case series	39 Patients	Statistically significant improvement after physical therapy on the DHI, ABC, PDS, the DGI, and the CS
		Brown et al,[31] 2001	Case series	24 Patients	Statistically significant improvement after physical therapy on the DHI, ABC, DGI, timed up &go measures, and the CS scores
		Regauer et al,[32] 2020	Systematic review	20 Randomized and 2 nonrandomized controlled trials	Interventions included: VR, CAVR, TCVR, CRM, and MT. VR and VR in addition to CRM and MT are effective in treating patients with VDB
		Liu et al,[33] 2020	Clinical trial	19 Patients	Significant decrease of the DHI and HAMA scores Significant increase of the ALFF values in the left posterior cerebellum
	Ginkgo biloba	Sokolova et al,[42] 2014	Randomized controlled trial	160 Patients	Both drugs were similarly effective in the treatment of vertigo, but EGb761 was better tolerated
		Hamann et al,[43] 2006	Systematic review		Preclinical and double-blind clinical studies show that EGB761 promotes compensation and is effective in the treatment of vertigo syndromes
		Lindner et al,[44] 2019	Preclinical study	40 Rats	Group A: significant reduction of nystagmus scores, of postural asymmetry, and increased motility in the open field when compared with controls Groups B and C: fast recovery of postural asymmetry

Ginkgo biloba in combination with neurofeedback	Decker et al,[45] 2021	Randomized controlled trial	120 Patients	Statistically significant improvement in the fall risk in balance-related situations and proprioceptive components of the gSBDT-CS in the active group
Zinc	Ferreira et al,[51] 2009	Case-control	16 Patients	Hypozincemia affects the function of the vestibulo-ocular, vestibulocerebellar, and vestibulocortical pathways
Acupuncture	Chiu et al,[78] 2015	Randomized controlled trial	60 Patients	Acupuncture reduced discomfort and VAS of both vertigo and dizziness after 30 min treatment in the emergency department

Abbreviations: ABC, Activities-Specific Balance Confidence Scale; ALFF, amplitude of low-frequency fluctuations; CAVR, computer-assisted vestibular rehabilitation; CRM, canalith repositioning maneuvers; CS, Composite Score; DGI, Dynamic Gait Index; DHI, Dizziness Handicap Inventory; FTSTS, Five Times Sit-to-Stand; gSBDT-CS, Geriatric Standard Balance Deficit Test Composite Score; HAMA, Hamilton Anxiety Scale; MSQ, Motion Sensitivity Quotient; MT, manual therapy; PDS, Perception of Dizziness Symptoms; TCVR, Tai Chi vestibular rehabilitation; VR, vestibular rehabilitation; VAS, visual analog scale; VDB, vertigo, dizziness, and balance disorders.

Table 3
Summary of alternative treatments of hearing loss

Symptom	Alternative Medicine Interventions	Study	Study Nature	Sample Size	Key Findings
Hearing loss	*Ginkgo biloba*	Koo et al,[41] 2016	Randomized controlled trial	56 Patients	Association between systemic steroids and EGb761 showed no superiority when compared with steroids alone in pure tone threshold The words recognition score improved in combination therapy
	Acupuncture	Zhang et al,[76] 2015	Meta-analysis	12 Randomized controlled trials	Manual acupuncture combined with conventional medicine comprehensive treatment was better than conventional medicine alone in treating patients with SSNHL
		Chen et al,[77] 2019	Meta-analysis	20 Randomized controlled trials	EA, EA + conventional medicine, and MA + conventional medicine were superior to conventional medicine alone for the treatment of SSNHL
	HBOT	Huang et al,[82] 2021	Randomized controlled trial	102 Patients	IVS + HBOT: better hearing recovery rate compared with the control group within the first 7 days No significant improvement of tinnitus
		Alimoglu et al,[83] 2011	Clinical trial	217 Patients	Patients receiving oral steroids + HBOT had higher chances to recover than patients receiving oral or IV steroids or HBOT alone
		Rhee et al,[84] 2018	Meta-analysis	19 Clinical trials	Patients with severe to profound hearing loss may benefit from the adjunction of HBOT to conventional medical treatment
		Bayoumy et al,[85] 2019	Review	68 Studies	HBOT can be used as an optional therapy in patients with acute hearing loss (idiopathic or acoustic trauma)
		Eryigit et al,[86] 2018	Systemic review	16 Studies	No significant difference was found between the intervention and control groups. However, patients with severe to profound hearing loss may benefit from the combination of steroids and HBOT

Abbreviations: EA, electroacupuncture; HBOT, hyperbaric oxygen therapy; IV, intravenous; IVS, intravenous steroid; MA, manual acupuncture.

habituation exercises in vestibular dysfunction. The investigators concluded that both practices were effective in reducing dizziness. Furthermore, greater improvement in the Motion Sensitivity Quotient was seen with yogasanas and greater improvement in the Dizziness Handicap Inventory (DHI) with stabilization and habituation exercises.[17] Based on the limited available data, yoga may have a beneficial effect on dizziness and tinnitus, but more confirmatory studies are needed to evaluate their efficacy.

NEUROFEEDBACK

Several neuromodulation techniques,[18] including neurofeedback, have been used to target tinnitus.[19] Neurofeedback is a form of biofeedback that measures the patient's brain activity and then generates audiovisual feedback in real time so the patient can reinforce his or her brain activity consciously via operant conditioning.[20] Interestingly, as reported in a randomized controlled study, an increase in alpha activity via neurofeedback training led to a decrease in tinnitus-related distress and loudness.[21,22] Similar results were found in a randomized controlled study comparing continuous with intermittent neurofeedback. This study showed that continuous feedback is superior to intermittent feedback in the long term; the TFI score significantly improved after all the sessions and patients felt more relaxed.[23] Targeting larger tinnitus-implicated areas in the brain might lead to even better outcomes; therefore, individualized neurofeedback training could potentially be a promising therapeutic option in the treatment of tinnitus.[24]

HYPNOSIS

Although the studies testing the effect of hypnosis on patients with tinnitus have been scarce, the few available ones demonstrated a positive result in the treatment of troublesome tinnitus. The largest study using Ericksonian hypnosis (EH) included 393 patients with subacute and chronic tinnitus who were treated within an inpatient closed group over 28 days, and compared with a waiting-list control group. The severity of the tinnitus was measured by Tinnitus Questionnaire (TQ) up to 12-month follow-up. Considering that the minimal clinically important difference of TQ changes was estimated to a reduction of at least 5 points,[25] significant improvement in TQ was observed compared with the waiting-list group with a mean reduction of 15.9 and 14.1 in the subacute and chronic tinnitus groups, respectively.[26] Two other trials by Maudoux and colleagues[27] and Yazıcı and colleagues,[28] verifying the effect of EH in an outpatient setting, have achieved similar results with less overall session time and a significant reduction in THI scores compared with admission, thus showing hypnosis efficacy. This area is still underresearched; however, preliminary results are promising.

PHYSICAL THERAPY

Studies have shown that patients with vestibular dysfunction improve with vestibular rehabilitation (VR).[29-31] In a systemic review, with 1876 patients, Regauer and colleagues[32] concluded that VR in any modality (**Table 2**), except Tai Chi and manual therapy, was superior to usual care in treating older patients with vertigo, dizziness, and balance disorders. Moreover, Liu and colleagues[33] investigated the effect of VR on brain activity in patients with vestibular migraine (VM), using resting-state functional MRI. The results showed a significant decrease in the DHI scores and an increase in the 36-Item Short Form Health Survey scores after VR training. The amplitude of low-frequency fluctuation was significantly higher in the left posterior cerebellum compared to baseline in patients with VM, asserting that the cerebellum may play a role in vestibular compensation.[33] These studies demonstrated the benefits of VR in improving vestibular symptoms and QOL.

SUPPLEMENTS
Ginkgo biloba

There are several contradictory studies on the effectiveness of Ginkgo biloba (GB) as a treatment for tinnitus. The active ingredient has been identified as EGb761.[3] In the studies that do not show superiority of GB over placebo, the herbal supplement was used in its nonstandardized form (other than GB extract EGb761) or with a lower dose than clinically indicated (<240 mg twice daily).[34] Otherwise, most studies have shown the efficacy of GB extract EGb761 as a treatment for patients with tinnitus.[35–38] A randomized placebo-controlled trial investigating the benefit of EGb761 in patients with dementia with tinnitus showed a direct positive effect on the severity of tinnitus, and an indirect positive effect by improving depression, anxiety, and cognition.[36] In a meta-analysis of 5 trials, Spiegel and colleagues[37] reported that EGb761 displayed significant therapeutic outcomes over placebo after 20 weeks of treatment in terms of tinnitus and dizziness in patients with dementia (at the end of the treatment, the 11-point box scales for tinnitus and dizziness were reduced by 1.06 and 0.77, respectively). EGb761 improves cerebral and cochlear blood flow[39] as well as mitochondrial functioning[40]—the desired effect in elderly patients with impaired perfusion and mitochondrial function. Furthermore, Radunz and colleagues[38] demonstrated an improvement in tinnitus severity and loudness after a 3-month period of treatment with GB and/or hearing aids, with no synergism between the treatments.

EGb761 was also tested in a randomized placebo-controlled trial in patients with idiopathic SSNHL. Although adjuvant systemic steroids with EGb761 showed no superiority when compared with steroids alone in pure tone threshold, the words recognition score improved in combination therapy.[41] Finally, in a randomized, double-blind trial, Sokolova and colleagues[42] found that EGb761 was as effective as betahistine in the treatment of unspecified vertigo in all outcome measures. EGb761 was also found to be superior to placebo in vestibular and nonvestibular vertigo. This superiority was measured by different means such as vertigo score (intensity, duration, frequency), global assessment of patients (visual analog scale [VAS]), caloric test, and sway amplitude in the craniocorpography and posturography.[43] In addition, following a unilateral labyrinthectomy in rats, oral supplementation with EGb761 was shown to be effective on the compensation of static and dynamic vestibular function (nystagmus, postural asymmetry, and locomotor behavior).[44] A bimodal therapy consisting of the combination of EGb761 with vibrotactile neurofeedback resulted in improvement in age-related vertigo and dizziness after 6 weeks of treatment. In addition, no safety issues were reported.[45] These results should be confirmed in future clinical trials.

Zinc

Studies have shown that the inner ear, especially the stria vascularis, has a high zinc content, which protects the cochlea from injury due to reactive oxygen species, and that a low serum level of zinc could lead to otologic disorders, such as tinnitus, imbalance, and hearing loss.[34,46] In a large study, using data from the Korea National Health and Nutrition Examination Survey, Jun and colleagues[47] found that serum zinc levels were significantly lower in patients with severe tinnitus only and that low serum zinc levels were not correlated to tinnitus in the other subpopulation (mild tinnitus, moderate tinnitus, and control group). Similarly, Berkiten and colleagues[48] showed by using the tinnitus severity index questionnaire that lower serum zinc levels were associated with increased severity and loudness of tinnitus. In addition, they demonstrated that serum zinc levels decrease as age increases and that an increase in hearing thresholds is associated with low serum zinc levels.[48] In 2 randomized placebo-controlled trials, zinc supplementation was not more effective than placebo in treating elderly patients with tinnitus.[49,50]

In a study by Ferreira and colleagues,[51] which included patients with zinc deficiency, it was demonstrated that hypozincemia possibly affected the function of vestibulo-ocular, vestibulocerebellar, and vestibulocortical pathways when tested using videonystagmography. The investigators suggested that zinc may affect the functioning of the vestibular system.[51] Overall, the advantage of supplementing zinc in the treatment of migrainous ear disorders remains an item of debate and requires further assessments.

Vitamin B and Antioxidants

Recent studies have shown a correlation between migraine headache and various vestibular disorders (Meniere disease [MD],[52] benign paroxysmal positional vertigo,[53] and mal de debarquement syndrome[54]). As such, it has been shown that treating MD with a migraine diet and lifestyle modifications (preventing dehydration, starvation, and sleep disturbances; avoiding certain foods such as chips, cheese, chocolate, nuts, processed meats, certain fruits, and pickled fruits or vegetables), as well as supplementation with vitamin B_2 and magnesium can control vestibular and cochlear symptoms.[55] Similarly, patients with tinnitus can benefit by preventing dehydration and avoiding certain foods such as caffeine, alcohol, processed meats, monosodium glutamate (found in soy sauce or pickled foods), aspartame, avocado, and chocolate.[56,57] Furthermore, Lee and Kim[58] reported that less vitamin B_2 intake in young ages was associated with tinnitus, whereas less intake of vitamin B_3 in the elderly was significantly associated with tinnitus-related annoyance. The investigators recommended that supplementation with vitamin B_2 and B_3 might be considered in conjunction with conventional pharmacologic therapy or CBT while managing tinnitus in patients.[58] Vitamin B_{12} is an essential cofactor for myelin sheath formation, thus preventing neuronal dysfunction peripherally and centrally. Seidman and Babu[4] believe that there might be an association between vitamin B_{12} deficiency and increased prevalence and severity of tinnitus in the elderly, because supplementation with vitamin B_{12} showed some relief. Consistently, in a randomized, double-blind clinical trial, patients with tinnitus and cobalamin (vitamin B_{12}) deficiency, receiving vitamin B_{12}, showed a significant improvement in the VAS and tinnitus severity index (TSI) after treatment with vitamin B_{12}.[59] It has been also demonstrated that following 1 month of treatment with vitamin B complex, the amplitude of the distortion product otoacoustic emissions increased with clinical improvement, especially in patients with tinnitus.[60] Similarly, using the UK Biobank resource, Dawes and colleagues conducted a study to evaluate the role of diet in tinnitus and hearing disorders. There were associations between a high intake of vitamin B_{12} and protein with a reduced likelihood of tinnitus, whereas high calcium, iron, and fat intakes were associated with an increased likelihood of tinnitus.[61]

Besides B vitamins, and based on the theory that reactive oxygen species contributed to tinnitus, Ekinci and Kamasak[62] supported the use of antioxidants. A clinical trial demonstrated that supplementing patients with low plasma coenzyme Q10 (CoQ10) levels and chronic tinnitus with CoQ10 may decrease tinnitus.[63] In addition, it has been reported in 2 meta-analyses that CoQ10 supplementation significantly reduced the duration and frequency of migraine headache attacks, without a significant effect on severity, when compared with the control group.[64,65] Patients with tinnitus, vertigo, and poor hearing may benefit from supplementation with some vitamins and certain antioxidants.

Melatonin

The precise mechanism of action of melatonin on tinnitus is not well known, but it is thought that its favorable outcomes are possibly related to the regulation of the labyrinthine perfusion, reduction of the muscular tone and sympathetic drive, antidepressive effects, and antioxidant effects.[66,67] Rosenberg and colleagues[68] performed the first randomized, double-blinded, placebo-controlled trial evaluating the efficacy of melatonin as a treatment of tinnitus. The investigators found that patients with high THI scores and/or difficulty sleeping would benefit from melatonin.[68] Abtahi and colleagues[69] demonstrated that melatonin may outperform sertraline in treating tinnitus. The investigators found that after 3 months of 3 mg melatonin once daily or 50 mg sertraline once daily, the THI scores significantly decreased in both groups; however, the decrease was significantly more for melatonin (reduction of THI score from 45 to 30 in melatonin group and from 45 to 37 in sertraline group). These results asserted that both drugs are effective, but melatonin was more helpful especially because no side effects,[69] apart from nightmares, have been reported to date.[34] Along with these findings, Albu and Chirtes[66] demonstrated that after 3 months of treatment, patients receiving intratympanic (IT) dexamethasone plus melatonin or only melatonin attained statistically significant improvement on the tinnitus loudness score, tinnitus awareness score, THI, Pittsburgh Sleep Quality Index, and Beck Depression Inventory, favoring the IT dexamethasone plus melatonin in patients with acute unilateral tinnitus.[66] Therefore, it would be desirable to redirect the available evidence through high-quality clinical trials, especially given that in all studies the efficacy of melatonin in tinnitus and associated sleep disturbances has been recognized.[70,71] It is likely that improvement of sleep may be the primary reason melatonin improves QOL in patients with tinnitus. Melatonin may be beneficial for patients with tinnitus who also suffer from sleep-onset delay.

ACUPUNCTURE

Acupuncture has been widely used to treat tinnitus in Eastern Asian countries.[34] It seems that deep acupuncture (needles inserted approximately 10 to 30 mm deep) improved tinnitus symptoms by modulating the sympathetic and parasympathetic nervous system balance.[72] Another study using infrared thermography test preacupuncture and postacupuncture treatment in patients with tinnitus showed that the efficacy of acupuncture is due to an improvement of cochlear blood flow in both ears even if acupuncture was applied on one side.[73] As such, multiple studies have demonstrated the superiority of acupuncture as a treatment of tinnitus when compared with placebo or conventional medication.[74,75] Additionally, 2 meta-analyses showed a better effect of acupuncture combined with conventional medicine (such as systemic or intratympanic steroids, hyperbaric oxygen, and vasodilators) than conventional medicine alone in the treatment of SSNHL and sudden deafness.[76,77] Finally, a controlled clinical trial demonstrated that acupuncture reduces the discomfort and VAS of dizziness and vertigo, after 30 minutes of treatment in the emergency department.[78]

HYPERBARIC OXYGEN THERAPY

Cochlear migraine (fluctuating or SSNHL) is a new concept that was first described in 2018.[79,80] One of the etiologic hypothesis has been attributed to an abnormal blood flow to the cochlea.[81] Thus, based on the principle of hypoxia of the inner ear, several studies supported the implementation of hyperbaric oxygen therapy (HBOT) in combination with steroids as a treatment of SSNHL,[82–85] specifically in patients with severe or profound hearing impairment.[86] At present, there is mixed evidence in support of HBOT for SSNHL. If there is a benefit, it is best provided early after the onset.

SUMMARY

Several CIM treatment options may be beneficial for migrainous tinnitus, vertigo, and ear symptoms. Although many physicians may be hesitant to consider these treatment modalities, CIM should be used as a complementary approach combined with conventional treatment, especially with patients who did not sufficiently benefit from medical therapy. More randomized controlled studies are needed to define the efficacy of the various CIM therapies on otologic migraine. These studies are best performed by collaboration of neurotologists and CIM specialists. In general, most treatments are well-tolerated with limited side effects. Therefore, CIM should be in the repertoire of every clinician treating otologic migraine.

REFERENCES

1. Goshtasbi K, Abouzari M, Risbud A, et al. Tinnitus and subjective hearing loss are more common in migraine: a cross-sectional NHANES analysis. Otol Neurotol 2021;42:1329–33.
2. Park HL, Lee HS, Shin BC, et al. Traditional medicine in China, Korea, and Japan: a brief introduction and comparison. Evidence-Based Complement Altern Med 2012;2012:e429103.
3. Asher BF, Seidman M, Snyderman C. Complementary and alternative medicine in otolaryngology. Laryngoscope 2001;111:1383–9.
4. Seidman MD, Babu S. Alternative medications and other treatments for tinnitus: facts from fiction. Otolaryngol Clin North Am 2003;36:359–81.
5. Clarke TC, Black LI, Stussman BJ, et al. Trends in the Use of complementary health approaches among adults: United States, 2002–2012. Natl Health Stat Rep 2015;10:1–16.
6. Wenzel A. Basic Strategies of Cognitive Behavioral Therapy. Psychiatr Clin North Am 2017;40:597–609.
7. Abouzari M, Goshtasbi K, Sarna B, et al. Adapting personal therapies using a mobile application for tinnitus rehabilitation: a preliminary study. Ann Otol Rhinol Laryngol 2021;130:571–7.
8. Andersson G. Psychological aspects of tinnitus and the application of cognitive-behavioral therapy. Clin Psychol Rev 2002;22:977–90.
9. McKenna L, Vogt F, Marks E. Current validated medical treatments for tinnitus. Otolaryngol Clin North Am 2020;53:605–15.
10. Cima RFF, Maes IH, Joore MA, et al. Specialised treatment based on cognitive behaviour therapy versus usual care for tinnitus: a randomised controlled trial. Lancet 2012;379:1951–9.
11. Beukes EW, Manchaiah V, Allen PM, et al. Internet-based interventions for adults with hearing loss, tinnitus, and vestibular disorders: a systematic review and meta-analysis. Trends Hearing 2019;23:1–22.
12. Andersson G. Clinician-supported internet-delivered psychological treatment of tinnitus. Am J Audiol 2015;24:299–301.

13. Fuller T, Cima R, Langguth B, et al. Cognitive behavioural therapy for tinnitus. Cochrane Database Syst Rev 2020;1:CD012614.

14. Nolan DR, Gupta R, Huber CG, et al. An effective treatment for tinnitus and hyperacusis based on cognitive behavioral therapy in an inpatient setting: a 10-year retrospective outcome analysis. Front Psychiatry 2020;11:25.

15. Köksoy S, Eti C, Karataş M, et al. The effects of yoga in patients suffering from subjective tinnitus. Int Arch Otorhinolaryngol 2018;22:009–13.

16. Niedziałek I, Raj-Koziak D, Milner R, et al. Effect of yoga training on the tinnitus induced distress. Complement Therapies in Clin Pract 2019;36:7–11.

17. Gazbare PS, Rawtani ND, Rathi M, et al. Effect of yogasanas versus gaze stability and habituation exercises on dizziness in vestibular dysfunction. Neurol India 2021;69:1241.

18. Peter N, Kleinjung T. Neuromodulation for tinnitus treatment: an overview of invasive and non-invasive techniques. J Zhejiang Univ Sci B 2019;20:116–30.

19. Guillard R, Fraysse MJ, Simeon R, et al. A portable neurofeedback device for treating chronic subjective tinnitus: feasibility and results of a pilot study. Prog Brain Res 2021;260:167–85.

20. Enriquez-Geppert S, Smit D, Pimenta MG, et al. Neurofeedback as a treatment intervention in ADHD: current Evidence and practice. Curr Psychiatry Rep 2019;21:46.

21. Güntensperger D, Thüring C, Kleinjung T, et al. Investigating the efficacy of an individualized alpha/delta neurofeedback protocol in the treatment of chronic tinnitus. Neural Plast 2019;2019:3540898.

22. Güntensperger D, Kleinjung T, Neff P, et al. Combining neurofeedback with source estimation: Evaluation of an sLORETA neurofeedback protocol for chronic tinnitus treatment. RNN 2020;38:283–99.

23. Emmert K, Kopel R, Koush Y, et al. Continuous vs. intermittent neurofeedback to regulate auditory cortex activity of tinnitus patients using real-time fMRI - A pilot study. NeuroImage: Clin 2017;14:97–104.

24. Riha C, Güntensperger D, Oschwald J, et al. Application of Latent Growth Curve modeling to predict individual trajectories during neurofeedback treatment for tinnitus. Prog Brain Res 2021;263:109–36.

25. Adamchic I, Tass PA, Langguth B, et al. Linking the Tinnitus Questionnaire and the subjective Clinical Global Impression: which differences are clinically important? Health Qual Life Outcomes 2012;10:79.

26. Ross UH, Lange O, Unterrainer J, et al. Ericksonian hypnosis in tinnitus therapy: effects of a 28-day inpatient multimodal treatment concept measured by Tinnitus-Questionnaire and Health Survey SF-36. Eur Arch Otorhinolaryngol 2007;264:483–8.

27. Maudoux A., Bonnet S., Lhonneux-Ledoux F., et al., Ericksonian hypnosis in tinnitus therapy. *B-ENT*, 3, 2007, 75–77.

28. Yazici ZM, Sayin I, Gökkuş G, et al. Effectiveness of Ericksonian hypnosis in tinnitus therapy: preliminary results. B-ENT 2012;8:7–12.

29. Brown KE, Whitney SL, Marchetti GF, et al. Physical therapy for central vestibular dysfunction. Arch Phys Med Rehabil 2006;87:76–81.

30. Whitney SL, Wrisley DM, Brown KE, et al. Physical therapy for migraine-related vestibulopathy and vestibular dysfunction with history of migraine. Laryngoscope 2000;110:1528–34.

31. Brown KE, Whitney SL, Wrisley DM, et al. Physical therapy outcomes for persons with bilateral vestibular loss. Laryngoscope 2001;111:1812–7.

32. Regauer V, Seckler E, Müller M, et al. Physical therapy interventions for older people with vertigo, dizziness and balance disorders addressing mobility and participation: a systematic review. BMC Geriatr 2020;20:494.
33. Liu L, Hu X, Zhang Y, et al. Effect of vestibular rehabilitation on spontaneous brain activity in patients with vestibular migraine: a resting-state functional magnetic resonance imaging study. Front Hum Neurosci 2020;14:227.
34. Luetzenberg FS, Babu S, Seidman MD. Alternative treatments of tinnitus: alternative medicine. Otolaryngol Clin North Am 2020;53:637–50.
35. Barth SW, Lehner MD, Dietz GPH, et al. Pharmacologic treatments in preclinical tinnitus models with special focus on Ginkgo biloba leaf extract EGb 761®. Mol Cell Neurosci 2021;116:103669.
36. Brüggemann P, Sória MG, Brandes-Schramm J, et al. The influence of depression, anxiety and cognition on the treatment effects of ginkgo biloba extract egb 761® in patients with tinnitus and dementia: a mediation analysis. J Clin Med 2021;10:3151.
37. Spiegel R, Kalla R, Mantokoudis G, et al. Ginkgo biloba extract EGb 761 alleviates neurosensory symptoms in patients with dementia: a meta-analysis of treatment effects on tinnitus and dizziness in randomized, placebo-controlled trials. Clin Interv Aging 2018;13:1121–7.
38. Radunz CL, Okuyama CE, Branco-Barreiro FCA, et al. Clinical randomized trial study of hearing aids effectiveness in association with Ginkgo biloba extract (EGb 761) on tinnitus improvement. Braz J Otorhinolaryngol 2020;86:734–42.
39. Wagner H, Ulrich-Merzenich G. Evidence and rational based Research on Chinese drugs. Vienna: Springer Science & Business Media; 2013.
40. Eckert A, Keil U, Scherping I, et al. Stabilization of mitochondrial membrane potential and improvement of neuronal energy metabolism by Ginkgo biloba extract EGb 761. Ann N Y Acad Sci 2005;1056:474–85.
41. Koo JW, Chang MY, Yun SC, et al. The efficacy and safety of systemic injection of Ginkgo biloba extract, EGb761, in idiopathic sudden sensorineural hearing loss: a randomized placebo-controlled clinical trial. Eur Arch Otorhinolaryngol 2016; 273:2433–41.
42. Sokolova L, Hoerr R, Mishchenko T. Treatment of vertigo: a randomized, double-blind trial comparing efficacy and safety of ginkgo biloba Extract EGb 761 and Betahistine. Int J Otolaryngol 2014;2014:682439.
43. Hamann K-F. Ginkgo special extract EGb 761® in vertigo: a systematic review of randomised, double-blind, placebo-controlled clinical trials. Internet J Otorhinolaryngol 2006;6:258–63.
44. Lindner M, Gosewisch A, Eilles E, et al. Ginkgo biloba Extract EGb 761 improves vestibular compensation and modulates cerebral vestibular networks in the rat. Front Neurol 2019;10:147.
45. Decker L, Basta D, Burkart M, et al. Balance training with vibrotactile neurofeedback and ginkgo biloba extract in age-related vertigo. Front Neurol 2021;12: 691917.
46. Yeh C-W, Tseng L-H, Yang C-H, et al. Effects of oral zinc supplementation on patients with noise-induced hearing loss associated tinnitus: a clinical trial. Biomed J 2019;42:46–52.
47. Jun HJ, Ok S, Tyler R, et al. Is hypozincemia related to tinnitus?: a population study using data from the korea national health and nutrition examination survey. Clin Exp Otorhinolaryngol 2015;8:335.
48. Berkiten G, Kumral TL, Yıldırım G, et al. Effects of serum zinc level on tinnitus. Am J Otolaryngol 2015;36:230–4.

49. Coelho C, Witt SA, Ji H, et al. Zinc to treat tinnitus in the elderly: a randomized placebo controlled crossover trial. Otol Neurotol 2013;34:1146–54.
50. Person OC, Puga ME, da Silva EM, et al. Zinc supplementation for tinnitus. Cochrane Database Syst Rev 2016;2016:CD009832.
51. Ferreira GDP, Cury MCL, Oliveira J A de, et al. Vestibular evaluation using videonystagmography of chronic zinc deficient patients due to short bowell syndrome. Braz J Otorhinolaryngol 2009;75:290–4.
52. Sarna B, Abouzari M, Lin HW, et al. A hypothetical proposal for association between migraine and Meniere's disease. Med Hypotheses 2020;134:109430.
53. Bruss D, Abouzari M, Sarna B, et al. Migraine features in patients with recurrent benign paroxysmal positional vertigo. Otol Neurotol 2021;42:461–5.
54. Ghavami Y, Haidar YM, Ziai KN, et al. Management of mal de debarquement syndrome as vestibular migraines. Laryngoscope 2017;127:1670–5.
55. Abouzari M, Abiri A, Djalilian HR. Successful treatment of a child with definite meniere's disease with the migraine regimen. Am J Otolaryngol 2019;40:440–2.
56. Seidman MD, Standring RT, Dornhoffer JL. Tinnitus: current understanding and contemporary management. Curr Opin Otolaryngol Head Neck Surg 2010;18: 363–8.
57. Ahmad N, Seidman M. Tinnitus in the older adult. Drugs Aging 2004;21:297–305.
58. Lee DY, Kim YH. Relationship between diet and tinnitus: korea national health and nutrition examination survey. Clin Exp Otorhinolaryngol 2018;11:158–65.
59. Singh C, Kawatra R, Gupta J, et al. Therapeutic role of Vitamin B12 in patients of chronic tinnitus: a pilot study. Noise Health 2016;18:93–7.
60. Hameed HM, Eleue AH, Al Mosawi AMT. The use of distortion product otoacoustic emissions (DPOAE) records to estimate effect of vitamin B complex on changing severity of tinnitus. Ann Med Surg 2018;36:203–11.
61. Dawes P, Cruickshanks KJ, Marsden A, et al. Relationship between diet, tinnitus, and hearing difficulties. Ear & Hearing 2020;41:289–99.
62. Ekinci A, Kamasak K. Evaluation of serum prolidase enzyme activity and oxidative stress in patients with tinnitus. Braz J Otorhinolaryngol 2020;86:405–10.
63. Khan M, Gross J, Haupt H, et al. A pilot clinical trial of the effects of coenzyme Q10 on chronic tinnitus aurium. Otolaryngol Head Neck Surg 2007;136:72–7.
64. Sazali S, Badrin S, Norhayati MN, et al. Coenzyme Q10 supplementation for prophylaxis in adult patients with migraine—a meta-analysis. BMJ Open 2021;11: e039358.
65. Parohan M, Sarraf P, Javanbakht MH, et al. Effect of coenzyme Q10 supplementation on clinical features of migraine: a systematic review and dose-response meta-analysis of randomized controlled trials. Nutr Neurosci 2020;23:868–75.
66. Albu S, Chirtes F. Intratympanic dexamethasone plus melatonin versus melatonin only in the treatment of unilateral acute idiopathic tinnitus. Am J Otolaryngol 2014; 35:617–22.
67. Pirodda A, Raimondi MC, Ferri GG. Exploring the reasons why melatonin can improve tinnitus. Med Hypotheses 2010;75:190–1.
68. Rosenberg SI, Silverstein H, Rowan PT, et al. Effect of melatonin on tinnitus. Laryngoscope 1998;108:305–10.
69. Abtahi S, Hashemi S, Mahmoodi M, et al. Comparison of melatonin and sertraline therapies on tinnitus: a randomized clinical trial. Int J Prev Med 2017;8:61.
70. Miroddi M, Bruno R, Galletti F, et al. Clinical pharmacology of melatonin in the treatment of tinnitus: a review. Eur J Clin Pharmacol 2015;71:263–70.
71. Merrick L, Youssef D, Tanner M, et al. Does melatonin have therapeutic use in tinnitus? Southampt Med J 2014;107:362–6.

72. Tu J, Kim M, Yang J, et al. Influence of acupuncture on autonomic balance in adult tinnitus patients: an exploratory study. CURR MED SCI 2019;39:947–53.
73. Cai W, Chen A-W, Ding L, et al. Thermal effects of acupuncture by the infrared thermography test in patients with tinnitus. J Acupuncture Meridian Stud 2019; 12:131–5.
74. Naderinabi B, Soltanipour S, Nemati S, et al. Acupuncture for chronic nonpulsatile tinnitus: a randomized clinical trial. Caspian J Intern Med 2018;9:38–45.
75. Pang P, Shi Y, Xu H, et al. Acupuncture methods put to the test for a tinnitus study: a Bayesian analysis. Complement Ther Med 2019;42:205–13.
76. Zhang X, Xu H, Xu W, et al. Acupuncture therapy for sudden sensorineural hearing loss: a systematic review and meta-analysis of randomized controlled trials. PLoS One 2015;10:e0125240.
77. Chen S, Zhao M, Qiu J. Acupuncture for the treatment of sudden sensorineural hearing loss: a systematic review and meta-analysis. Complement Ther Med 2019;42:381–8.
78. Chiu C-W, Lee C-T, Hsu P-C, et al. Efficacy and safety of acupuncture for dizziness and vertigo in emergency department: a pilot cohort study. BMC Complement Altern Med 2015;15:173.
79. Lin HW, Djalilian HR. The Role of Migraine in Hearing and Balance Symptoms. JAMA Otolaryngol Head Neck Surg 2018;144:717–8.
80. Benjamin T, Gillard D, Abouzari M, et al. Vestibular and auditory manifestations of migraine. Curr Opin Neurol 2022;35:84–9.
81. Abouzari M, Goshtasbi K, Chua JT, et al. Adjuvant migraine medications in the treatment of sudden sensorineural hearing loss. Laryngoscope 2021;131: E283–8.
82. Huang C, Tan G, Xiao J, et al. Efficacy of hyperbaric oxygen on idiopathic sudden sensorineural hearing loss and its correlation with treatment course: prospective clinical research. Audiol Neurotol 2021;26:479–86.
83. Alimoglu Y, Inci E, Edizer DT, et al. Efficacy comparison of oral steroid, intratympanic steroid, hyperbaric oxygen and oral steroid + hyperbaric oxygen treatments in idiopathic sudden sensorineural hearing loss cases. Eur Arch Otorhinolaryngol 2011;268:1735–41.
84. Rhee T-M, Hwang D, Lee J-S, et al. Addition of hyperbaric oxygen therapy vs medical therapy alone for idiopathic sudden sensorineural hearing loss: a systematic review and meta-analysis. JAMA Otolaryngol Head Neck Surg 2018; 144:1153–61.
85. Bayoumy AB, de Ru JA. The use of hyperbaric oxygen therapy in acute hearing loss: a narrative review. Eur Arch Otorhinolaryngol 2019;276:1859–80.
86. Eryigit B, Ziylan F, Yaz F, et al. The effectiveness of hyperbaric oxygen in patients with idiopathic sudden sensorineural hearing loss: a systematic review. Eur Arch Otorhinolaryngol 2018;275:2893–904.

Natural Alternatives and the Common Cold and Influenza

Varun S. Patel, MD, Michael D. Seidman, MD*

KEYWORDS

• Viral illness • Influenza • Herbal remedies • Dietary supplements • COVID treatment

KEY POINTS

- Complementary and integrative medicine has penetrated the traditional health care market as an alternative option for treating the symptoms of colds and influenza.
- Herbal products have a host of functions that fight against viral illnesses. Generally, these products can upregulate immune function and reduce inflammation.
- Many complementary medicines are available for management of the common cold and influenza, such as immune formulas, vitamin supplements, and probiotics.
- Diet and drinking play an important role for homeostasis and balance of the immune system. More specifically, they can affect the pH of the blood system, thereby creating an incompatible environment for viruses, bacteria, and other pathogens.
- Other adjunct options are available for supportive treatment of the common cold and influenza.

Recent years have shown that upper respiratory viruses can have a significant impact on patient quality of life and can affect communities around the world. The World Health Organization estimates that influenza alone can lead to 150,000 hospitalizations and 30,000 deaths annually.[1] Many traditional therapies exist for treating the symptoms of these infections. However, not all of them are universally effective. Complementary and integrative medicine (CIM) has penetrated the traditional health care market as an alternative option for treating the symptoms of cold and influenza.[2] CIM has been shown to help with other disease processes also, such as back pain, tinnitus, and anxiety.[3,4] These therapies have proliferated with the anticipation of providing more effective control of symptomatology without significant adverse risk. The purpose of this article is to outline CIM therapies for treating the symptoms of viral respiratory illnesses.

AdventHealth Medical Group – Otolaryngology-Head and Neck Surgery, 410 Celebration Place, Suite 305, Celebration, FL 34747, USA
* Corresponding author.
E-mail address: Michael.seidman.md@adventhealth.com

Otolaryngol Clin N Am 55 (2022) 1035–1044
https://doi.org/10.1016/j.otc.2022.06.009

HERBAL PRODUCTS

Herbal products have a host of functions that fight against viral illnesses. Generally, these products can upregulate immune function and reduce inflammation. Additionally, they can provide a biochemical milieu that facilitates protective mechanisms focusing on stress reduction and mitigation of infection.[5] For instance, *maoto* is a traditional Japanese medicine composed of 4 medicinal herbs. When *maoto* (0.9 and 1.6 kg/d) was orally administered to mice, a significant antipyretic effect was shown compared with water-treated controls.[6] One of the components of *maoto*, *Ephedrae herba* extract (100–400 µg/mL), has been shown to inhibit the growth of the influenza virus by suppressing cellular components such as lysosomes.[7]

Another popular herbal remedy is glycyrrhizin, a component of licorice root, which provides expectorant properties and may help with gastric ulceration and constipation. It has been shown to inhibit penetration of viruses by altering cell membrane fluidity and decreasing membrane permeability.[8] It has previously been used as an adjunct treatment to prevent hepatitis B infection by suppressing the surface antigen production. It has been reported that glycyrrhizin possesses anti-inflammatory and antioxidant properties, and furthermore, stimulates interferon production. Such antioxidant properties have shown benefit even beyond the treatment of infectious diseases, such as reversing acquired hearing loss.[9,10]

Korean red ginseng, a traditional herb in Chinese medicine, has commonly been used to help with disease recovery. In a study of staff at a geriatric hospital compared with the general population, those treated with red ginseng had significantly reduced symptoms of the common cold and influenza. The rate of influenza-like symptoms was 1.38% in those who consumed red ginseng versus 5% in the general population. One potential mechanism of action is that red ginseng suppresses the degradation of the immune system elicited by stress factors. It has also been shown to enhance the immune activity of mucous membranes and protect subjects from viral infections.[11] It additionally has been demonstrated to significantly regulate the autonomic-endocrine system of the human body.

Another popular remedy option includes *Uncaria tomentosa* (cat's claw). Most recently, the herbal treatment has been used to help patients infected with severe acute respiratory syndrome corona virus 2 (SARS-CoV 2). *U tomentosa* is a vine indigenous to the Peruvian Amazon and tropical areas of South and Central America. Extracts from this plant have been shown to have inhibitory effects on viral replication, and specifically prevent viral attachment to host cells.[12] Other claims include a boost in T and B cell lymphocytes, increase in phagocytic function, improvement in wound healing, and enhancement of cartilage restoration.

Hypericum perforatum (commonly referred to as St. John's Wort), can be topically or systemically applied to help with viral and other cold-like infections. In addition to treating mild-to-moderate depression and helping with wound healing, St. John's Wort inhibits 5-lipoxygenase inhibitor, a key enzyme in leukotriene biosynthesis. Hence, it may reduce inflammatory biomarkers. It also impairs interactions with coactosin-like protein and nuclear membrane translocation.[13] More recent studies have also established its efficacy in preventing SARS-CoV 2 by boosting the innate immune response.[14] The usual dosage is 300 mg 3 times a day with food, with a potential effect of photosensitivity. St. John's wort is commonly also used to treat mild-to-moderate depression. However, 1 downside is that it can interfere with commonly used anesthetics and result in death. Thus, it is critical to learn about the potential for interactions.

One of the most reputable references with regard to the medicinal use of herbs is the "Complete German Commission E." This commission provides monographs on hundreds of herbs, rating them as either positive or negative. Typically, an herb that is rated positively has reasonable scientific support and data to validate its use. An herb with a negative rating may be ineffective, unsafe, or simply not studied to the extent that sufficient information is available. The herb *Echinacea* provides a good example of some of the issues involved in herbal remedies. *Echinacea* is a popular herb with a reputation for combating the common cold and influenza-like illnesses. It is a commonly used herb by professional singers at the first sign of a sniffle, cough, or general malaise. What most people do not realize is that there are at least 9 different subtypes of *Echinacea*, including *Echinacea purpurea, Echinacea pallida*, and *Echinacea angustafolia*. Not only does each subtype have different health benefits, but those benefits vary depending on the part of the plant used. The leaf of *E purpurea,* for example, has been shown to enhance T and B cell functions, whereas the root of that same plant does not. Conversely, *E pallida* root has been shown to enhance T and B cell function, but the leaf of that same plant does not. Meanwhile, *E angustafolia* is rated as a negative herb by the commission. Yet while visiting numerous health food stores, there were more than 100 bottles of *Echinacea* on the shelves, and 95% of them contained *E angustafolia*.[15]

Why would the market be filled with *E angustafolia* if it is a negatively rated herb? One explanation is that manufacturers are not doing their homework. Another possibility is that it is a much less expensive or more available herb. Nutritional products that contain *E purpurea* leaf and *pallida* root are to be considered, both of which have been clearly shown in scientific studies to enhance and activate T and B cell functions, encourage phagocytosis, and have antiviral properties. Unfortunately, if a study is conducted with a product made from *E angustafolia,* the results may indicate that it does not work in treating cold or influenza symptoms. Studies like this cast doubt on all herbal remedies.[16–19]

Traditional Chinese medicine also plays an important supportive role in the treatment of the common cold and influenza. Generally, these treatments are prescribed based on symptomatology rather than disease process. Shigao (*gypsum fibrosum*) is used to reduce fever. Caihu (*bupleurum chinesenes DC*) and Jinjie (*herba schizonepetae*) are used as analgesics. Fangfeng (*radix saposhnikiviae*) and Zhishuye (*folium perillae*) are used for chills and cough. Different solutions can be mixed to provide optimal results based on patient symptoms. Two authentic randomized control trials were used to examine children with influenza virus who were treated with *Eshuyou* oral decoction.[20] Those who had received the oil had better effects than ribavirin for recovery within 3 days of treatment, although not statistically significant.

Regardless of the many benefits that herbal treatments can provide, herbal remedies can have suboptimal interactions with certain drugs. *Echinacea,* for example, may interfere with Neoral, prednisone, Imuran, and methotrexate. Furthermore, consumers and physicians should understand that immune-stimulants, like *Echinacea* and the herb goldenseal, should not be used for prolonged periods of time. There are also contraindications for patients who have immune disorders or severe infections, such as tuberculosis.

DIETARY SUPPLEMENTS

Several complementary medicines are available for management of the common cold and influenza. For instance, *Peak365Nutrition* developed a proprietary "Natural Shield Advanced Immune Support Formula," which provides the body with ingredients known by herbal experts to promote healthy immune function. Its primary function is to further boost the body's natural immune system so that it may fight off cold and influenza. Of note, it includes 554% of the daily value of vitamin C, and an adequate amount of zinc. Other additional herbs included are *E purpurea*, Goldenseal and Elder Flower. **Table 1** highlights the various ingredients included in the supplement and its percentage daily values. These supplements can be used in adults and in children weighing at least 50 pounds. Limited clinical trials (unpublished, Michael D. Seidman, 2021) have demonstrated that this formulation reduces the symptoms associated with the common cold and influenza to 2 to 4 days in 88% of users.

Zinc is a commonly used remedy, and as such has been included in dietary supplements. Zinc plays an important role in the components of structural and regulatory proteins, such as transcription factors. Through this mechanism, it helps with the body's cellular and humoral immune response. It exerts its greatest effect through Th lymphocytes. Reduced zinc contents disturb the balance between Th1 and Th2 lymphocytes, with a shift toward Th2.[21] Zinc supplementation helps maintain this balance, increasing interferon release from blood cells. Interferon has been shown to have antiviral, immune-regulatory and anticancer properties. In addition, zinc helps with release of thymulin from the thymic cells. Studies have shown that zinc supplementation of 20 mg/d for 5 weeks in children can increase the percentage of CD4+ and CD8+ cells.[21] Other studies have illustrated that 12.8 mg or 13.3 mg of zinc acetate administered every 2 to 3 hours during cold-like symptoms can reduce the duration and severity of symptoms. More specifically, it could reduce the duration of nasal discharge from 5 to 3 days overall. The supplement is relatively safe, with adverse effects listed as altered taste and mouth irritation.

Vitamin C has also shown to have significant beneficial effects in fighting off the common cold and other viral infections. The recommended dosage per the European Union is 90 mg/d for men and 80 mg/d for women. Vitamin C boosts the immune system through development of T lymphocytes, leukocyte chemotaxis, and protection of the endothelium.[22] It has been shown to increase certain enzymes such as superoxide

Table 1 Supplement facts		
	Amount Per Serving	**% Daily Value***
Vitamin C (ascorbic acid)	333 mg	555%
L-Arginine (Hcl)	133.3 mg	*
Echinacea purpurea leaf (Echinacea purpurea)	75 mg	*
Echinacea padilla root (Echinacea padilla)	75 mg	*
Goldenseal root (Hydrasris Canadensis)	75 mg	*
Calcium (from ascorbate)	33 mg	3%
Astragalus root (Astragalus membranaceus)	33.3 mg	*
Quercitin	33.3 mg	*
Citrus bioflavonoids	33.3 mg	*
Zinc (from monomethinonate)	12 mg	80%
Elder flowers (Sambucus nigra)	10 mg	*
Linden flowers (Tilia europaea)	10 mg	*
Meadowsweet (Filipendula ulmania)	10 mg	*

* unspecified value.
Serving size: 2 capsules.
Servings per container: 30.
Other ingredients: vegetarian capsules.

dismutase. Additionally, it may reduce reactive oxidative species generation and inflammation via modulation of nuclear transcription factors. More recently, in relation to the SARS-CoV 2 pandemic, vitamin C was studied in chick embryo tracheal organ cultures and found to increase resistance to viral infection by supporting the innate and adaptive immune systems. Vitamin C was shown to reduce inflammatory mediators such as interleukin (IL)-6, which is elevated in hypertensive and obese adult patients.[23] Another study has noted the role of vitamin C in treating the symptoms of SARS-CoV 2 infection by boosting free radical oxygen and nitrogen-scavenging properties along with anti-inflammatory effects.[24] Further studies are warranted to more fully delineate the effects of vitamin C on preventing and/or treating SARS-CoV 2 symptoms.

Another category of dietary supplements includes probiotics. Although traditionally thought to improve gut health and facilitate a balance of healthy gastrointestinal organisms, probiotics have also been shown to help reduce cold and influenza-like symptoms. A double-blind, placebo-controlled study of 326 children evaluated the effect of *Lactobacillus acidophilus* in combination with *Bifidobacterium animalis* on symptomatology.[25] Relative to the placebo group, the probiotic-treated group demonstrated reduction in fever of 53% and in coughing of 41.4%. Additionally, the use of probiotics was associated with a reduced use of antibiotics by 68.4%. A possible mechanism involves immune-enhancing effects through modulation of toll-like receptors.[25] Another study demonstrated that the combination of probiotics with vitamins and minerals reduced the severity and duration of common cold symptoms.[26] A potential mechanism is by stimulating dendritic cell regulatory function. Other studies have alluded how changing the intestinal microflora can affect overall immune status. For instance, live probiotic culture can induce mucin expression and phagocytosis and modulate cytokine profiles.[27] These effects are also noted when consuming even parts of the probiotic cells such as peptidoglycan or DNA, without the live bacteria.

Several ingredients in whole grain contain immune-modulating agents. These grains are especially high in metal ions such as iron, zinc, and copper. Deficiencies in metal ions have been associated with poor health outcomes, such as increased risk of infection and increased morbidity.[28] Copper deficiency has been associated with anemia, low body temperatures, low white cell blood count, and thyroid disease. Therefore, proper homeostasis of metal ions is critical for proper immune function. Furthermore, selenium has also been shown to support the immune system by reducing the level of free radical levels.[29] In an observational study of 50 hospitalized patients with SARS-CoV 2 infection, selenium deficiency was found in 42% of patients.[30] Deficiency in these cases could be associated with increased levels of proinflammatory molecules.

THE EFFECT OF DIET

Diet and drinking play an important role for homeostasis and balance of the immune system. More specifically, they can affect the pH of the blood system, thereby creating an incompatible environment for viruses, bacteria, and other pathogens. Controversial theories exist that alkaline diets and drinks can induce low-grade levels of metabolic alkalosis, which can be a hindrance for viruses.[6] Ways to increase blood pH are to include alkaline diets into the body (ie, soft drinks, and grain products) and reduce acidic diets (ie, meats, fish, dairy, and eggs). A review of the literature, however, did not find any scientific-based evidence regarding alkaline diets and the prevention and treatment of viral illnesses.

Other diets, however, have been studied in regards to their effect on treatment of viruses and other pathogens. In particular, the Mediterranean diet has been thoroughly studied. This diet is rich in vegetables, beans, nuts, olive oil, and seeds. The effects of this type of diet include an increase in dietary polyphenols, which has antioxidant properties, blocks proinflammatory cytokines, reduces oxidative stress, and leads to an overall reduced bio-inflammatory state.[31] The diet has also been shown to reduce insulin resistance, lower blood pressure, and reduce cholesterol levels. More recently, it has been shown to have a beneficial effect against the SARS-CoV 2 virus. One ecological study across regions of Europe showed a negative association between the Mediterranean diet and SARS-CoV 2-related death rates.[32] Lending further credence to this study is that it was completed before any traditional medical therapies against the SARS-CoV 2 virus were implemented.

In contrast to the Mediterranean diet, the Western diet has been shown to have the opposite effects against overall health and comorbidity. This diet contains caloric intake high in sugars, saturated fats, and refined carbohydrates. Ingestion of saturated fats and fatty acids has been shown to induce proliferation of toll-like receptors, neutrophils, and dendritic cells, leading to a state of chronic inflammation.[33] More specifically, saturated fats and fatty acids promote adhesion and transmigration of leukocytes from the microcirculation to the tissues, structural changes to the body's microcirculation, and other changes in vascular caliber. Furthermore, the cyclooxygenase enzyme, which promotes the synthesis of prostaglandins and thromboxanes, is upregulated by fatty acids. In contrast, omega-3 fatty acids can act as an anti-inflammatory mediator by downregulating certain pathways involved in the synthesis of IL-1 and IL-6. In a meta-analysis of 3 randomized control trials involving patients with acute respiratory distress syndrome, consumption of omega-3 fatty acids was associated with a lower risk of developing organ failure, time on ventilator support, and overall morbidity.[34] Currently, studies are underway to further assert the effect of omega-3 fatty acids on hospitalized patients with the SARS-CoV 2 virus.

OTHER OPTIONS

Herbal products, dietary supplements, and dietary intake comprise the major CIM treatment options for the common cold and influenza. However, other adjunct options exist, although they are less popular and not as well studied. For instance, acupuncture has been noted in the literature to be a possible treatment option for symptomatic relief of viral infections such as SARS-CoV 2. This treatment option is commonly used in China. Acupuncture has demonstrated its ability to suppress inflammatory cytokines such as IL-6 and tumor necrosis factor (TNF)-alpha, and activate cholinergic anti-inflammatory pathways during viral infections.[35] In addition, acupuncture may enhance the ratio of CD4+ T cells to CD8+ T cells in experimental rat studies.[36] In a recent study, the treatment of acupuncture combined with routine regimens was examined in patients with SARS-CoV 2. In this study, all patients who received both acupuncture along with traditional medical therapies were cured and discharged with improved symptoms of chest distress, anxiety, loss of appetite, and insomnia.[37] Additionally, it is widely used and has shown strong benefit for allergic symptoms, which early on may mimic typical upper respiratory infection symptoms.[38,39]

Earthing (also known as grounding) may also play an important role in mediating the immune system during active viral or pathogenic infection. Earthing is described as the connection of the human body to earth through various methods (ie, walking on the ground bare foot, tending to a garden without gloves, leaning against a tree). It is well established that the earth's surface contains free circulating electrons to which humans previously were well connected with (prior to the time of modern innovation). Modern innovations such as wearing shoes and sleeping on a mattress have halted this connection with the earth. One theory hypothesizes that earthing of the human body helps reduce free radical production.[40] One recent double-blinded study showed that grounding for 1 hour altered the number of circulating neutrophils and lymphocytes and altered the balance of circulating cytokines.[41] These changes in the immune system may prove to reduce the symptomatology period of viral illnesses. Other studies have showed that earthing can improve blood pressure, reduce blood viscosity, reduce muscle soreness, and improve heart rate variability. However, further studies are needed to establish a clear link between viral illness and treatment with earthing mechanisms.

Exercise may also play an important role in improving quality of life during active viral infections. For instance, progressive muscle relaxation exercises may reduce anxiety and improve sleep quality in patients infected with SARS-CoV 2.[42] This is a deep relaxation technique based on the idea that muscle strain can be a physiologic response to human stress and mental thoughts. Therefore, relaxation of muscle groups may be associated with reduced human stress and a more relaxed state of mind, ultimately helping with the psychological symptoms of viral infections. Other studies have also demonstrated that relaxation techniques can also help improve the human physiologic state by reducing blood pressure, heart rate, and lactic acid production.

SUMMARY

The use of CIM has increased significantly over the past several decades, and more recently, with the SARS-CoV 2 pandemic worldwide. It is estimated that one-third of the US population uses some form of alternative medicine.[43] Physicians should consider integrative medicine therapies in addition to traditional forms of medicine when caring for patients in order to achieve best results. However, it is important to research and study these therapies for any risks, side effects, or harmful effects. Therefore, communication with patients and other health care providers is of utmost importance. This will ensure effective and positive patient care experiences. Further randomized clinical trials are necessary to further establish the role of various alternative options for the prevention and treatment of viral illnesses.

CLINICS CARE POINTS

- When *maoto* (0.9 and 1.6 kg/d) was orally administered to mice, a significant antipyretic effect was shown compared with water-treated controls.[6] One of the components of *maoto*, *Ephedrae Herba* extract (100–400 μg/mL), has been shown to inhibit the growth of the influenza virus by suppressing cellular components such as lysosomes.

- Extracts from *U tomentosa* (cat's claw) have been shown to have inhibitory effects on viral replication, and specifically prevent viral attachment to host cells.

- *H perforatum* (commonly referred to as St. John's wort), can be topically or systemically applied to help with viral and other cold-like infections. In addition to treating mild-to-moderate depression and helping with wound healing, St. John's wort inhibits 5-lipoxygenase inhibitor, a key enzyme in leukotriene biosynthesis.

- *Peak365Nutrition* developed a proprietary "Natural Shield Advanced Immune Support Formula," which provides the body with ingredients known by herbal experts to promote healthy immune function.

- Vitamin C and zinc have also shown to have significant beneficial effects in fighting off the common cold and other viral infections.
- Acupuncture has been noted in the literature to be a possible treatment option for symptomatic relief of viral infections such as SARS-CoV 2. Acupuncture has demonstrated its ability to suppress inflammatory cytokines such as IL-6 and TNF-alpha, and activate cholinergic anti-inflammatory pathways during viral infections.

DISCLOSURE

M.D. Seidman is the founder of Peak365Nutrition and Body Language Vitamin Co and has financial interest in these companies. He has lectured at various venues on alternative and complementary medicine.

REFERENCES

1. Hamilton MA, Liu Y, Calzavara A, et al. Predictors of all-cause mortality among patients hospitalized with influenza, respiratory syncytial virus, or SARS-CoV-2. Influenza Other Respir Viruses 2022. https://doi.org/10.1111/irv.13004.
2. Seidman MD, van Grinsven G. Complementary and integrative treatments. Otolaryngol Clin North Am 2013;46(3):485–97.
3. Luetzenberg FS, Babu S, Seidman MD. Alternative treatments of tinnitus. Otolaryngol Clin North Am 2020. https://doi.org/10.1016/j.otc.2020.03.011.
4. Seidman MD, Babu S. Alternative medications and other treatments for tinnitus: facts from fiction. Otolaryngol Clin North Am 2003;36(2):359–81.
5. Papadopoulos NG, Megremis S, Kitsioulis NA, et al. Promising approaches for the treatment and prevention of viral respiratory illnesses. J Allergy Clin Immunol 2017;140(4):921–32.
6. Mousa HAL. Prevention and treatment of influenza, influenza-like illness, and common cold by herbal, complementary, and natural therapies. J Evid Based Complement Altern Med 2016;22(1):166–74.
7. Nagai T, Kataoka E, Aoki Y, et al. Alleviative effects of a kampo (a Japanese herbal) medicine "maoto (ma-huang-tang)" on the early phase of influenza virus infection and its possible mode of action. Evid Based Complement Altern Med 2014, 1–12.
8. Gomaa AA, Abdel-Wadood YA. The potential of glycyrrhizin and licorice extract in combating COVID-19 and associated conditions. Phytomedicine Plus 2021;1(3): 100043.
9. Darrat I, Ahmad N, Seidman K, et al. Auditory research involving antioxidants. Curr Opin Otolaryngol Head Neck Surg 2007;15(5):358–63.
10. Seidman MD. Effects of dietary restriction and antioxidants on presbyacusis. Laryngoscope 2000;110(5):727–38.
11. Kaneko H, Nakanishi K. Proof of the mysterious efficacy of ginseng: basic and clinical trials: clinical effects of medical ginseng, Korean red ginseng: specifically, its anti-stress action for prevention of disease. J Pharmacol Sci 2004;95(2): 158–62.
12. Yepes-Pérez AF, Herrera-Calderon O, Quintero-Saumeth J. *Uncaria tomentosa* (cat's claw): a promising herbal medicine against SARS-CoV-2/ACE-2 junction and SARS-CoV-2 spike protein based on molecular modeling. J Biomol Struct Dyn 2020;40(5):2227–43.
13. Feißt C, Pergola C, Rakonjac M, et al. Hyperforin is a novel type of 5-lipoxygenase inhibitor with high efficacy in vivo. Cell Mol Life Sci 2009;66(16):2759–71.

14. Boozari M, Hosseinzadeh H. Natural products for COVID -19 prevention and treatment regarding to previous coronavirus infections and novel studies. Phytotherapy Res 2020;35(2):864–76.
15. Blumenthal M, Busse WR, Bundesinstitut für Arzneimittel und Medizinprodukte. The complete German Commission E monographs, therapeutic guide to herbal medicines. American Botanical Council; 1998.
16. Seidman M. Nutrition and health; fact or fantasy [Los Angeles, CA]. American Academy of Otolaryngology - Head & Neck Surgery Conference 2004.
17. Benninger MS, Murry T. The singer's voice. San Diego (CA): Plural Pub; 2008.
18. Sataloff RT, Benninger MS. Sataloff's comprehensive textbook of otolaryngology, head and neck surgery. Vol. 4, laryngology. Jaypee Brothers Medical Publishing (P), Ltd; 2016.
19. Campbell K. Pharmacology and ototoxicity for audiologists. Clifton Park (NY): Thomson/Delmar Learning; 2007.
20. Wu T, Yang X, Zeng X, et al. Traditional Chinese medicine in the treatment of acute respiratory tract infections. Respir Med 2008;102(8):1093–8.
21. Skrajnowska D, Bobrowska-Korczak B. Role of zinc in immune system and anti-cancer defense mechanisms. Nutrients 2019;11(10):2273.
22. Holford P, Carr AC, Jovic TH, et al. Vitamin C—an adjunctive therapy for respiratory infection, sepsis and COVID-19. Nutrients 2020;12(12):3760.
23. Feyaerts AF, Luyten W. Vitamin C as prophylaxis and adjunctive medical treatment for COVID-19? Nutrition 2020;79–80:110948.
24. Rawat D, Roy A, Maitra S, et al. Vitamin C and COVID-19 treatment: a systematic review and meta-analysis of randomized controlled trials. Diabetes Metab Syndr Clin Res Rev 2021;15(6):102324.
25. Leyer GJ, Li S, Mubasher ME, et al. Probiotic effects on cold and influenza-like symptom incidence and duration in children. Pediatrics 2009;124(2):e172–9.
26. Winkler P, Vrese MD, Laue C, et al. Effect of a dietary supplement containing probiotic bacteria plus vitamins and minerals on common cold infections and cellular immune parameters. Int J Clin Pharmacol Ther 2005;43(07):318–26.
27. Zhang H, Yeh C, Jin Z, et al. Prospective study of probiotic supplementation results in immune stimulation and improvement of upper respiratory infection rate. Synth Syst Biotechnol 2018;3(2):113–20.
28. Maares M, Haase H. Zinc and immunity: an essential interrelation. Arch Biochem Biophys 2016;611:58–65.
29. Chen O, Mah E, Dioum E, et al. The role of oat nutrients in the immune system: a narrative review. Nutrients 2021;13(4):1048.
30. Avery J, Hoffmann P. Selenium, selenoproteins, and immunity. Nutrients 2018; 10(9):1203.
31. Bonaccio M, Pounis G, Cerletti C, et al. Mediterranean diet, dietary polyphenols and low grade inflammation: results from the MOLI-SANI study. Br J Clin Pharmacol 2016;83(1):107–13.
32. Singh B, Eshaghian E, Chuang J, et al. Do diet and dietary supplements mitigate clinical outcomes in COVID-19? Nutrients 2022;14(9):1909.
33. Rogero M, Calder P. Obesity, inflammation, toll-like receptor 4 and fatty acids. Nutrients 2018;10(4):432.
34. Pontes-Arruda A, DeMichele S, Seth A, et al. The use of an inflammation-modulating diet in patients with acute lung injury or acute respiratory distress syndrome: a meta-analysis of outcome data. J Parenter Enteral Nutr 2008;32(6): 596–605.

35. Li J, Wu S, Tang H, et al. Long-term effects of acupuncture treatment on airway smooth muscle in a rat model of smoke-induced chronic obstructive pulmonary disease. Acupuncture Med 2016;34(2):107–13.

36. Liu YM, Liu XJ, Bai SS, et al. The effect of electroacupuncture on T cell responses in rats with experimental autoimmune encephalitis. J Neuroimmunology 2010; 220(1–2):25–33.

37. Han Z, Zhang Y, Wang P, et al. Is acupuncture effective in the treatment of COVID-19 related symptoms? Based on bioinformatics/network topology strategy. Brief Bioinform 2021;22(5). https://doi.org/10.1093/bib/bbab110.

38. Taw MB, Reddy WD, Omole FS, et al. Acupuncture and allergic rhinitis. Curr Opin Otolaryngol Head Neck Surg 2015;23(3):216–20.

39. Asher BF, Seidman MD, Reddy WD, et al. Integrative medical approaches to allergic rhinitis. Curr Opin Otolaryngol Head Neck Surg 2015;23(3):221–5.

40. Oschman JL. Can electrons act as antioxidants? A review and commentary. J Altern Complement Med 2007;13(9):955–67.

41. Mousa HA. Health effects of alkaline diet and water, reduction of digestive-tract bacterial load, and earthing. Altern Ther Health Med 2016;22(Suppl 1):24–33..

42. Özlü B, Öztürk Z, Karaman Özlü Z, et al. The effects of progressive muscle relaxation exercises on the anxiety and sleep quality of patients with COVID-19: a randomized controlled study. Perspect Psychiatr Care 2021;57(4):1791–7.

43. Asher BF, Seidman M, Snyderman C. Complementary and alternative medicine in otolaryngology. Laryngoscope 2001;111(8):1383–9.

Integrative Approach to Managing Obstructive Sleep Apnea

Kathleen R. Billings, MD[a,b],*, John Maddalozzo, MD[a,b]

KEYWORDS

- Obstructive sleep apnea • Integrative medicine
- Complementary and integrative medicine • Continuous positive airway pressure

KEY POINTS

- Conventional therapies for obstructive sleep apnea (OSA), including continuous positive airway pressure and oral appliances, offer the best opportunity for symptomatic improvement and reduction in OSA overall health impact.
- Integrative medicine brings conventional and complementary approaches together in a coordinated way.
- With rising obesity rates, weight loss and lifestyle programs seem to be the most favorable integrative methods to combine with conventional OSA therapies.
- Complementary and alternative approaches to OSA management are varied and, in conjunction with conventional methods, may offer some reduction in the apnea-hypopnea index (AHI).
- Studies of complementary and integrative management options alone have not demonstrated sustainable reductions in the AHI.

OVERVIEW

Obstructive sleep apnea (OSA) is a common disorder affecting 14% of men and 5% of women when defined by the apnea-hypopnea index (AHI) greater than 5 events/h and symptoms of daytime sleepiness.[1-3] Adult OSA is associated with several adverse effects if left untreated, including daytime sleepiness, reduced quality of life (QoL), increased cardiovascular morbidity and mortality, and increased risk of motor vehicle accidents.[4-7] The conventional treatment of OSA includes noninvasive options, that is, continuous positive airway pressure (CPAP) and dental appliances and invasive

[a] Division of Pediatric Otolaryngology-Head and Neck Surgery, Ann & Robert H. Lurie Children's Hospital of Chicago, 225 E Chciago Ave, Box #25, Chicago, IL, 60611, USA; [b] Department of Otolaryngology-Head and Neck Surgery, Northwestern University Feinberg School of Medicine, 675 N St Clair St, Chicago, IL, 60611, USA
* Corresponding author. Division of Otolaryngology-Head and Neck Surgery, Ann & Robert H. Lurie Children's Hospital of Chicago, 225 East Chicago Ave, Box #25, Chicago, IL 60611.
E-mail address: kbillings@luriechildrens.org

Otolaryngol Clin N Am 55 (2022) 1045–1054
https://doi.org/10.1016/j.otc.2022.06.010   oto.theclinics.com
0030-6665/22/© 2022 Elsevier Inc. All rights reserved.

options, including a variety of surgical procedures aimed at addressing site-specific areas of upper airway obstruction. The goal of any treatment is reduction in sleep disruption and the AHI, with resultant improved overall health and QoL.

CONVENTIONAL TREATMENT APPROACHES AND OUTCOMES FOR OBSTRUCTIVE SLEEP APNEA

The gold standard treatment of OSA is CPAP.[1,8] CPAP is effective in preventing upper airway collapse, correcting oxyhemoglobin saturation, and reducing cortical arousals associated with apnea/hypopnea events. Despite improvements in mask design and flow technology to address issues with PAP mask tolerance, a large number of patients struggle to adhere to long-term PAP therapy.[9-11] Nonadherence rates with PAP therapy are reported to range from 20% to 40%, and patients with moderate to severe sleep apnea with poor compliance may continue to experience significant sequelae secondary to OSA.[12] With rising rates of OSA in adults related to increased rates of obesity and an aging population, both risk factors for OSA,[13] poor adherence to PAP therapy highlights the importance of a multifaceted approach in the care of patients with OSA.

Mandibular advancement devices (MADs), and other oral appliances, offer an alternative, noninvasive option for OSA management.[9] MADs consist of superior and inferior plates that are interconnected and work by displacing the mandible forward during sleep, thereby opening the posterior pharyngeal space. Kashida *and colleagues*[14] described MADs as a first-line therapy or alternative to PAP therapy in patients with mild to moderate OSA, and a second-line therapy for those with severe OSA who have failed PAP therapy. Reduction in the AHI and Epworth Sleepiness Scale (ESS) has been demonstrated with MADs, when compared with no interventions.[9,15,16] There are several side effects associated with MADs and close monitoring with a dentist specializing in sleep medicine is recommended, as the appliance may need to be replaced or adjusted over time with extended use.[9] Patients fitted with an oral appliance should undergo a polysomnogram (PSG) with the appliance in place after final adjustments to the fit have been performed. In addition, some patients may benefit from MAD use in conjunction with PAP treatment. Noninvasive options for OSA management are shown in **Box 1**.

A variety of surgical options to open the airway are available for the management of OSA. Carberry and colleagues[13] suggested that surgeries that target the anatomy of the upper airway could be a useful adjunct to improve the efficacy of other treatments such as CPAP and MADs. Clinical success for upper airway surgery is typically defined as a greater than 50% reduction in the AHI to less than 20 events/h, but the success rates of surgery range from 5% to 78%.[17] Surgical options (**Box 2**) are varied

---

Box 1
Noninvasive Obstructive Sleep Apnea Options

Noninvasive Obstructive Sleep Apnea Management

Continuous positive airway pressure

Mandibular advancement devices

Weight loss (dietary and exercise regimens)

Positional devices for sleep

Adjuvant nasal therapies (eg, nasal steroids)

Box 2
Surgical Options for Obstructive Sleep Apnea*

Surgical Obstructive Sleep Apnea Management

Tonsillectomy

Adenoidectomy

Uvulopalatopharyngoplasty (UPPP); modified or variant UPPP

Maxillomandibular advancement

Expansion sphincteroplasty

Lingual tonsillar reduction

Midline glossectomy

Transoral robotic surgery of tongue base reduction procedures

Hypoglossal nerve stimulator

*not comprehensive, other options for surgery available at discretion of treating physician

---

and target patient-specific areas of upper airway obstruction, either alone or in combination with other procedures. The disadvantages of surgical procedures include their cost, varied and unpredictable efficacy, pain, infections, and anesthetic complications.[13] Surgical procedures may facilitate comfort with adjunctive CPAP use in some patients.

INTEGRATIVE TREATMENT APPROACHES AND OUTCOMES FOR OBSTRUCTIVE SLEEP APNEA

Complementary and integrative medicine (CIM) approaches are defined as a group of diverse medical and health care systems, practices, and products that are not presently considered to be part of conventional medicine.[18] The five subgroups of CIM therapies are shown in **Box 3**. Complementary interventions are used along with conventional treatments, whereas alternative approaches are used instead of conventional medicine. The term integrative refers to practice that includes two or more disciplines or distinct approaches to care.[19] Integrative health brings conventional and complementary approaches together in a coordinated way. As per web-based content,[20] integrative health emphasizes multimodal interventions, including combinations of conventional medicine, lifestyle changes, physical rehabilitation, psychotherapy, and complementary health approaches. The emphasis is on treating the

---

Box 3
Five Categories of Complementary and Integrative Medicine Approaches

Complementary and Integrative Medicine Approaches

Alternative medical systems (eg, acupuncture, Ayurveda)

Mind–body interventions (eg, meditation)

Biologically based therapies (eg, herbal supplements)

Manipulative and body-based methods (eg, chiropractic therapy, osteopathic medicine)

Energy therapies (eg, magnetic therapy)

---

whole person rather than one organ system. People who choose CIM are potentially seeking ways to improve their health and well-being or to relieve symptoms associated with chronic illnesses or the side effects of conventional treatments. In the United States, the increased use of acupuncture, deep breathing exercises, massage therapy, naturopathy, and yoga were seen in adults between the years 2002 and 2007.[18]

Integrative Therapies for Obstructive Sleep Apnea

Epidemiologic studies have shown a strong association between excess weight and OSA in that most individuals with moderate to severe OSA also have an elevated body mass index.[21,22] Integrative therapies aimed at lifestyle changes and weight loss should play a role in managing obese patients with OSA, regardless of the conventional treatment being used. The pathophysiology of OSA, as it relates to obesity, can involve excess pharyngeal adipose tissue, which leads to airway narrowing, and excess abdominal wall and chest wall fat, which reduces lung volumes[21,23] A longitudinal prospective cohort study, the Wisconsin Sleep Disorder Study, found that weight loss of about 10% predicted a 26% reduction in the AHI.[21,24] Garvey and colleagues[25] suggested that for clinically significant and meaningful improvement in OSA, the weight loss goal should be at least 7% to 10%. Lifestyle modifications with reduced calorie intake and increased physical activity form the foundation of all weight loss interventions and have been demonstrated to result in weight-independent benefits in OSA.[26]

A randomized control trial (RCT) comparing the effectiveness of an intensive weight loss program for severe OSA in patients on CPAP showed a significant reduction in weight loss in the intervention group, when compared with the control group (received standard lifestyle recommendations).[1] The AHI decreased more in the intervention group (-23.72 vs -9 events/h) at 3 months, but there was no difference between the groups at 12 months. There were improvements in the lipid profiles, glycemic control, and inflammatory markers in the intervention group, and the authors highlighted the importance of incorporating weight loss programs in the treatment of those with severe OSA on CPAP with the aim of improving their general health status.

Another study demonstrated the clinical importance of lifestyle modifications in addition to CPAP treatment in patients with OSA. Igelstrom and colleagues[27] performed an RCT comparing overweight patients with moderate–severe OSA who were assigned to a CPAP and behavioral sleep medicine (BSM) interventions targeting physical activity and eating behavior experimental group or a CPAP and advice about weight loss control group. There was a mean improvement in the AHI by 9.7 events/h in the experimental group, and 40% ($n = 14$) of patients in the experimental group had reduced severity of their OSA compared with 16.7% ($n = 6$, $P = .02$) in the control group. Despite improvements with BSM, the number of patients studied was small, and the sustainability of the impact of BSM on weight loss and AHI was not demonstrated in this 6-month trial. The authors commented that behavioral changes may not cure OSA but may be clinically relevant to the individual by reducing the disease severity and thereby the risk of comorbidities.

In Saunder and colleagues[21] review of surgical and nonsurgical weight loss for those with OSA, diet, physical activity, and behavioral modifications were described as the cornerstone of weight management. The authors cite a previous meta-analysis[28] suggesting that significant weight loss was observed with any low-carbohydrate or low-fat diet and that the best diet for any given patient was the one they could adhere to. Despite diet and weight loss interventions, many patients require additional interventions, such as anti-obesity medications and weight loss (bariatric) surgery.[21] Pharmaceuticals used for weight loss, and the range of bariatric surgery options and outcomes are well reviewed by the authors, although these additional options fall into conventional medicine approaches.

Integrative Medical Systems

Nonconventional CIM approaches, which can be used in the management of patients with OSA, include alternative medical systems, such as acupuncture and Ayurveda. Acupuncture originated in China thousands of years ago and has been used to treat a variety of maladies. Even today, it is one of the potential treatment options for those with chronic pain who are seen by the pain management services at many institutions. Evidence has shown that the effects of acupuncture include the release of serotonin from the caudal raphe nucleus and endogenous opioid systems[29,30] For those with OSA, the activation of these pathways stimulates upper airway motor neurons allowing for increased muscle tone in the area, thereby preventing pharyngeal collapse. Several studies have analyzed the utility of acupuncture in treating OSA[29–31]

A meta-analysis evaluating the efficacy of acupuncture for OSA management included nine RCTs.[29] The cumulative analysis showed acupuncture significantly reduced the AHI in those with OSA, especially in moderate to severe cases. Results of the studies were not able to demonstrate a clinically significant threshold of AHI improvement and could not determine the curative effect of acupuncture for OSA treatment. The quality of evidence of included studies was mainly low to very low. One of the RCTs included in the meta-analysis was a study by Freire and colleagues.[30] The authors designed a randomized, placebo-controlled trial looking at the efficacy of treating moderate OSA with acupuncture. Patients enrolled in the study received acupuncture or sham acupuncture once a week for 10 weeks. A control group received no acupuncture. The sham group was stimulated with the same number of needles, but not in regions related to any acupoints, and the needles were not manipulated. The AHI and the number of respiratory events decreased significantly in the acupuncture group but not in the sham group. The sham group did not differ from the control group in any of the posttreatment PSG measurements. All the acupuncture patients had improved mental health scores on the posttreatment ESS and short form 36 (SF-36) questionnaires, and the authors noted the potential of acupuncture for a profound placebo effect.

Another RCT[31] studied the impact of acupuncture on OSA severity and blood pressure control in patients with hypertension ($n = 26$). The control group received sham acupuncture. The study did not demonstrate a reduction in OSA severity, daytime or nocturnal blood pressure, or QoL. The authors suggested that the number of treatment sessions were limited and may have impacted their results when compared with previous studies.

The utility of Chinese therapeutic massage (*Tui Na*) was investigated in a 1-year, single-blinded, randomized trial in 20 patients.[32] The treatment was given at multiple acupoints twice weekly for 10 weeks. The authors suggested that *Tui Na* of the neck and pharynx could affect muscles of the throat beneficially, thereby improving the stability of the upper airway. Some improvement in the AHI, QoL, sleep architecture, snoring intensity, and excessive daytime sleepiness was noted in their analysis.

Ayurveda is an ancient, holistic healing system developed over 1000 years ago in India. As per online content,[33,34] it is based on the concept of wellness and health being dependent on a manageable delicate balance between the spirit, mind, and body, with the goal to promote health and fight disease. These therapies seem to be targeted at some of the symptoms of sleep disturbances/OSA, such as cardiovascular issues, fatigue, headaches, and low productivity. The impact of Ayurveda on lowering the AHI in patients with OSA has not been specifically investigated.

Given the lack of existing evidence showing a long-term benefit to these therapies, they cannot be recommended as a primary treatment of OSA. As an adjunct to improving the comfort and QoL of patients, acupuncture and other complementary therapies are intriguing options, although the widespread availability of this resource in the United States is unclear and possibly limited in some regions.

Mind–Body Interventions

Mind–body interventions are the most common CIM therapies used in the United States and include meditation, relaxation, breathing techniques, T'ai chi and qigong (TCQ), hypnosis, and biofeedback.[35] T'ai Chi is a traditional Chinese martial art commonly used for health benefits. Qigong exercises form a basis for T'ai Chi and regulate mind, body, and breathing, and these exercises have been shown to improve fatigue, anxiety, depressive symptoms, and sleep disorders.[36] In an RCT performed in patients with mild to moderate OSA by Gokmen and colleagues,[36] an intervention group (n = 25) received TCQ training under a physiotherapist supervision along with a home exercise program, and the control group (n = 25) received a home exercise program. The intervention group was noted to have reduced AHI and daytime sleepiness, and improved subjective sleep quality when compared with the control group. Long-term outcomes were not analyzed.

Another study investigated the efficacy of mind–body (Baduanjin) exercise on self-reported sleep quality and QoL in elderly subjects with sleep disturbances.[37] These exercises involve coordinating one's breathing with physical movement slowly and gently, and the actions are less physically and cognitively demanding than other mind–body interventions. The authors noted an improved self-reported sleep quality in the intervention group, but no difference in QoL between the intervention and control groups. No AHI data were reported.

Biologically Based Therapies, Herbal and Dietary Supplements

As per Zhou and colleagues,[38] traditional Chinese medicine uses an overall therapeutic approach to treat and prevent inflammatory responses and oxidative stress with the aim of improving the patient's QoL. Traditional Chinese medicine offers a variety of active ingredients, which can act on targets simultaneously, rather than a single step Western medicine approach. The efficacy and safety of Chinese medicine for OSA was studied in a protocol for systematic review and meta-analysis by Bao and colleagues,[39] as a means of providing a reliable reference for the clinical application of Chinese medicine for OSA. The limitations of the analyses included differences in the doses of Chinese medicine used in the studies and the condition of the patient's disease.

The most common biologic products used to treat sleep disturbances, although not specifically OSA, include herbal tea, melatonin, chamomile, St. John's wort, lavender, and valerian.[40] Melatonin is a natural hormone produced and secreted by the pineal gland causing an increase in hypothalamus aminobutyric and serotonin. Increased secretion occurs during dark hours. Melatonin has been shown to help regulate the circadian rhythm and has been studied for treatment of delayed sleep phase syndrome and insomnia. Caution with use is recommended because of several drug interactions. Melatonin, chamomile, lavender, and valerian have a sedative effect and are not specifically recommended for the treatment of OSA.

The efficacy of oral dietary supplements has largely been based on subjective reports, and safety is assumed based on lack of reported adverse effects. Meoli and *colleagues*[41] discussed the efficacy of herbal lubricating nasal spray in their analysis. No significant objective difference in snoring intensity or frequency was seen, but bed partners reported a lessening in snoring intensity in 65% of patients. Physicians should question their patients about the use of these products, given the lack of published scientific evidence of objective benefits for these treatments in managing OSA. Patients should be counseled as to their potential risks and benefits, and the role of these remedies as a complement to conventional therapies not as an alternative should be reinforced.

Manipulative and Body-Based Methods

Manipulative and body-based practices focus primarily on the structures and systems of the body, including the bones and joints, the soft tissues, and the circulatory and lymphatic systems.[42,43] Practices include chiropractic and osteopathic manipulation, therapeutic massage, and yoga. Acupuncture and TCQ are also considered in this category. Intraoral myofascial therapy for the sphenopalatine ganglion (SPG) is widely used in osteopathic practice for the management of nasal obstruction, chronic rhinitis, and snoring. A proof-of-concept study to determine if manipulation of the SPG would improve pharyngeal stability in OSA was performed on nine subjects by Jacq *and colleagues.*[44] The findings of the study did not demonstrate efficacy of this treatment of OSA.

There is evidence that playing certain types of wind instruments was associated with improving the AHI and reducing the risk of developing OSA. In a systematic review by De Jong *and colleagues,*[45] the investigators suggested that by training and strengthening the muscles of the upper airway, patients could decrease airway collapsibility and effectively reduce progression and development of OSA. Instruments are accessible, inexpensive, and could be an adjunctive treatment of OSA, but the study suggested more validated studies were needed, as most of the existing literature did not report on the AHI of patients analyzed.

Energy Therapies

Energy treatments are aimed at healing imbalances in the energy fields purported to be in and around the human body. Examples of energy therapies include Reiki, a spiritual, vibrational healing practice, and healing touch, hands used to facilitate physical, emotional, mental, and spiritual health.[46] These therapies are used by some individuals for managing insomnia and fatigue. There specific use for OSA management has not been investigated.

SUMMARY

Conventional treatments of OSA, including CPAP, oral appliances, and various surgical interventions in appropriately selected patients, are the mainstay of OSA management. Particularly with the rising rates of obesity, integrative approaches to improve weight loss and lifestyle habits are essential to managing patients with OSA to aid in achieving longer term success. CIM therapies, as part of an integrative approach to treating OSA, may result in improving symptoms of sleep disturbances and QoL, but they may not be associated with sustainable reductions in the AHI when used alone. As more and more patients seek CIM treatments, physicians should be aware of their role and utility in treating patients with OSA.

DISCLOSURES/CONFLICTS

The authors have no disclosures or conflicts of interest.

REFERENCES

1. Lopez-Padros C, Salord N, Alves C, et al. Effectiveness of an intensive weight-loss program for severe OSA in patients undergoing CPAP treatment: randomized controlled trial. J Clin Sleep Med 2020;16(4):503–14.
2. Peppard PE, Young T, Palta M, et al. Increased prevalence of sleep-disordered breathing in adults. Am J Epidemiol 2013;177(9):1006–14.
3. Gavrey JF, Pengo MF, Drakatos P, et al. Epidemiological aspects of obstructive sleep apnea. J Thorac Dis 2015;7(5):920–9.
4. MacKay S, As Carney, Catcheside PG, et al. Effect of multilevel upper airway surgery vs medical management on the apnea-hypopnea index and patient-reported daytime sleepiness among patients with moderate or severe obstructive sleep apnea: the SAMS randomized clinical trial. JAMA 2020;324(12):1168–79.
5. Kie C, Zhu R, Tian Y, et al. Association of obstructive sleep apnoea with the risk of vascular outcomes and all-cause mortality: a meta-analysis. BMJ Open 2017;7(12):e013983.
6. Patil SP, Ayappe IA, Caples SM, et al. Treatment of adult obstructive sleep apnea with positive airway pressure: an American Academy of Sleep Medicine systematic review, meta-analysis, and GRADE assessment. J Clin Sleep Med 2019;15(2):301–34.
7. Tregear S, Reston J, Schoelles K, et al. Obstructive sleep apnea and risk of motor vehicle crash: a systematic review and meta-analysis. J Clin Sleep Med 2009;5(6):573–81.
8. McDaid C, Duree KH, Griffin SC, et al. A systematic review of continuous positive airway pressure for obstructive sleep apnea-hypopnoea syndrome. Sleep Med Rev 2009;13(6):427–36.
9. Suurna MV, Frieger AC. Obstructive sleep apnea: Non-positive airway pressure treatments. Clin Geriatr Med 2021;37:429–44.
10. Rotenberg BW, Marariu D, Pang KP. Trends in CPAP adherence over twenty years of data collection: a flattened curve. J Otolaryngol Head Neck Surg 2016;45:43.
11. Sawyer AM, Gooneratne NS, Marcus CL, et al. A systematic review of CPAP adherence across age groups: clinical and empiric insights for developing CPAP adherence interventions. Sleep Med Rev 2011;15(6):343–56.
12. Kent D, Stanley J, Aurora N, et al. Referral of adults with obstructive sleep apnea for surgical consultation: an American Academy of Sleep Medicine systematic review, meta-analysis, and GRADE assessment. J Clin Sleep Med 2021;17(12):2507–31.
13. Carberry JC, Amatoury J, Eckert DJ. Personalized management approach for OSA. Chest 2018;153(3):744–55.
14. Kashida CA, Littner MR, Morgenthaler T, et al. Practice parameters for the indications for polysomnography and related procedures: an update for 2005. Sleep 2005;28(4):499–521.
15. Blanco J, Zamarron C, Abeleira Pazos MT, et al. Prospective evaluation of an oral appliance in the treatment of obstructive sleep apnea syndrome. Sleep Breath 2005;9:20–5.
16. Petri N, Svanholt P, Solow B, et al. Mandibular advancement appliance for obstructive sleep apnea: results of a randomized placebo-controlled trial using parallel group design. J Sleep Res 2008;17:221–9.
17. Dorrity J, Wirtz N, Frymovich O, et al. Genioglossal advancement, hyoid suspension, tongue base radiofrequency, and endoscopic, partial midline glossectomy for obstructive sleep apnea. Otolaryngol Clin North Am 2016;49(6):1399–414.

18. Sood A, Narayanan S, Wahner-Roedler DL, et al. Use of complementary and alternative medicine treatments by patients with obstructive sleep apnea hypopnea syndrome. J Clin Sleep Med 2007;3(6):575–9.

19. Frish NC, Rabinowitsch D. What's in a definition? Holistic nursing, integrative health care, and integrative nursing: report of an integrated literature review. J Holist Nurs 2019;37(3):260–72.

20. Complementary, alternative, or integrative health: what's in a name?. Available at: www.nccih.nih.gov. Accessed January 30 2022.

21. Saunders KH, Igel LI, Tchang BG. Surgical and nonsurgical weight loss for patients with obstructive sleep apnea. Otolaryngol Clin North Am 2020;53:409–20.

22. Young T, Peppard PE, Taheri S. Excess weight and sleep-disordered breathing. J Appl Physiol 1985;99(4):1592–9.

23. Joosten SA, Hamilton GS, Naughton MT. Impact of weight loss management in OSA. Chest 2017;152(1):194–203.

24. Peppard PE, Young T, Palta M, et al. Longitudinal study of moderate weight change and sleep-disordered breathing. JAMA 2000;284(23):3015–21.

25. Garvey WT, Garber AJ, Mechanik JI, et al. American association of clinical endocrinologists and American College of Endocrinology position statement on the 2014 advanced framework for a new diagnosis of obesity as a chronic disease. Endocr Pract 2014;20(9):977–89.

26. Tham KW, Ching Lee P, Lim CH. Weight management in obstructive sleep apnea: medical and surgical options. Sleep Med Clin 2019;14:143–53.

27. Igelstrom H, Asenlof P, Emtner M, et al. Improvement in obstructive sleep apnea after a tailored behavioral sleep medicine intervention targeting healthy eating and physical activity: a randomized controlled trial. Sleep Breath 2018;22:653–61.

28. Johnston BC, Kanters S, Bandayrei K, et al. Comparison of weight loss among named diet programs in overweight and obese adults: a meta-analysis. JAMA 2014;312(9):923–33.

29. Wang L, Xu J, Zhan Y, et al. Acupuncture for obstructive sleep apnea (OSA) in adults: a systematic review and meta-analysis. Biomed Res Internat 2020; ID6972327:1–10.

30. Friere AO, Sugai GCM, Chrispin FS, et al. treatment of moderate obstructive sleep apnea syndrome with acupuncture: a randomized, placebo-controlled pilot trial. Sleep Med 2007;8:43–50.

31. Silva MV, Lustosa TC, Arai VJ, et al. Effects of acupuncture on obstructive sleep apnea severity, blood pressure control and quality of life in patients with hypertension: a randomized controlled trial. J Sleep Res 2020;29:e12954.

32. Lu CN, Friedman M, Lin HC, et al. Alternative therapy for patients with obstructive sleep apnea/hypopnea syndrome: a 1-year, single-blind, randomized trial of Tui Na. Altern Ther Health Med 2017;23(4):16–24.

33. Ayurveda for sleep apnea: natural remedies to cease snoring and ensure a deep slumber. Available at: www.netmeds.com. Accessed February 19 2022.

34. 5 Ayurvedic remedies for sleep apnea. Available at: www.shankara.com. Accessed February 19 2022.

35. Wahbeh H, Elsas SM, Oken BS. Mind-body interventions: applications in neurology. Neurology 2008;70(24):2321–8.

36. Gokman GY, Akkoyunlu ME, Kilic L, et al. The effect of T'ai Chi and Qigong training on patients with obstructive sleep apnea: a randomized controlled study. J Altern Complement Med 2019;25(3):317–25.

37. Fan B, Song W, Zhang J, et al. The efficacy of mind-body (Baduanjin) exercise on self-reported sleep quality and quality of life in elderly subjects with sleep disturbances: a randomized controlled trial. Sleep Breath 2020;24:696–701.
38. Zhou M, Liang Q, Pei Q, et al. Chinese herbs medicine Huatan Huoxue prescription for obstructive sleep apnea hypopnea syndrome as complementary therapy: a protocol for a systematic review and meta-analysis. Medicine 2020;99:e21070.
39. Bao JL, Gao X, Han YB, et al. Efficacy and Safety of Chinese medicine for obstructive sleep apnea. Medicine 2021;100(3):1–4.
40. Gooneratne NS. Complementary and alternative medicine for sleep disturbances in older adults. Clin Geriatr Med 2008;24(1):121–viii.
41. Meoli AL, Rosen CL, Kristo D, et al. Nonprescription treatments of snoring or obstructive sleep apnea: an evaluation of products with limited scientific evidence. Sleep 2003;26(5):619–24.
42. Manipulative and body-based practice: an overview. Available at: www.healthyplace.com. Accessed February 6 2022.
43. Jacq O, Arnulf I, Similowski T, et al. Upper airway stabilization by osteopathic manipulation of the sphenoplatine ganglion versus sham manipulation in OSAS patients: a proof-of-concept, randomized, crossover double-blind, controlled study. Complement Altern Med 2017;17(546):1–10.
44. De Jong JC, Maroda AJ, Camacho M, et al. The impact of playing a musical instrument on obstructive sleep apnea: a systematic review. Ann Otol Rhinol Laryngol 2020;129(9):924–9.
45. What is energy medicine?. Available at: www.nm.org. Accessed February 6 2022.

Complementary/Integrative Medicine for Pediatric Otitis Media

Ajay S. Nathan, MS[a], Jessica R. Levi, MD[a,b],*, Robert O'Reilly, MD[c]

KEYWORDS

- Otitis media • Pediatrics • Homeopathy • Supplements • Eastern medicine
- Osteopathy • Chiropractic • Alternative medicine

KEY POINTS

- Complementary/integrative medicine can be useful in the treatment of otitis media (OM), especially during the watchful waiting periods and in combination with conventional therapy.
- Prevention is important, principally through avoidance of risk factors. However, products such as echinacea and xylitol used correctly have stronger evidence supporting their use for prevention.
- Homeopathic treatments also have evidence for use in combination with conventional therapy, as it may help decrease pain and lead to a faster resolution of disease.
- Probiotics are a promising area for future research, as research is conflicting and limited at this point.
- Many studies have been performed for traditional Chinese and Japanese medicine in OM, but conclusions are limited due to language barriers, methodological concerns, and formulation variability.

INTRODUCTION

Acute otitis media (AOM), one of the most common diseases of childhood, has a peak incidence between 6 and 15 months of age. Almost half of all pediatric antibiotic prescriptions are written for otitis media (OM), which also prompts more physician visits than any other childhood illness.[1] The American Academy of Pediatrics (AAP)[2] and the American Academy of Otolaryngology and Head and Neck Surgery define AOM[3] as (1) a history of acute onset of signs and symptoms, (2) the presence of middle ear effusion, and (3) signs and symptoms of middle ear inflammation. It is differentiated

[a] Boston University School of Medicine, 72 East Concord Street, Boston, MA, USA; [b] Department of Otolaryngology/Head and Neck Surgery, Boston Medical Center, BCD Building, 5th Floor, 800 Harrison Avenue, Boston, MA 02118, USA; [c] Perelman School of Medicine at the University of Pennsylvania, 3400 Civic Center Boulevard, Philadelphia, PA 19104, USA
* Corresponding author.
E-mail address: Jessica.Levi@bmc.org

Otolaryngol Clin N Am 55 (2022) 1055–1075
https://doi.org/10.1016/j.otc.2022.06.018   oto.theclinics.com
0030-6665/22/© 2022 Elsevier Inc. All rights reserved.

from both recurrent acute otitis media (ROM), AOM occurring at least three times within 6 months, and chronic otitis media with effusion (COM), the presence of middle ear fluid in the absence of symptoms for greater than 8 weeks.

80% of AOM episodes resolve spontaneously within three days. In 2004 and 2013, the American Academy of Family Physicians (AAFP)[4] and AAP[5] released recommendations highlighting initial watchful waiting for children with OM. Unwilling to let a child's illness run its course and seeing a persistence of symptoms, many families seek alternative modes of treatment, which can fall under the umbrella term of complementary and alternative medicine (CAM), but a less negative term complementary/integrative medicine (CIM) is preferred.

CIM may be defined as "anything not in the realm of modern or evidence-based medicine," which can include treatments based on historical or cultural traditions or those emphasizing self-treatment and prevention.[6,7] Evaluating the efficacy of CIM for OM is fraught with difficulty, including language barriers and lack of randomization. Regardless, CIM, with its numerous modalities,[7] is quite common: in a Centers for Disease Control and Prevention (CDC) National Health Statistics survey in 2007, 4 out of 10 adults had used some form of CIM in the last year, and the children of these adults were twice as likely to have also used CIM compared with other US children.[8] Perhaps most relevant, in a 2009 survey of 840 children in Italy, 46% of those aged 1 to 7 years with 3 or more episodes of AOM in 6 months had used some component of CIM.[9]

In this article, we discuss therapeutic options relating to CIM for pediatric OM. We review the evidence by category and provide a summary of studies discussed in **Table 1**. Overall, the literature shows that while many of these modalities are promising, few have been assessed with large, high-quality randomized controlled trials (RCTs), emphasizing the need for further research.

THERAPEUTIC OPTIONS
Prevention

One of the first tenets of many CIM modalities is prevention, and numerous risk factors for OM have been identified. Well-documented studies demonstrate increased rates of OM with bottle-feeding compared with breastfeeding.[10] In addition, smoking around children, large daycare settings, and pacifier use can also play a role (**Table 2**).[11]

Nutrition has been implicated in the pathogenesis of OM. In a study by Lasisi and colleagues,[12] patients with COM and ROM were found to have retinol/vitamin A levels that were lower than age-matched controls. These findings are supported by a 2009 meta-analysis by Elemraid and colleagues,[13] who found some evidence that deficiencies of zinc and/or vitamin A may lead to increased rates of OM. However, Abba and colleagues[14] reviewed 12 RCTs in which placebo was compared with zinc and found conflicting reports regarding the efficacy of supplementation.

Vaccines also play an important role in the prevention of OM. In 2001, the CDC recommended that the seven-valent pneumococcal conjugate vaccine (PCV7, the initial Prevnar vaccine) be administered to all young children. Research has shown an overall decrease in rates of OM caused by pneumococcus.[15–17] Subsequently, higher-valent vaccines with protection against additional serotypes were developed and replaced PCV7 beginning in 2009 because of the residual burden of pneumococcal diseases. In the United States, a second-generation Prevnar Vaccine, the 13-valent pneumococcal conjugate vaccine (PCV13) was recommended in 2010 for universal immunization of children through age 5. These vaccines have had a significant worldwide impact on AOM, although their impact must be studied locally because of the regional variance in strains.

Table 1
Complementary and alternative medicine studies reviewed in this article

Category	First Author, Year	Study Type	Number Participants (Age)	Study Group(s)	Main Finding(s) Relating to AOM
Homeopathy	Harrison[23] 1999	Open RCT	33 (18 m–8 y)	Homeopathy vs. Watchful Waiting	• Significantly more patients in homeopathic group had normal tympograms at end of study period
Homeopathy	Jacobs[24] 2001	Double-Blind, Placebo Controlled RCT	75 (18 m–6 y)	Homeopathy vs. Control	• Insufficient sample size to statistically determine treatment failure rates, although trend toward significance in homeopathy group • Significantly lower symptom scores recorded by diary in homeopathy group
Homeopathy	Frei[25] 2001	Observational	230 (0–16 y)	Time to pain control with homeopathy (no comparison)	• 39% of patients achieved pain control within 6 h of first homeopathic dose, 33% of patients within 12 h, and the remaining 28% went on to receive antibiotics
Homeopathy	Wustrow[26] 2005	Self-Selection Prospective Trial	390 (1–10 y)	"Conventional treatment" vs. Homeopathy	• Significantly less analgesics required in homeopathy group with no change in time to recovery
Homeopathy	Taylor[27] 2011	Open RCT	119 (6 m–11 y)	Homeopathic ear drops vs. No treatment	• Fewer antibiotic prescriptions filled in homeopathy group

(continued on next page)

Table 1
(continued)

Category	First Author, Year	Study Type	Number Participants (Age)	Study Group(s)	Main Finding(s) Relating to AOM
Homeopathy	Sinha et al.,[28] 2012	Double-Blind, Placebo Controlled RCT	81 (2–6 y)	"Conventional treatment" vs. Homeopathy	• Homeopathy group significantly less likely to require antibiotics by day three for treatment failure • No significant difference in overall cure rate between the two groups
Natural health	Uhari, 1996	Double-Blind, Placebo Controlled RCT	306 (?)	Xylitol gum vs. Control	• Xylitol as syrup or gum was effective in reducing the occurrence of AOM • Less antibiotics were prescribed to the Xylitol group compared with control
Natural health	Uhari, 1998	Double-Blind, Placebo Controlled RCT	857 (?)	Xylitol (syrup and gum) vs. Control (syrup and gum)	• Xylitol as syrup or gum was effective in reducing the occurrence of AOM Less antibiotics were prescribed to the Xylitol group compared with control
Natural health	Tapiainen et al.,[38] 2002	Double-Blind, Placebo Controlled RCT	1277 (10 m–7 y)	Xylitol (gum or syrup) vs. Control	• Xylitol administered only during active respiratory tract infection failed to prevent AOM
Natural health	Cohen[30] 2004	Double-Blind, Placebo Controlled RCT	430 (1–5 y)	Herbal preparation (echinacea, vitamin C) vs. Control	• Herbal preparation group had a significant reduction in incidence of AOM

Category	Author/Year	Study Type	N (age)	Intervention	Findings
Natural health	Hautalahti [39] 2007	Double-Blind, Placebo Controlled RCT	663 (7 m–7 y)	Xylitol (gum or syrup) vs. Control	• Three times daily dosing (rather than five times daily as done in other studies) failed to prevent AOM
Natural health	Wahl et al.,[31] 2008	Double-Blind, Placebo Controlled RCT	90 (1–5 y)	Echinacea ± Osteopathic Manipulative Treatment vs. Placebo	• Echinacea group had a borderline increased risk of at least one episode of AOM during 6-month period
Natural health	Schapowal [32] 2015	Meta-Analysis of RCTs	2458 (N/A)	Pooled analysis of Echinacea vs. Control for prevention of upper respiratory infection in 6 studies	• Complications from upper respiratory infections including AOM were significantly less frequent with echinacea treatment
Natural health	Azarpazhooh [40] 2016	Meta-Analysis of RCTs	3405 (N/A)	Pooled analysis of Xylitol vs. Control for prevention of AOM in healthy children in 5 studies	• Xylitol can reduce the occurrence of AOM among healthy children (and not otitis prone children) with no acute upper respiratory tract infection with no difference in side effects
Natural health	Ogal et al.,[33] 2021	Double-Blind, Placebo Controlled RCT	200 (4–12 y)	Echinacea vs. Vitamin C (placebo)	• Complications from upper respiratory infections including AOM were significantly less frequent with echinacea treatment
Probiotics (oral)	Hatakka [43] 2001	Double-Blind, Placebo Controlled RCT	571 (1–6 y)	Lactobacillus rhamnosus GG milk vs. Control	• Consistent trends toward significance for reduction in respiratory infections Lactobacillus GG group • Significantly fewer sick absences from daycare in Lactobacillus GG group

(continued on next page)

Table 1
(continued)

Category	First Author, Year	Study Type	Number Participants (Age)	Study Group(s)	Main Finding(s) Relating to AOM
Probiotics (oral)	Hatakka [44] 2007	Double-Blind, Placebo Controlled RCT	309 (10 m–6 y)	Probiotic capsule (*L rhamnosus* GG, *L rhamnosus* LC *Bifidobacterium breve; Propionibacterium freudenreichii* ssp. *shermanii* JS) vs. Control	• Probiotics did not reduce the occurrence or recurrence of AOM episodes • *Streptococcus pneumoniae* or *Haemophilus influenzae* colonization were unaffected, but probiotics increased the prevalence of *Moraxella catarrhalis*
Probiotics (oral)	Stecksén-Blicks [45] 2009	Double-Blind, Placebo Controlled RCT	248 (1–5 y)	*L rhamnosus* LB21 with 2.5 mg fluoride vs. Control	• Reduction in days of antibiotic therapy and days with otitis media in probiotic group • No change in number of sick absences from daycare
Probiotics (oral)	Rautava [46] 2009	Double-Blind, Placebo Controlled RCT	81 (<2 m)	*L rhamnosus* GG and *Bifidobacterium lactis* milk vs. Control	• Significant reduction in the number of episodes of otitis media in the first 7 months of life in the probiotics group • Decrease in the amount of antibiotics prescribed in the probiotics group
Probiotics (oral)	Cohen et al., [47] 2013	Double-Blind, Placebo Controlled RCT	224 (7–13 m)	*S thermophilus* NCC *S salivarius* DSM, *L rhamnosus* LPR and PreB (Raftilose/Raftiline) vs. Control	• No significant difference in incidence of AOM episodes, ROM, or antibiotics use for AOM

Probiotics (nasal)	Roos [41] 2001	Double-Blind, Placebo Controlled RCT	108 (6 m–6 y)	Nasal spray composed of 5 strains of Strep from healthy children (2 × S sanguis, 2 × S mitis and 1 × S oralis) vs. Control	• Significantly more children in the probiotic group had no AOMs at follow-up
Probiotics (nasal)	Marchisio et al., [48] 2015	Double-Blind, Placebo Controlled RCT	100 (1–5 y)	S salivarius 24 SMB nasal spray vs. Control	• No significant difference in number of AOM episodes or antibiotics use at follow-up between groups • Subgroup analysis of colonized children only (revealed by nasopharyngeal swab) yielded significantly reduced AOM episodes and antibiotic prescriptions compared with placebo
Osteopathy	Mills [49] 2003	Open RCT	57 (6 m–4 y)	Standard care + OMT vs. Standard Care	• OMT intervention group had fewer episodes of AOM, fewer surgical procedures, and more frequent normal tympanograms
Osteopathy	Degenhardt [51] 2006	Cohort Study	8 (7 m–35 m)	Recurrence of symptoms over one year with OMT with concurrent medical management (no comparison)	• Five out of eight patients with recurrent otitis media had no recurrence of symptoms
Osteopathy	Steele et al., [50] 2014	Open RCT	52 (6 m–24 m)	Standard care + OMT vs. Standard Care	• Greater proportion of resolution of middle ear effusion in OMT group at 3 weeks

(continued on next page)

Table 1
(continued)

Category	First Author, Year	Study Type	Number Participants (Age)	Study Group(s)	Main Finding(s) Relating to AOM
Chiropractics	Froehle [52] 1996	Cohort Study	46 (<5 y)	Observing AOM Improvement with Chiropractic Treatments	• 93% of AOM improved, 75% within 10 days, 43% after 1–2 treatments
Chiropractics	Fallon [54] 1997	Cohort Study	332 (27 d–5 y)	Observing AOM and COM Improvement with Chiropractic Treatments	• Children who had AOM received 4.0 ± 1.03 adjustments and had normal tympanograms after 6.67 ± 1.9 days and normal otoscopic exams in 8.35 ± 1.96 days • Children who had COM received 5.0 ± 1.53 adjustments and had normal tympanogram after in 10.18 ± 3.39 days and normal otoscopic exams in 8.57 ± 1.96 days • AOM recurrence rate of 11% in 6 months
Chiropractics	Zhang [53] 2004	Cohort Study	21 (9 m–9 y)	Observing AOM Improvement with Low-Force Chiropractic Treatments	• 95% had return of normal-appearing tympanic membranes and decrease in fevers after 2 weeks
Traditional Chinese and Japanese medicine	Zhang [59] 2000	Double Blind RCT	104 (5 y–63 y)	Eryanling decoction vs. Cephalexin	• Significantly faster recovery initiation time in herbal medicine group compared with antibiotic group

Traditional Chinese and Japanese medicine	Sun[60] 2005	Double Blind RCT	90 (2 y–70 y)	Qingqiao Capsule vs. Cefaclor	• Significantly greater proportion of resolution of middle ear effusion in herbal medicine group compared with antibiotic group
Traditional Chinese and Japanese medicine	Maruyama[66] 2009	Observational	24 (6–33 m)	Clinical course of otitis-prone patients given juzen-taiho-to (JTT) over 3 months	• The frequency of AOM decreased significantly with herbal medicine • Duration of fever, administration of antibiotics, and number of hospital visits showed decreases after herbal medicine was initiated • At the end of the study period, 66.7% of patients experienced purulent otitis media after stopping the medicine, which decreased again after re-starting the medication
Traditional Chinese and Japanese medicine	Sanchez-Araujo, 2011	Placebo-Controlled RCT in Dogs	14 (N/A)	Acupuncture vs. Sham Acupuncture (control)	• Significantly more dogs with ROM were free of otitis after 1 year and four sessions of acupuncture compared with control

Table 2
Risk factors for recurrent acute otitis media (AOM): Uhari M et al. 1996

Risk Factor	Risk for	RR	P Value
Family history of AOM	AOM	2.6	<0.001
Daycare outside home	AOM	2.5	0.003
Not breastfeeding at all	Recurrent AOM	2.1	<0.001
At least one sibling	Recurrent AOM	1.9	0.001
Child care outside home	Recurrent AOM	1.8	0.004
Parental smoking	AOM	1.7	<0.001
Family daycare	AOM	1.6	0.002
Pacifier use	AOM	1.2	0.008
Breast feeding <3 months	AOM	1.2	0.003

The incidence of AOM may also be reduced by prevention of preceding upper respiratory infections or other viral illnesses such as influenza. A study by Block and colleagues[18] compared live attenuated influenza vaccine (approved for children greater than 2 years old) with placebo and found the overall efficacy against influenza-associated AOM was 85.0%. Finally, the prevention of gastroesophageal reflux, due to its potential role in OM pathogenesis, may also play a role in the prevention of OM, although further research is needed.[19]

Symptomatic Relief

Symptomatic relief of AOM is of paramount importance to families, especially with watchful waiting recommendations. Warm compress, steam, saltwater gargling, and over-the-counter decongestant nasal sprays may provide relief. Others find herbal eardrops helpful, although their compositions are quite variable (eg, *Calendula flores* [marigold], garlic [*Allium sativum*], mullein [*Verbascum thapsus*], St. John's wort [*Hypericum perforatum*], lavender, vitamin E). Sarrell and colleagues[20] compared Otikon Otic Solution, a naturopathic herbal extract containing *A. sativum*, *V. thapsus*, *C. flores*, and *H. perforatum*, with anesthetic ear drops (containing ametocaine and phenazone) and found comparable rates of analgesia in patients with AOM. A Cochrane review in 2006 found favorable results for naturopathic eardrops in review of three trials, but ultimately deemed that there was insufficient evidence to determine the effectiveness of naturopathic eardrops at this time.[21]

Homeopathy

Homeopathy is based on the principle of "like treats like" and uses minute amounts of natural substances to treat disease. Its use is individualized and includes belladonna, chamomilla, and hepar sulphuricum (Appendix 1). Remedies used for OM are generally regarded as "safe," but there are reports of initial symptoms worsening in 10% to 20% of patients.[22]

In a small, non-blinded, RCT by Harrison and colleagues,[23], more children with OM with effusion randomized to receive "homeopathic therapy" had normal tympanograms compared with watchful waiting (75% vs. 31%, $p = 0.015$). Since then, there have been five other clinical trials in homeopathy. Jacobs and colleagues[24] randomized 75 children diagnosed with AOM to receive either "homeopathic therapy" or placebo three times daily for 5 days. The homeopathic group had a decrease in symptoms at 24 and 64 h after treatment compared with placebo ($p < 0.05$). Frei and Thurneysen[25] looked at symptomatic improvement among 230 children with AOM. They found that 72% of patients were able to achieve pain control with homeopathic treatment within 12 h, whereas the other 28% went on to receive standard antibiotic treatment. They also found homeopathic remedies were 14% less expensive than traditional remedies.

Wustrow and colleagues[26] looked at symptomatic improvement in 390 children with AOM self-selected to receive either "conventional treatment" (decongestant nose drops, mucolytics, analgesics, and antibiotics) or homeopathic remedies (Otovowen). Patients in the conventional group took more analgesics (66.8% vs. 53.2%; $p = 0.007$) and had better pain control than patients taking homeopathic remedies. Time to recovery was similar in the two groups. Taylor and Jacobs[27] found fewer patients who administered a homeopathic eardrop during a watchful waiting period for AOM filled an antibiotic prescription compared with those who administered no ear drops during the same period. In 2011, an RCT comparing homeopathic treatment to "conventional treatment" (antipyretics, analgesics, and anti-inflammatory medications) found the homeopathy group was less likely to require antibiotics for treatment failure but there was no significant difference in cure rate between the two groups.[28]

Natural Health Products

Natural health products such as echinacea, cod liver oil, and xylitol are generally regarded safe, though efficacy is unclear, and some patients experience gastrointestinal symptoms. Although many natural health products are available (Appendix 2), one of the most taken is echinacea, used to prevent or treat the common cold. There are at least nine subtypes of Echinacea according to the German Commission E. Only *Echinacea pallidum* root and *E purpurea* leaf have demonstrated efficacy in treating symptoms of upper respiratory infection, although other echinacea products are commonly sold in the United States.[29]

In addition, Cohen and colleagues[30] looked at a mixture containing echinacea (with propolis and vitamin C) and found it reduced the number of AOM episodes per child by 68% ($p < 0.001$) compared with placebo among 430 children. In contrast, Wahl and colleagues[31] found borderline increased incidence of AOM in the echinacea group compared with placebo. Since then, larger RCTs have been performed, as well as a 2015 and 2021 meta-analysis.[32,33] These studies have added significant evidence of the protective effects of echinacea in reducing the risk of upper respiratory tract infections and associated incidents of OM, with negligible adverse effects.

Xylitol, a natural sugar found in many fruits and chewing gum, is also thought to have preventative properties in OM. Xylitol can inhibit the growth of *S. pneumoniae* and the attachment of both *S. pneumoniae* and *H. influenzae* to nasopharyngeal cells in vitro.[34] The first major RCT showed xylitol (8.4 g/d in divided doses five times daily) reduced the occurrence of AOM by 41% (95% confidence interval [CI]: 4.6% to 55.4%), with the additional benefit that the xylitol group required fewer antibiotics during the study period (18.5% vs. 28.9%, $p = 0.032$).[35] The most common side effects were abdominal pain and diarrhea. The same group also showed a 40% reduction of OM in patients receiving xylitol gum, 30% reduction with syrup, and 20% reduction with xylitol lozenge, compared with controls.[36] Interestingly, xylitol was ineffective in children with indwelling tympanostomy tubes.[37] Also, there was no therapeutic benefit of multiple forms of xylitol compared with placebo when used during active respiratory tract infections.[38] To address the frequent daily dosing in most trials, Hautalahti and colleagues [39]looked at three times daily xylitol for 3 months (9.6 g/d divided into three doses) and found no preventive effect over control solutions/gum in preventing OM. A recent Cochrane review examined Xylitol in five RCTs and found it could help reduce the risk of AOM in healthy children with no active upper respiratory tract infection from 30% to 22%.[40] This review also noted chewing gum and lozenges to be more effective than syrup, although these are not safe for children <2 years old who are at the greatest risk for OM.

Probiotics

Probiotics are microorganisms (most commonly lactobacilli and/or bifidobacteria) that can confer health benefits by restoring microbial balance. Probiotics are thought to reduce upper respiratory tract colonization with pathogenic bacteria by enhancing the phagocytic activity of leukocytes and stimulating antibody production.[41] They are considered safe in immunocompetent individuals but have the potential to interact with other medications. Probiotics for AOM can be administered orally or trans-nasally. No study has directly compared these, although the evidence somewhat favors trans-nasal.[42]

In an oral route RCT by Hatakka and colleagues,[43] 571 children were randomized to receive milk with or without *Lactobacillus rhamnosus* for 7 months. There was a significant decrease in the number of days absent from daycare in the probiotic group but only a slight trend toward fewer episodes of AOM. Hatakka and colleagues[44] randomized children to receive a probiotic capsule or placebo daily for 24 weeks. There was a large dropout rate, and they found probiotics did not reduce the occurrence or recurrence of OM and actually increased nasopharyngeal prevalence of *M. catarrhalis.* Later studies have conflicted with these results. Stecksén-Blicks and colleagues[45] showed milk supplemented with probiotics and fluoride consumed once daily had preventive effects on OM (0.4 days of OM vs. 1.3 days of OM, $p < 0.05$). Similarly, Rautava and colleagues[46] looked at daily supplementation of formula with probiotics of infants younger than 2 months compared with placebo until the age of 12 months. There was a significant reduction in the number of episodes of OM in the first 7 months of life (22% vs. 50%; $p = 0.014$) and a decrease in the amount of antibiotics prescribed (31% vs. 60%; $p = 0.015$). Finally, in a 2013 placebo-controlled RCT, Cohen and colleagues[47] examined a combination of probiotics with prebiotics and found no significant difference in incidence of AOM episodes ($p = 0.39$), ROM ($p = 0.889$), or antibiotic use ($p = 0.45$).

Promoting balanced flora in the nasopharynx to prevent colonization by pathogenic strains (and subsequent OM) may be better achieved through administering probiotics trans-nasally. This was examined by Roos and colleagues,[41] who found preventive effects on AOM and COM (42% without recurrence in the five-strain *Streptococcus* probiotic nasal spray group vs. 22% in the placebo group, $p = 0.02$). In a similar RCT in 2015, there was no significant differences in the number of AOM episodes or antibiotic treatment compared with control. Interestingly, when only the sub-group of children who had been successfully colonized with the probiotic flora (confirmed by nasopharyngeal microbiological analysis) were compared with those not colonized, they found that the number of colonized children experienced significantly fewer AOM episodes (42.8 vs. 13.6 %; $p = 0.03$) and were treated with less antibiotics (67.8 vs. 95.5 %; $p = 0.029$).[48]

Osteopathy

Osteopathy emphasizes that a body with normal structural relationship and good nutrition can heal itself, sometimes in combination with other therapies including chiropractic and craniosacral therapy. Therefore, treatment of OM may include the correction of cervical and cranial "osteopathic restrictions," particularly regarding the movement of the temporal bones.

An RCT by Mills and colleagues[49] evaluated osteopathic procedures (OMT) including myofascial release, articulation, balanced membranous tension, balanced ligamentous tension, facilitated positional release, and/or counter strain on "areas of restriction" for treatment of OM. Children with ROM were randomized to receive standard care, including antibiotics, with or without OMT over 6 months. Patients in the OMT group had fewer episodes of AOM per month ($p = 0.04$) and less need for tympanostomy tubes ($p = 0.03$). There was no difference in antibiotic use, parental satisfaction, or hearing results. There was a large dropout rate (25%), making conclusions difficult. Similarly, Steele and colleagues[50] performed a similar RCT in 2014 with OMT for 1 month with and without standard of care on patients with diagnosis of AOM and abnormal tympanogram. Based on tympanograms there was greater improvement in middle ear effusion in the OMT group by the third week (68.4% resolution vs. 42.1%; $p = 0.02$). Finally, a small cohort study was performed by Degenhardt and Kuchera[51] where children with ROM were given weekly OMT and antibiotics for 3 weeks and then evaluated 1 year later. Five of eight subjects had no documented episode of AOM at the 1-year follow-up. Without a control group, it is difficult to interpret these results.

Chiropractics

Chiropractic practitioners use manipulation to attempt to improve innervation and function of the tensor veli palatini, which they propose helps treat or prevent OM. Unfortunately, clinical trials evaluating the effectiveness of chiropractics in treating AOM are limited and possess significant methodological flaws. There are three major noncontrolled clinical trials evaluating its use, which mainly examine time to AOM recovery with chiropractic manipulation.[52–54] Children may be at increased risk for injury following rapid rotational movements or forces secondary to anatomic immaturity. Serious adverse events have been reported such as paraplegia and death.[55]

Traditional Chinese and Japanese Medicine

Traditional Chinese medical (TCM) practices encompass diverse healing modalities, and two forms, acupuncture and Chinese herbal medicine, are approved by the World Health Organization as therapies to treat AOM and COM. Acupuncture (with needles) may require numerous sessions to judge its efficacy[56] and could be difficult to tolerate for children. Instead, alternative modalities such as acupressure or laser acupuncture can be employed. Although there is little understanding of its mechanism in treating OM, it is theorized that acupuncture has immunomodulatory properties that may play a role in the clearance of middle ear fluid. In a study in 2011, 31 dogs with ROM were randomized to either conventional medicine with sham acupuncture or actual acupuncture in 4 sessions. Over the subsequent year, 93% of the dogs in the acupuncture group were free of otitis, compared with 50% (7) in the sham group ($p < 0.01$).[57] In addition, acupuncture has been shown to be effective for general acute pain control in children with minimal side effects (most commonly dizziness).[58]

Many herbs exist in TCM, though few studies are in pediatrics. Eryanling (EYL) liquid is one of the few herbal medicines that was tested on its own in comparison to antibiotics. It was found to be superior in symptom recovery time (MD -7.90; $p = 0.0001$), but with otherwise no difference in tympanogram or audiometry readings.[59] In one trial of a combination herbal medicine, the Qingqiao capsule (QQC), patients with OM were randomized to receive either QQC or cefaclor. Those receiving QQC had improved hearing ($p < 0.01$), but no difference in ear pain.[60] Other RCTs that compare herbal medicine, such as Longdan-xiegan decoction and Sinupret in combination with standard antibiotic treatment, were generally found to improve recovery time but have significant methodologic errors including lack of blinding.[61] Herbal compounds (eg, borneol-walnut oil [62] and Tongqiao[63]) have also been studied in OM but conclusions are limited by small sample size, lack of randomization, and unclear outcome measures. Furthermore, most research is not in English which adds difficulty to interpretation.

Although Japanese traditional medicine (Kampo) bears many resemblances to TCM, needles are not inserted as deeply, which may make it easier for children to tolerate. The herbs are different also. It has been suggested that Saireito enhances of mucociliary clearance[64] and prevents endotoxin-induced otitis.[65] Maruyama and colleagues examined Juzen-taiho-to (JTT and TJ-48), in 24 otitis-prone infants. Infants receiving JTT had fewer hospital visits, antibiotics, and fevers than before JTT administration; 95% had *no* OM while taking JTT. Interestingly, 66.7% (16 of 24) had purulent OM following discontinuation of JTT ($p = 0.004$), and rates of OM decreased again with JTT resumption ($p = 0.005$).[66]

Other Therapies

Aromatherapy may treat OM. Lavender (*Lavandula officinalis*) essence may help to reduce inflammation and pain associated with OM. Other oils include chamomile (*Matricaria recutita*), cajuput, evening primrose oil (*Oenothera biennis*), fatty acid, flax oil, and borage. Aromatherapy has not been well studied to date.

Ayurvedic medicine, developed in ancient India, is based on the principle of balance and means "knowledge for long life". In OM, Ayurvedic physicians massage the lymph nodes outside the ears to open the Eustachian tubes. A drink made with the herb amala (which contains vitamin C and may possess antiviral and antibacterial properties) is given. Again, more research is needed.

DISCUSSION

Overall, research in CIM is limited for multiple reasons. It is generally not regulated by the FDA, and there are no patents for CIM modalities, eliminating economic incentives for research. The National Center for Complementary and Integrative Health does sponsor and conduct research, but funding for a particular domain depends on the Center's overall research priorities. For AOM, any interventions are difficult to evaluate secondary to the disease's rapid resolution and natural history, and many studies have significant methodological flaws, making definitive conclusions difficult. Studies of cost-effectiveness of such treatments need to be performed, and safety profiles, drug interactions, and effects in immunocompromised patients are not yet known.

Based on the literature it is possible homeopathy leads to a more rapid reduction of symptoms, shorter duration of pain, and a reduction in antibiotic use. However, to accurately assess the efficacy and safety of these treatments, larger blinded randomized controlled studies are required. Similarly, natural health products also have higher quality evidence in preventing upper respiratory tract infections and the complications associated with them, such as AOM. Echinacea has shown particular promise, with a large meta-analysis of 6 RCTs showing significantly fewer episodes of AOM when preventative echinacea was taken.[32] Xylitol has a similar strength of evidence, although its use may be impractical as most studies report a five-times-a-day dosing schedule that could limit full compliance.

There is conflicting evidence on the effectiveness of probiotics in preventing AOM. Overall, trials in this category were of poorer quality and were difficult to compare given the heterogeneity of the study design and the probiotic strains.[42] This has led to inconsistent results, which limits recommendations on their use. One direction for future work is to analyze only those patients with successful colonization of the nasopharynx with the probiotic strains, as done by Marchisio and colleagues[48] to assess the true magnitutde of therapeutic effect.

Research on osteopathy for AOM is limited, hindered by small study groups and the lack of control groups. Similarly, the effectiveness of chiropractic medicine is unclear because the few existent studies possess significant methodological shortcomings. In addition, the risks of chiropractic treatment, especially in children, outweigh the potential benefits.

Finally, a relatively large body of research exists for both Chinese and Japanese traditional medicine. Some herbal formulations have promising evidence, especially if used in combination with conventional therapy, though their production is not standardized and thus safety is unclear. Furthermore, very few studies are in English, and all are limited by methodologic concerns including a combined study group of children and adults, which limits conclusions for pediatric populations.

SUMMARY

According to the AAFP and AAP, management of AOM begins with watchful waiting. It is important to emphasize prevention with the elimination of risk factors such as secondhand smoke and supine bottle-feeding, as well as maintaining nutrition and vaccinations. Herbal eardrops may help to relieve symptoms. Homeopathic treatments may help decrease pain and may lead to a faster resolution of disease. Probiotics, echinacea, and xylitol may be beneficial in preventing OM and decreasing antibiotic use. Of all the CIM therapies, only echinacea and xylitol have been studied in well-designed, randomized, blinded trials. Probiotics and traditional Chinese and Japanese medicine are areas with promising emerging research, and larger, well-designed trials are needed to confirm their safety and efficacy.

CLINICS CARE POINTS

- Many integrative medicine methodologies have shown some positive trends in small groups, but few have shown benefit in double-blind randomized controlled studies and, thus, remain speculative

- Although most complementary/integrative medicine therapies are safe, especially when used in combination with standard treatment, it is best to consult a physician when making treatment decisions for full guidance on the risks and benefits of any treatment option.

- More severe cases of otitis media, such as those with complications or those that fail to improve with observation or complementary/integrative medicine (after 48 to 72 h) should be treated with antibiotics and, in some cases, surgical intervention.

DISCLOSURE

This research received no specific grant from any funding agency in the public, commercial, or not-for-profit sectors. The authors declare that they have no financial conflicts of interest.

REFERENCES

1. Stool SE, Field MJ. The impact of otitis media. Pediatr Infect J 1989;8:S11–4.

2. Lieberthal AS, Carroll AE, Chonmaitree T, et al. The diagnosis and management of acute otitis media. Pediatrics 2013;131(3):e964–99.

3. Rosenfeld RM, Tunkel DE, Schwartz SR, et al. Clinical practice guideline: tympanostomy tubes in children (update). Otolaryngol Neck Surg 2022;166(1_suppl): S1–55.

4. Harmes KM, Blackwood RA, Burrows HL, et al. Otitis Media: Diagn Treat 2013; 88(7):6.

5. Subcommittee on Management of Acute Otitis Media. Diagnosis and management of acute otitis media. Pediatrics 2004;113(5):1451–65.

6. Complementary, Alternative, or Integrative Health: What's In a Name? NCCIH. Available at: https://www.nccih.nih.gov/health/complementary-alternative-or-integrative-health-whats-in-a-name. Accessed April 21, 2022.

7. Seidman MD, van Grinsven G. Complementary and integrative treatments. Otolaryngol Clin North Am 2013;46(3):485–97.

8. Barnes PM, Bloom B, Nahin RL. Complementary and alternative medicine use among adults and Children: United States, 2007: (623942009-001). Natl Health Stat Report 2008. https://doi.org/10.1037/e623942009-001.

9. Marchisio P, Bianchini S, Galeone C. Use of complementary and alternative medicine in children with recurrent AOM in Italy. Int J Immunopathol Pharmacol 2011; 24:441–9.

10. Sabirov A, Casey M JR, Murphy TF. Breast-feeding is associated with a reduced frequency of AOM and high serum antibody levels against NTHi and outer membrane protein vaccine antigen candidate P6. Pediatr Res 2009;66:565–70.

11. Uhari M, Mantysaari K, Niemela M. A meta-analytic review of risk factors for AOM. Clin Infect Dis 1996;22:1079–83.

12. Lasisi AO. The role of retinol in the etiology and outcome of suppurative otitis media. Eur Arch Otorhinolaryngol 2009;266:647–52.

13. Elemraid MA, Mackenzie IJ, Fraser WD. Nutritional factors in the pathogenesis of ear disease in children: a systematic review. Ann Trop Paediatr 2009;29:85–99.

14. Abba K, Gulani A, Sachdev HS. Zinc supplements for preventing otitis media. Cochrane Database Syst Rev 2010;2:CD006639.

15. Feikin DR, Kagucia EW, Loo JD, et al. Serotype-specific changes in invasive pneumococcal disease after pneumococcal conjugate vaccine introduction: a pooled analysis of multiple surveillance sites. PLoS Med 2013;10(9):e1001517.

16. Hsu KK, Pelton SI. Heptavalent pneumococcal conjugate vaccine: current and future impact. Expert Rev Vaccin 2003;2(5):619–31.

17. Centers for Disease Control and Prevention (CDC). Progress in introduction of pneumococcal conjugate vaccine–worldwide, 2000-2008. MMWR Morb Mortal Wkly Rep 2008;57(42):1148–51.

18. Block SL, Heikkinen T, Toback SL. The efficacy of live attenuated influenza vaccine against influenza-associated acute otitis media in children. Pediatr Infect J 2011;30:203–7.

19. Lechien JR, Hans S, Simon F, et al. Association between laryngopharyngeal reflux and media otitis: a systematic review. Otol Neurotol 2021. https://doi.org/10.1097/MAO.0000000000003123.

20. Sarrell EM, Mandelberg A, Cohen HA. Efficacy of naturopathic extracts in the management of ear pain associated with AOM. Arch Pediatr Adolesc Med 2001;155:796–9.

21. Foxlee R, Johansson A, Wejfalk J, et al. Topical analgesia for acute otitis media. Cochrane Database Syst Rev 2006;(3):CD005657.

22. Dantes F, Rampes H. Do homeopathic medicines provoke adverse effects? Br Homeopath J 2000;89:S35–8.
23. Harrison H, Fixsen A, Vickers A. A randomized comparison of homoeopathic and standard care for the treatment of glue ear in children. Complement Ther Med 1999;7:132–5.
24. Jacobs J, Springer DA, Crothers D. Homeopathic treatment of AOM in children: a preliminary randomized placebo-controlled trial. Pediatr Infect J 2001;20:177–83.
25. Frei H, Thurneysen A. Homeopathy in AOM in children: treatment effect or spontaneous resolution? Br Homeopath J 2001;90:178–9.
26. Wustrow TP. Naturopathic therapy for acute otitis media. An alternative to the primary use of antibiotics. HNO 2005;53:728–34.
27. Taylor JA, Jacobs J. Homeopathic ear drops as an adjunct to standard therapy in children with acute otitis media. Homeopathy 2011;100(3):109–15.
28. Sinha MN, Siddiqui VA, Nayak C, et al. Randomized controlled pilot study to compare Homeopathy and Conventional therapy in Acute Otitis Media. Homeopathy 2012;101(1):5–12.
29. Asher BF, Seidman M, Snyderman C. Complementary and alternative medicine in otolaryngology. Laryngoscope 2001;111(8):1383–9.
30. Cohen HA, Varsano I, Kahan E. Effectiveness of an herbal preparation containing Echinacea, propolis, and vitamin C in preventing respiratory tract infections in children: a randomized, double-blind, placebo-controlled, multicenter study. Arch Pediatr Adolesc Med 2004;158:217–21.
31. Wahl RA, Aldous MB, Worden KA, et al. Echinacea purpurea and osteopathic manipulative treatment in children with recurrent otitis media: a randomized controlled trial. BMC Complement Altern Med 2008;8(1):56.
32. Schapowal A, Klein P, Johnston SL. Echinacea reduces the risk of recurrent respiratory tract infections and complications: a meta-analysis of randomized controlled trials. Adv Ther 2015;32(3):187–200.
33. Ogal M, Johnston SL, Klein P, et al. Echinacea reduces antibiotic usage in children through respiratory tract infection prevention: a randomized, blinded, controlled clinical trial. Eur J Med Res 2021;26(1):33.
34. Kontiokari T, Uhari M, Koskela M. Effect of xylitol on growth of nasopharyngeal bacteria in vitro. Antimicrobial Agents Chemother 1995;39(8):1820–3.
35. Uhari M, Kontiokari T, Koskela M. Xylitol chewing gum in prevention of AOM: double-blind randomised trials. Br Med J 1996;313:1180–4.
36. Uhari M, Kontiokari T, Niemela M. A novel use of xylitol sugar in preventing AOM. Pediatrics 1998;102:879–84.
37. Uhari M, Tapiainen T, Kontiokari T. Xylitol in preventing acute otitis media. Vaccine 2000;19(Supplement 1):S144–7.
38. Tapiainen T, Luotonen L, Kontiokari T, et al. Xylitol administered only during respiratory infections failed to prevent acute otitis media. Pediatrics 2002;109(2):E19.
39. Hautalahti O, Renko M, Tapiainen T. Failure of xylitol given three times a day for preventing AOM. Pediatr Infect J 2007;26:423–7.
40. Azarpazhooh A, Lawrence HP, Shah PS. Xylitol for preventing acute otitis media in children up to 12 years of age. Cochrane Database Syst Rev 2016;2016(8):CD007095.
41. Roos K, Hakansson EG, Holm S. Effect of recolonisation with "interfering" alpha streptococci on recurrences of acute and secretory otitis media in children: randomised placebo controlled trial. BMJ 2001;322:210–2.

42. Chen TY, Hendrickx A, Stevenson DS, et al. No evidence from a systematic review for the use of probiotics to prevent otitis media. Acta Paediatr 2020; 109(12):2515–24.

43. Hatakka K, Savilahti E, Ponka A. Effect of long-term consumption of probiotic milk on infections in children attending day care centres: double blind, randomised trial. Br Med J 2001;322:1327–9.

44. Hatakka K, Blomgren K, Pohjavuori S. Treatment of AOM with probiotics in otitis-prone children-a double-blind, placebo-controlled randomised study. Clin Nutr 2007;26:314–21.

45. Stecksén-Blicks CTS, Sjöström I. Effect of long-term consumption of milk supplemented with probiotic lactobacilli and fluoride on dental caries and general health in preschool children: a cluster-randomized study. Caries Res 2009;43:374–81.

46. Rautava S, Salminen S, Isolauri E. Specific probiotics in reducing the risk of acute infections in infancy—a randomised, double-blind, placebo-controlled study. Br J Nutr 2009;101:1722–6.

47. Cohen R, Martin E, de La Rocque F, et al. Probiotics and prebiotics in preventing episodes of acute otitis media in high-risk children: a randomized, double-blind, placebo-controlled study. Pediatr Infect Dis J 2013;32(8):810–4.

48. Marchisio P, Santagati M, Scillato M, et al. *Streptococcus salivarius* 24SMB administered by nasal spray for the prevention of acute otitis media in otitis-prone children. Eur J Clin Microbiol Infect Dis 2015;34(12):2377–83.

49. Mills MV, Henley CE, Barnes LL. The use of osteopathic manipulative treatment as adjuvant therapy in children with recurrent AOM. Arch Pediatr Adolesc Med 2003; 157:861–6.

50. Steele KM, Carreiro JE, Viola JH, et al. Effect of osteopathic manipulative treatment on middle ear effusion following acute otitis media in young children: a pilot study. J Osteopath Med 2014;114(6):436–47.

51. Degenhardt BF, Kuchera ML. Osteopathic evaluation and manipulative treatment in reducing the morbidity of otitis media: a pilot study. J Am Osteopath Assoc 2006;106:327–34.

52. Froehle RM. Ear infection: a retrospective study examining improvement from chiropractic care and analyzing for influencing factors. J Manipulative Physiol Ther 1996;19:169–77.

53. Zhang JQ, Synder BJ. Effect of toftness chiropractic adjustments for children with acute otitis media. J Vertebr Subluxation Res 2004;29:1–4.

54. Fallon JM. The role of the chiropractic adjustment in the care and treatment of 332 children with otitis media. J Clin Chiropract Pediatr 1997;2:167–83.

55. Lee KP, Carlini WG, McCormick GF. Neurologic complications following chiropractic manipulation: a survey of California neurologists. Neurology 1995;45: 1213–5.

56. Luetzenberg FS, Babu S, Seidman MD. Alternative treatments of tinnitus. Otolaryngol Clin North Am 2020;53(4):637–50.

57. Sánchez-Araujo M, Puchi A. Acupuncture prevents relapses of recurrent otitis in dogs: a 1-year follow-up of a randomised controlled trial. Acupunct Med 2011; 29:21–6.

58. Tsai SL, Reynoso E, Shin DW, et al. Acupuncture as a nonpharmacologic treatment for pain in a pediatric emergency department. Pediatr Emerg Care 2018. https://doi.org/10.1097/PEC.0000000000001619.

59. Zhang H, Li S, Liu R. Clinical and experimental study on treatment of acute catarrhal otitis media with eryanling oral liquid. Zhongguo Zhong Xi Yi Jie He Za Zhi 2000;20:743–6.

60. Sun YD, Chen LH, Hu WJ. Evaluation of the clinical efficacy of Qingqiao capsule in treating patients with secretory otitis media. Chin J Integr Med 2005;11:243–8.

61. Son MJ, Kim YE, Song YI, et al. Herbal medicines for treating acute otitis media: A Systematic review of randomised controlled trials. Complement Ther Med 2017; 35:133–9.

62. Liu SL. Therapeutic effects of borneol-walnut oil in the treatment of purulent otitis media. Zhong Xi Yi Jie He Za Zhi 1990;10(93–5):69.

63. Liao Y, Huang Y, Ou Y. Clinical and experimental study of Tongqiao tablet in treating catarrhal otitis media. Zhongguo Zhong Xi Yi Jie He Za Zhi 1998;18:668–70.

64. Sugiura Y, Ohashi Y, Nakai Y. The herbal medicine, sairei-to, enhances the mucociliary activity of the tubotympanum in the healthy guinea pig. Acta Otolaryngol Suppl 1997;531:17–20.

65. Sugiura Y, Ohashi Y, Nakai Y. The herbal medicine, sairei-to, prevents endotoxin-induced otitis media with effusion in the guinea pig. Acta Otolaryngol Suppl 1997; 531:21–33.

66. Maruyama Y, Hoshida S, Furukawa M. Effects of Japanese herbal medicine, Juzen-taiho-to, in otitis-prone children—a preliminary study. Acta Otolaryngol 2009;129:14–8.

APPENDIX 1: LIST OF COMMON HOMEOPATHIC REMEDIES USED TO TREAT OTITIS MEDIA AND CONDITIONS THEY ARE USED FOR. MOST COMMONLY USED ARE INDICATED BY AN **

List of common homeopathic remedies used to treat otitis media and conditions they are used for. Most commonly used are indicated by an **.

** *Aconitum/Aconite/Aconitum napellus*: For throbbing ear pain that comes on suddenly after exposure to cold or wind and in children with high fever and whose ears are bright red or tender to the touch. Better in the initial stages of an ear infection.

** *Belladonna*: For throbbing and sharp pain accompanied by fever, intense heat, and flushing in the outer ear and along the side of the face. Some suggest it is better for the right ear. It comes from an extract from a poisonous plant of the nightshade family and should be used with caution.

Capsicum: Treats heat and inflammation and significant pain.

** *Chamomilla*: For children with otitis media who are irritable, in great pain, and can't be consoled.

Ferrum phosphoricum: In early otitis media, this is a common remedy used; gradual onset of symptoms; patient has flushed face, doesn't like noise, wants to lie still.

Hepar Sulphuricum: Pain in ears especially with swallowing; yellowish-green discharge, wind or draft aggravates pain.

Kali muraticum: Popping and crackling sound heard in ear when swallowing and with nose blowing, hearing may be decreased, feeling of fullness and congestion in the ear. Also used to clear Eustachian tubes when fluid persists after AOM.

Lycopedium: For right-sided ear pain that is worse in the late afternoon and early evening; fullness of the ears, ringing or buzzing of the ears.

Magnesia phosphorica: Earache, especially after exposure to cold wind and drafts. May not be an infection at all, but rather nerve irritation, more right ear than left; pain relieved by heat, feels better with rubbing.

Mercurius: Good for chronic ear infections; for pain that is worse at night and may extend down into the throat; relief comes from nose blowing; earache may occur when damp or fog or weather changes occur, may salivate or sweat.

** *Pulsatilla*: For infection following exposure to cold or damp weather; the ear is often red and may have a yellowish/greenish discharge from ear or nose; ear pain may worsen after sleep and with warmth, may be alleviated by cool compresses.

Silica: For chronic or late stage infection when the child feels chilly, weak, and tired; sweating may also be present.

Verbascum: Especially left-sided otitis media, may have a cough or laryngitis as well.

APPENDIX 2: LIST OF COMMON NATURAL HEALTH PRODUCTS USED TO TREAT OTITIS MEDIA

List of common natural health products used to treat otitis media.

Chamomile (*Matricaria chamomilla*): It is thought to have antiviral properties and has been used for infant colic, digestive upset, and diarrhea. The oil fraction is believed to have the anti-infective properties, whereas the flavonoids are thought to be anti-inflammatory. There is little evidence for its use in otitis media. It comes as a tincture (1–3 mL tid; infants: 1–3 drops/lb body weight tid) and a tea (1 cup of boiling water over 1 heaping tbsp of flowers). Occasionally patients are allergic to it.

Cleavers: It is used to assist lymphatic clearance of debris during AOM or with serous otitis media. Tincture 0.5 to 2 mL three times daily. Tea is also used: 1 cup two or three times per day.

Cod liver oil: It is a source of omega-3 fatty acids and vitamins A and D. It has been shown that patients with ROM have low blood levels of some omega-3 fatty acids, vitamin A, and selenium. Safety of long-term consumption of cod liver oil is not known; studies have shown adverse health effects from polychlorinated biphenyls and dioxin residues found in fish oil.

Echinacea (Echinacea purpurea): Its activity is believed to be nonspecific activation of the immune system (including activating natural killer cells and macrophages and increasing circulating levels of alpha interferon), but there is some evidence that the caffeic esters are antibacterial and antiviral and the polyacetylenes may be bacteriostatic. It is most commonly used for treatment of upper respiratory infections, but it is not well studied for otitis media specifically. Dose of Echinacea: tinctures, either in alcohol or glycerites, are available. Children: 1–5 mL three to five times daily, infants: 1 or 2 drops/lb body weight tid. Tablets, capsules, and whole herb taken as tea or infusion are also used orally.

Elder flower/berry (*Sambucus nigra*), European alder (*Sambucus canadensis*), or American elder (*Caprifoliaceae*): It is used to dry excessive nasal secretions and also has antiviral activity, best during AOM, especially if an upper respiratory tract infection is present. Tincture 0.5–3 mL three times daily. Tea is also used: 1 cup 2 or three times per day.

Elecampane root (Inula helenium). Bacteriostatic and antiviral activity and may strengthen resistance of mucosal lining. Can be used in AOM or chronic serous otitis media. Tincture 0.5–2 mL three times daily.

Eucalyptus: Administered usually as steam inhalation and is used mostly late in the course of AOM.

Goldenseal (*Hydrastis canadensis*): It is used only during AOM when there is evidence of purulence. Tincture 0.5–2 mL three times daily.

Marshmallow (*Althea officinalis*): It is used for soothing inflamed mucous membranes and helps loosen and moisten thick mucus. In otitis media, it is used particularly to help open the Eustachian tube. Tincture: 1 drop per 2 pounds of body weight (up to 2 mL) three to six times daily. Decoction: 1 tbsp root simmered in 1 cup of water for 10 min; 1 to 3 tbsp of the strained liquid is taken two to six times daily. If taking with prescription medications, take the medications at least 1 h before or 2 h after taking marshmallow root, because the herb may decrease the absorption of drugs.

Mullein (*V. thapsus*): It decreases phlegm and strengthens the respiratory mucosa and acts topically as a local anti-inflammatory. It can be used as topical ear oil for otitis externa. For otitis media, it is chosen to unblock the Eustachian tube and to decrease inflammation. Tincture: 1 drop per 2 pounds of body weight every 4 h. Tea: 1 to 2 tsp herb/cup of boiling water, steeped covered 10 to 15 min, and strained; 1 to 4 cups per day.

Usnea (*Usnea barbata*): It has antiviral and antibacterial properties and is used during acute episodes of otitis media. Tincture 0.5–5 mL three times daily.

Xylitol: It is used as an artificial sweetener in chewing gum and has been shown to inhibit the growth of *Streptococcus pneumoniae* by changing the ultrastructure of the bacterial capsule. Many studies show effectiveness of xylitol (gum > syrup) in preventing otitis media when given five times daily. It can cause abdominal pain and loose stools, which leads to large dropout rates from many studies and difficulty drawing meaningful conclusions. It also prevents dental caries.

Guided Meditation (Hypnosis) and Whole Person Health

Robert A. Levine, PhD[a],*, Charlene S. Levine, LMT[a],
Michael D. Seidman, MD[b]

KEYWORDS

- Holistic • APRI system • Health care • Hypnosis • Guided meditation • ACL

KEY POINTS

- In whole person health, the general view is that imbalances in the whole being in mind-body-spirit are causal in many diseases, and balancing the whole person can help resolve ill-health.
- The power of the whole person health approach is that it promotes optimal health as a means of preventing the onset of chronic ill-health conditions and often reversing and eliminating them without prescription medicines.
- Stress is a silent killer, and the automatic generation of internal stress in response to circumstances or triggers results from hidden automatic patterns that reside in the subconscious mind.
- The Automatic Pattern Recognition and Interruption System (APRI) has many natural modalities that when used together create a powerful and freeing health-optimizing strategy when ill-health is caused by these unwanted patterns.
- Guided meditation, the foundation of the APRI system, helps the conscious and subconscious minds connect, so that unwanted subconscious automatic patterns can be interrupted, and people become free to achieve what they really want for their health and life.

WHOLE PERSON (HOLISTIC) HEALTH VERSUS CONVENTIONAL HEALTH-CARE APPROACHES

When thinking about "whole person health" or "holistic health," it is appropriate to focus on the mind–body–spirit connection and the role that the mind plays in contributing to health status.[1] Before the time of the French philosopher and scientist, René Descartes, in the 1600s, each person was viewed and treated by many civilizations as

a Community Wellness Resources LLC, 7040 Seminole Pratt Whitney Road, Suite 25-61, Loxahatchee, FL 33470, USA; b Advent Health Celebration, 400 Celebration Place, Celebration, FL 34747, USA
* Corresponding author.
E-mail address: bob@drboblevine.com

Otolaryngol Clin N Am 55 (2022) 1077–1086
https://doi.org/10.1016/j.otc.2022.07.001
0030-6665/22/© 2022 Elsevier Inc. All rights reserved.

an integrated whole in mind–body–spirit. Descartes was the first to initiate thinking that there are distinct domains of human "construction" and that the exactness of science was needed to explain the origins of ill-health; thus, the mind, body, and spirit became viewed as separate domains distinct from one another. In other words, health-care practitioners could work on the body domain without considering the mind or spirit domains. At this point, whole person health went on the decline. With the emphasis on attempting to resolve illness by focusing on the body, this has led conventional medicine to theorize that disease is caused by dysfunctions at the cellular level. In whole person health, the general view is that imbalances in the whole being in mind–body–spirit are causal in disease, and the effects of disease have to be reflected in cellular and fluid changes (where else could whole person disease imbalances show up?). In the last several decades, there has been an opening for whole person (holistic) health to play a role in helping to improve the health status of the world population. The world will be a better place when conventional care and holistic practices can be truly integrated.

Whole person health can contribute to healing chronic illness but is probably most valuable for society in helping create a lifestyle to optimize health and well-being. In conventional health care, more emphasis is placed on dealing with chronic illness once symptoms present, such as in cardiovascular disease,[2] diabetes,[3] migraine headaches,[4] or cancer.[5] In conventional care, we rely mostly on pharmaceuticals to manage symptoms. Pharmaceuticals, many with potent side effects, address symptoms of chronic illness rather than addressing the underlying source of ill-health. Holistic health attempts to balance the whole living being in mind, body, and spirit so that health status can be optimized, and ill-health can be minimized. When the whole being is balanced, cellular and fluid changes that were identified in conventional care as problematic can also come into balance in a disease-free state. As simple example is the use of statins by conventional medicine to lower cholesterol.[6] People are encouraged to be on statins for the rest of their lives when their cholesterol is high and other blood lipids are out of balance. In this case, many of the out-of-balance whole people exhibit lipid changes in the blood that over the long term can cause cellular changes detectable by conventional medicine. However, it has been shown that for many people, high cholesterol and lipid imbalances can be corrected through appropriate nutrition and exercise.[7] This example demonstrates that balancing the health of the whole person can reverse changes that are detectable by conventional medicine, and the long-term use of pharmaceuticals can be avoided. There are many diseases where balancing the whole person to improve/optimize health should be encouraged. A question that arises is, how do we reliably and easily achieve optimal balance of the whole person to prevent or resolve chronic illness without the use of pharmaceuticals? This question is addressed later in this article.

One of the main objectives of a whole person approach is to have individuals take responsibility for their health, learn healthy practices in the areas of nutrition, exercise, and mind health, and ultimately become their own healers whenever possible.[1] Of course, we can all take advantage of the power of conventional health care to assist with emergency medicine, surgeries, cosmetics, and others. However, conventional medicine has always been challenged when it comes to reversing and eliminating chronic ill-health conditions without long-term use of pharmaceuticals; this has created the need for whole person health. The power of the whole person health approach is that it promotes optimal health as a means of preventing the onset of chronic ill-health conditions and often reversing and eliminating them without the long-term use of prescription medicines (**Figs. 1–3**).

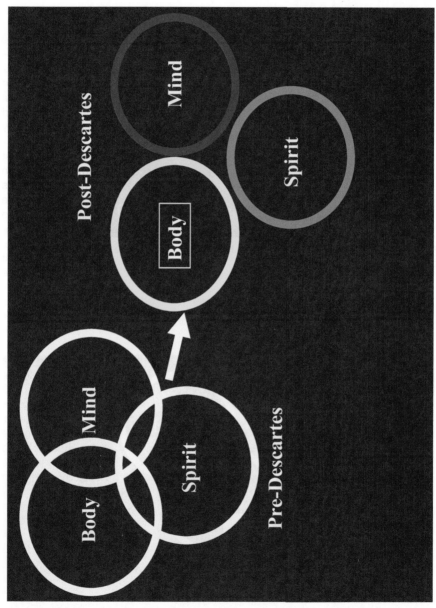

Fig. 1. Descartes (in 1600s) initiated thinking of distinct domains of human "construction" and the exactness of science.

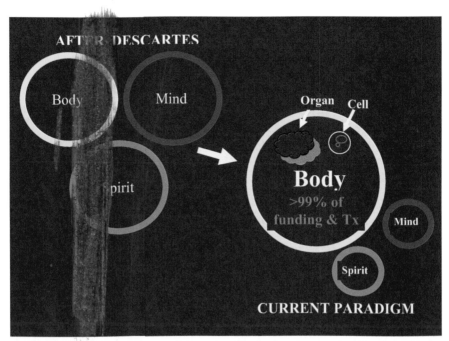

Fig. 2. Conventional Western medicine. Hypothesis: diseases are CAUSED by INTERNAL cellular/organ dysfuction.

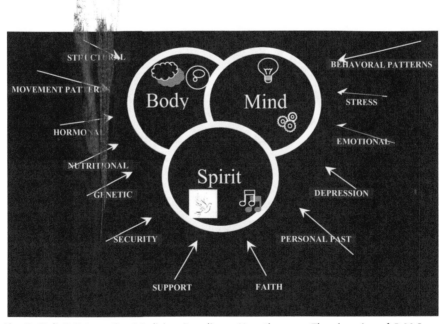

Fig. 3. Holistic/Integrative Medicine Paradigm—Hypotheses: • The domains of B-M-S are inseparable and out-of-balance in disease. • Optimal treatment involves addressing all domains TOGETHER.

THE POWER OF THE MIND AND PLACEBO

One of the hallmarks of holistic health is harnessing the power of the mind to facilitate healing and reversal of ill-health conditions. One of the best examples of mind power is with placebo. There are many definitions of placebo and most are related to "an inert or innocuous substance used especially in controlled experiments testing the efficacy of another substance (such as a drug)." A meta-analysis of 186 trials (16,655 patients) analyzing placebo effects concluded that approximately half of the overall treatment effect in RCTs seems attributable to contextual effects (placebo) rather than to the specific effect of treatments.[8] Would it be valuable to find a way to harness the power of placebo to be effective for an even higher percentage of people? It is in this area where we thought that harnessing the power of the mind, as discussed below, can provide dramatic benefit.

Why is it that some people have a placebo response that is identical to the beneficial effect of a pharmaceutical and others do not? In our view, the benefits of placebo happen because the people receiving placebo have a future vision that the treatment will be effective for them; they have no doubt this is the case and, what is key here, is that nothing in their mind is in the way of achieving the health benefit. Someone who does not respond to placebo may have a future vision that they are in trouble and the treatment will not work. You may have heard the phrase, what the mind focuses on expands. If people are able to freely focus on getting the benefit of placebo that can "expand," then the likelihood of a positive placebo response increases. Whereas, if people are focused on being anxious or worried that the treatment will not work for them, this may interfere with a positive placebo response. Perhaps when people learn how to harness and direct their mind power toward healing, the percentage of placebo responders will increase, and more importantly, people will be more healthy and vital.

HYPNOSIS, GUIDED MEDITATION, AND RELATED THERAPIES FOR HARNESSING MIND POWER

Hypnosis is one of the most misunderstood "therapies" in all of health care, and how hypnosis works is subject to much conjecture.[9] We will provide some simple explanations and models that will explain how hypnosis and related therapies are likely to work and why hypnosis is one of the most powerful health-improvement strategies. If you are still reading this, you are not one of the group of people that thinks hypnosis is to be feared because a person gives up control of their mind to another, hypnosis has little value in helping resolve chronic illnesses, or it is too new age and nonscientific. Some people are more accepting of hypnosis when they learn that hypnosis can be considered an umbrella over many other disciplines, including guided imagery, guided visualization, and guided meditation. Neurolinguistic programming can also be considered to be under the hypnosis umbrella. There are also an increasing number of clinical studies being published on the value of these hypnosis-related techniques (eg, see refs[10–12]). We practice guided meditation because we have developed specific language to help people harness mind power and achieve desired results, which is what all the practitioners of the previously mentioned techniques want to accomplish.

What does it mean to harness mind power? One can take a very simple view of the mind and divide it into the conscious and subconscious components. By definition, people at any given moment have no idea what is in their subconscious mind because it is below the conscious level; most people do not even know that they have a subconscious mind. In our clinical experience with thousands of individuals from all walks of life, it is apparent that the subconscious mind is the predominant controller of how life goes for people. For example, someone who is overweight and consciously does not want to eat the chocolate cake eats it anyway, as if they have no control. Well, they do not have conscious control. How did that happen? The subconscious mind dictated the action and overrode the conscious desire. However, any time the subconscious mind is aligned with the desire of the conscious mind, then conscious action can happen. The bottom line is the subconscious mind always wins and dictates the action (eg, thoughts, speaking, movement) when not aligned with the conscious mind.

Any hypnosis-related technique, when implemented properly, can harness mind power by connecting the conscious and subconscious minds. This allows for information that was buried in the subconscious to be revealed to the conscious mind, and there is the opportunity to reprogram the subconscious mind to support what people consciously want. Once the information reaches the conscious mind, mind–body connection experts can work with people to help them reprogram their subconscious mind using some of the techniques described below.

A dramatic demonstration of harnessing the power of the mind to affect the mind–body connection made national news in 2004 when we facilitated anesthesia for a patient undergoing anterior cruciate ligament (ACL) reconstruction. The patient (the lead editor of this book (M.D.S.)) had ACL surgery and used hypnosis (guided meditation) and acupuncture to provide anesthesia. No general or spinal anesthesia were used (see this 5-minute video; https://www.youtube.com/watch?v=7iOgxdWQauo&t=83s). To our knowledge, this was a surgical first in the United States and demonstrates that, with proper training, mind power can be harnessed to achieve a remarkable feat in the unified domain of mind–body–spirit.

AUTOMATIC PATTERNS IN THE SUBCONSCIOUS MIND THAT CONTROL LIFE ACTIVITIES

An important question is, what has the subconscious mind not aligned with conscious desires? We could write books on this topic, yet we can break it down simply by saying that the subconscious mind contains automatic patterns that drive actions, even when the actions are consciously not desired (eg, eat the cake). We could call these unwanted automatic patterns because they interfere or block actions that we want to take. If there is an automatic pattern buried in the subconscious mind that contradicts an action someone consciously wants to take, he or she will be unable to take that action. The subconscious mind always wins!

Some of the components that make up automatic patterns residing in the subconscious mind include the following:

- How and what we think of ourselves and others.
- How and what we say about ourselves and others.
- How we listen to others and our internal voice.
- How we move (walk, stand/sit, bend/reach).
- How, what, and when we eat.
- How we relate to ourselves.
- How we relate to others.
- Our view of the world.
- Parts of our belief systems.
- Repetitive activities that we do not want to do, yet cannot help (eg, excessive drinking, drugs, eating, smoking, and other uses of tobacco).
- How we automatically generate STRESS in response to circumstances.
- Everything, nearly every aspect of life, has a place in automatic patterns at certain times.

ORIGINS OF AUTOMATIC PATTERNS

Where do these automatic patterns that reside in the subconscious mind come from? In our experience, most of these automatic patterns in the subconscious mind are formulated early in life, usually before the age of 6 or 7. Some early traumatic event happens, and the child instantly invents some disempowering conclusion about themselves, which gets buried immediately in the subconscious mind; this becomes an automatic pattern that can express in a variety of ways (see example below). Note that there is a wide variety of traumatic events, many of which would not seem to be traumatic yet were for the individuals. Moreover, invented conclusions are not good or bad, true or false, right or wrong; they just happen. Once the disempowering-invented conclusion is buried in the subconscious and can drive an automatic pattern, the child at times will compensate for this during much of their life, without realizing that automatic patterns are driving life sometimes in unwanted ways. When driven by an automatic pattern, certain desired changes are difficult, if not impossible. People can feel trapped and feeling like there is no way out. We speculate that this inability to make changes and take certain desired actions leads people to think and feel there is something wrong with them, that they are on some level inadequate; this stays with them until the automatic pattern is interrupted.

How do children start the compensation process? The compensation process can take many forms. A simple example is a child aged younger than 6 or 7 years who has some traumatic experience that causes the child to invent the disempowering conclusion of being stupid and he or she consciously did not know they invented that conclusion; this conclusion became buried in the subconscious. There are many ways to compensate for having concluded being stupid. Some people might compensate throughout their teen and adult life by being funny all the time, even making fun at inappropriate times because of being driven by the automatic "stupid" pattern. Another compensation for people inventing the conclusion they are stupid is to drive themselves to academic excellence by getting advanced degrees (doctor, lawyer). Here is a practical tip. When someone consciously sets a high goal and achieves it, if there is no celebration of the achievement, then it is likely that the person was driven by an automatic pattern. When the person is driven by an automatic pattern that has them feel in some way inadequate, no amount of achievement will erase the effect of the pattern and have the person feel successful until the automatic pattern is interrupted. Here is where the harnessing the power of the mind is ever so valuable.

AUTOMATIC STRESS REACTIONS

Stress and anxiety are most likely the most prominent silent killers and are significant contributors to nearly all, if not all, ill-health conditions. It is hard to identify the long-term effects of stress and anxiety, much like cigarette smoking, because human beings can withstand a large magnitude of insults to health over decades before illness finally surfaces. Many people do not consider that their experience of stress is an automatic phenomenon. If it were not automatic, people would just say, "Oh, I'm through experiencing stress, and I'm now a stress-free person for the rest of my life." Unfortunately, it does not work that way. People experience stress because the expression of stress is automatic. It is the result of a subconsciously driven automatic pattern, which cannot be helped. If it could be helped, people would just let it go and be done with stress. There would never be any stress.

It is really important for people to understand that the stress that they experience is generated from within themselves. For example, if somebody is afraid to fly in an airplane, and somebody is very comfortable with it, the person who is afraid of that will experience stress, and the person who is very comfortable with flying an airplane will not experience stress. The person who is experiencing stress out of fear of flying an airplane, they are generating the stress from within themselves. Therefore, when somebody understands that they are generating their own stress in reaction to circumstances in their life—whether it is external circumstances, or whether it is the way they are thinking about things, the thoughts they are having—they are generating the stress. That is very powerful when people understand that, because once they understand that they are generating their own stress, they actually have some power to get relief from that stress. Because they are causing the stress, they can resolve it. Once people learn to get stress relief and spend very little time in stress, their health can improve because ill-health fades away. The automatic generation of internal stress in response to circumstances or triggers results from automatic patterns that reside in the subconscious mind. Thus, automatic stress reactions will continue to wreak havoc on human health until people learn how to be free of them.

AUTOMATIC PATTERN RECOGNITION AND INTERRUPTION SYSTEM©

To help people recognize when they are being affected by an unwanted automatic pattern keeping them from accomplishing desired results, we have developed the Automatic Pattern Recognition and Interruption (APRI) System©. The APRI System allows people to:

- identify their unique subconscious mind-driven automatic habits and patterns that are at the core of causing, maintaining, and/or worsening chronic ill-health conditions of all types, and
- interrupt those automatic patterns, which frees them to make rapid changes that improve health, performance, relationships, creativity, and productivity.

Representative modalities and approaches that are part of the APRI system include:

- *Guided meditation:* To recognize and interrupt automatic patterns, hidden in the subconscious mind.
- *Future Visioning:* To shift the focus from past results and failures to focusing on achieving rapid health improvement and other desired life results moving toward the future.
- *Muscle Stretching and Release:* Uses our *Effective Muscle Release©* process to identify and release overly contracted muscles that are stiff, have restricted mobility, cause pain, and create postural misalignments.
- *Repetitive Movements of Daily Living:* To have participants correct dysfunctional repetitive movement patterns (eg, walking, sitting/standing, bending/reaching) that may be reinforcing pain, postural misalignments, fatigue, and sleep disturbance.
- *Effective Communication Skills:* To eliminate miscommunication stress because most stress are triggered during communication.
- *Health Activities at Home/Work:* To empower participants to take responsibility, become their own healers, and accomplish rapid, sustained improvement in health and performance.
- *Long-term Support Tools:* To maintain and enhance long-term health improvement far beyond the end of programs.

These modalities have been used together in large in-person multisession group wellness programs that the lead author (R.A.L.) delivered to Chrysler, Dow, and other corporations. These clinical studies proved that the multimodal approach using these modalities was effective in significantly relieving chronic pain, stress, anxiety, sleep disturbance, and other measured outcomes. Guided meditation is the foundation of the APRI system because it helps people recognize and interrupt unwanted subconscious automatic patterns causing ill-health and holding people back from achieving what they want for their health and life. Guided meditation also provides effective accelerated learning and retention in the conscious and subconscious minds of all the information learned through the other modalities. In our clinical experience, the use of guided meditation or other hypnosis-related modalities is the fastest and most efficient way to support clients making desired changes and achieving desired results, including resolving ill-health and achieving optimal health. Whole person health in our hands relies on harnessing the power of the mind at the subconscious and conscious levels.

SUMMARY

Whole person (holistic) health deals with the mind–body–spirit connection as a unified domain. Balancing the whole person's health makes it possible for cells, tissues, and fluids that are out of balance in disease to come back into balance as the person heals from illness. Guided meditation is the hallmark of the APRI System because it allows for reprogramming and harnessing the power of the subconscious mind, which is a critical controller of life activities. The APRI System can facilitate rapid change in people, once they are freed up from subconscious mind constraints. The goal of the modern, transformed health-care system should be to combine the best of conventional care and whole person health to produce the best health care on the planet. We are not there yet, but we are on the way!

To find out more, go to www.DrBobTalks.com.

CLINICS CARE POINTS

Pearls:

- Multimodal care, where certain modalities are combined and used simultaneously in the same protocol can provide synergy for healing.

- Hypnosis/Guided Meditation has been shown to help a variety of conditions and is even more effective when combined with other natural therapies.

- Many people prefer natural therapies as a way of avoiding side effects from pharmaceuticals.

- Hypnosis supports people in harnessing the power of their mind, which has them gaining control of their mind.

Pitfalls:

- Unimodal care, where a single modality is used, or individual modalities are used sequentially rather than simultaneously, is far inferior to multimodal care.

- Patients might not want natural therapies and prefer to use pharmaceuticals to help improve their health.

- A small percentage of patients fear hypnosis allows someone else to control their mind.

REFERENCES

1. Collinge William. The American holistic health Association Complete Guide to Alternative medicine. New York: Warner Books; 1996.
2. Tan SY, Mei Wong JL, Sim YJ, et al. Type 1 and 2 diabetes mellitus: A review on current treatment approach and gene therapy as potential intervention. Diabetes Metab Syndr 2019;13(1):364–72.
3. Behera SS, Pramanik K, Nayak MK. Recent Advancement in the Treatment of Cardiovascular Diseases: Conventional Therapy to Nanotechnology. Curr Pharm Des 2015;21(30):4479–97.
4. Lipton RB, Silberstein SD. Episodic and chronic migraine headache: breaking down barriers to optimal treatment and prevention. Headache 2015;55(Suppl 2):103–22.
5. Baudino TA. Targeted Cancer Therapy: The Next Generation of Cancer Treatment. Curr Drug Discov Technol 2015;12(1):3–20.
6. Sirtori CR. The pharmacology of statins. Pharmacol Res 2014;88:3–11.
7. Varady KA, Jones Peter JH. Combination diet and exercise interventions for the treatment of dyslipidemia: an effective preliminary strategy to lower cholesterol levels? J Nutr 2005;135(8):1829–35.
8. Haflidadóttir Sigurlaug H, Juhl Carsten B, Nielsen Sabrina M, et al. Placebo response and effect in randomized clinical trials: meta-research with focus on contextual effects. Trials 2021;22:493.
9. Douglas Flemons. Toward a Relational Theory of Hypnosis. Amer J Clin Hypn 2020;62(4):344–63.
10. Leonard S Milling, Valentine Keara E, McCarley Hannah S, et al. A Meta-Analysis of Hypnotic Interventions for Depression Symptoms: High Hopes for Hypnosis? Am J Clin Hypn 2019;61(3):227–43.
11. Leonard S Milling, Valentine Keara E, LoStimolo Lindsey M, et al. Hypnosis and the Alleviation of Clinical Pain: A Comprehensive Meta-Analysis. Int J Clin Exp Hypn 2021;69(3):297–322.
12. Carlson Linda E, Toivonen Kirsti, Flynn Michelle, et al. The Role of Hypnosis in Cancer Care. Curr Oncol Rep 2018;20(12):93.

Acupuncture and the Otolaryngology-Head & Neck Surgery Patient

Chau T. Nguyen, MD[a],*, Malcolm B. Taw, MD[b]

KEYWORDS

- Acupuncture • Otolaryngology • Otology • Laryngology • Rhinology • Pediatrics
- Posttonsillectomy pain

KEY POINTS

- Acupuncture, a part of Traditional Chinese medicine (TCM), has been used for millennia to treat a variety of medical conditions including those related to ENT (Ear, nose, & throat).
- Acupuncture in ENT involves the placement of needles at specific points in the body to exert a desired physiologic effect restoring health and balancing homeostasis.
- The mechanism of action of acupuncture involves a complex interplay between local chemical mediators, regional pain modulation, central limbic processing, and expectation-induced placebo analgesia.
- Within the last twenty years, much research has been conducted on the role of acupuncture for post-tonsillectomy pain management, otologic disease, and rhinolaryngologic applications including tinnitus, imbalance, rhinitis, sinusitis, dysphonia, and dysphagia.

ACUPUNCTURE IN OTOLARYNGOLOGY

The use of acupuncture among US adults was estimated at nearly 40% in 2012.[1] A study from the United Kingdom in 2010 found 60% of otolaryngologic patients had used a form of complementary or integrative medicine, with greater than a third in the last year alone. Acupuncture was the second most common nonherbal therapy used after massage.[2]

Acupuncture, a therapeutic modality of traditional Chinese medicine (TCM), has been used for millennia in Asian countries. It involves the placement of needles into specific points along the body[3] and has been used as early as the fifth century BC for various otolaryngologic disorders.[4] According to TCM theory, energy or vitality

[a] Division of Otolaryngology-Head & Neck Surgery, Ventura County Medical Center, 300 Hillmont Avenue, Suite 401, Ventura, CA 93003, USA; [b] UCLA Center for East-West Medicine, 1250 La Venta Drive, Suite 101A, Westlake Village, CA 91361, USA
* Corresponding author.
E-mail address: chau.nguyen@ventura.org

Otolaryngol Clin N Am 55 (2022) 1087–1099
https://doi.org/10.1016/j.otc.2022.06.011
0030-6665/22/© 2022 Elsevier Inc. All rights reserved.
oto.theclinics.com

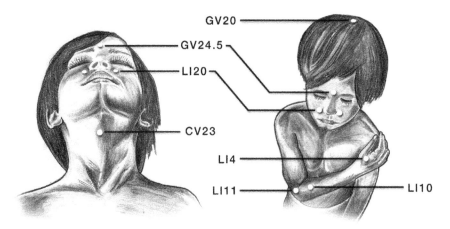

Fig. 1. Acupuncture points used for posttonsillectomy. (*From* Ochi JW. Acupuncture instead of codeine for tonsillectomy pain in children. Int J Pediatr Otorhinolaryngol. 2013 Dec;77(12):2058-62. https://doi.org/10.1016/j.ijporl.2013.10.008. Epub 2013 Oct 20. PMID: 24210291.)

called qi flows throughout the body along channels or meridians. Disruption of this flow may lead to impaired function and disease. Acupuncture seeks to restore health and homeostasis through accessing specific points along targeted meridians (**Fig. 1**).

MECHANISM OF ACTION

There are many proposed mechanisms of action for the effects of acupuncture. When a needle is inserted into an acupoint, the sensation elicited is often described as a deep ache, soreness, heaviness, or even numbness. This is referred to as "de qi" in TCM. From a neuroanatomic perspective, this sensation is generated from the activation of various sensory receptors, small fiber-innervated nociceptors and myelinated fiber-innervated mechanoreceptors.[5] Acupuncture stimulation may create a steady stream of impulses transmitted to the substantia gelatinosa in the spinal cord causing the gate for pain impulses to close.[6] It may work in a similar fashion to transcutaneous electrical nerve stimulation by selectively activating large diameter nonnoxious afferents (A-beta) to reduce nociceptor cell activity and sensitization at a segmental level in the central nervous system.[7] Brain imaging studies using functional MRI have shown that acupuncture modulates the limbic network, an important intrinsic regulatory system, with significant overlap to the default mode of the resting brain.[8] On a molecular level, the effect of acupuncture was blocked by naloxone,[9] suggesting a role of endorphins, and increased nitric oxide levels may promote its effect by increasing the local blood circulation.[10] Adenosine has also been found to play a key role. A study in 2010 demonstrated that acupuncture had no effect on adenosine A1 receptor knockout mice, whereas it relieved discomfort in two-thirds of normal mice with local adenosine levels 24 times greater than before treatment. A drug that prevented the uptake of adenosine, deoxycoformycin, increased the length of time adenosine remained in the tissues and the length of time the treatment was effective.[11] Finally, the role of the placebo response has been explored, with acupuncture possibly exerting specific neurophysiologic effects combined with expectation-induced placebo analgesia for pain conditions.[12]

Table 1
Clinical applications of acupuncture in otolaryngology

Pediatrics	Posttonsillectomy pain
Laryngology	Hoarseness SD Dysphagia poststroke
Otology	Tinnitus Cervical vertigo SSNHL Meniere disease Bell's palsy
Rhinology	AR Inferior turbinate hypertrophy Chronic sinusitis

OVERVIEW

Within otolaryngology, acupuncture has been used for a variety of conditions encompassing otology, laryngology, rhinology, and pediatrics.[13] Acupuncture has been used in pediatric pain conditions ranging from headache, to complex regional pain, cancer pain, and perioperative pain **Table 1**.[14]

POSTTONSILLECTOMY PAIN MANAGEMENT

In 2009, a study by Vokow and colleagues showed otolaryngologists to be the leading prescribers of opioids in the 0-to-9-year old age group.[15] Ever since the Food and Drug Administration ban in 2013 on codeine for posttonsillectomy pain in children,[16] there has been a renewed interest in effective nonopioid therapies.

One of the earliest studies on acupuncture for posttonsillectomy pain management was done by Dr James Ochi in 2013, who retrospectively reviewed 56 cases of children and adolescents after adenotonsillectomy during a 3 month period. These patients were asked to use acetaminophen and/or ibuprofen as analgesics at home, but no opioids, and were offered acupuncture in the office if their pain persisted. Thirty-one patients received acupuncture and the LI4 acupoint was always used, in addition to CV23, GV24.5, GV20, LI20, LI10, and LI11, depending on the response and author experience. The mean reported pain level before acupuncture was 5.52 out of 10 on the faces pain score-revised scale (SD = 2.28), falling to 1.92 (SD = 2.43) after acupuncture. The duration of effect varied, with 30% reporting pain relief greater than 60 hours and 30% less than 3 hours.[17]

A group from Stanford performed a randomized, double-blind, placebo-controlled trial of intraoperative acupuncture for posttonsillectomy pain and enrolled 59 children.[18] Through home surveys of patients, they found significant improvement in pain control in the acupuncture treatment-group, postoperatively ($P = .006$). There were no reported adverse effects. Another prospective, double-blind, randomized controlled trial included 46 patients, who were divided into 3 cohorts (true acupuncture vs control acupuncture vs Drug-based treatment). All patients received nonsteroidal anti-inflammatory drugs but the differences between both acupuncture groups and the drug group were significant ($P < .01$) with the longest effect found in the true acupuncture group.[19]

In 2018, a literature review of complementary and alternative medical treatment of posttonsillectomy pain and nausea found the greatest amount of evidence for

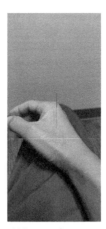

Fig. 2. Acupuncture needling at the LI4 acupoint.

acupuncture and honey. Both were deemed cost effective and safe.[20] Because patients, parents, and providers seek nonopioid alternatives, acupuncture may play a useful adjunct role. A survey of nearly 400 parents showed 98% chose acupuncture for their child when offered with tonsillectomy for pain relief.[21] A systematic review found most adverse events in pediatric acupuncture were categorized as mild, such as pain and bruising.[22]

In 2020, a prospective, randomized controlled trial was done on auricular acupuncture (Battlefield acupuncture protocol, BFA) for adult patients who underwent tonsillectomy at a tertiary care Naval Hospital. Ninety-nine patients completed the study and received either BFA or control (ear bandages). Pain scores for the acupuncture group following tonsillectomy were found to be significantly lower than the control group on the day of surgery (2.9, 4.3; $P = .01$) but there was no statistically significant difference in pain thereafter.[23] In a 2021 guideline on procedure-specific postoperative pain management recommendations for tonsillectomy, interventions that improved postoperative pain were paracetamol, nonsteroidal anti-inflammatory drugs, intravenous dexamethasone, ketamine (only assessed in children), gabapentinoids, dexmedetomidine, honey, and acupuncture (**Fig. 2**).[24]

LARYNGOLOGY APPLICATIONS

Researchers in Hong Kong performed a mixed-model, prospective randomized, placebo-controlled, blinded study evaluating wound healing and the local inflammatory milieu of the larynx in dysphonic patients with phonotrauma pathologic condition before and after acupuncture.[25] Anti-inflammatory cytokine interleukin (IL)-10 and proinflammatory cytokine IL-1β levels were measured in the laryngeal secretions of 17 subjects with vocal nodules, and were given acupuncture or sham acupuncture at voice-related acupoints. A significant increase in the anti-inflammatory cytokine IL-10 was found in the genuine acupuncture group (N = 9) but not in the sham acupuncture group (N = 8), whereas there was an inverse correlation of the proinflammatory IL-1β level for each group. The anti-inflammatory increase, however, was not seen at 24 hours. This same group investigated the effects of acupuncture on benign vocal fold pathologic condition including vocal fold nodules, polyps, and chronic laryngitis using the voice and endoscopic measurement and quality of life instrument, voice activity and participation profile.[26] Eighty-four patients had completed the study.

Three groups (genuine vs sham acupuncture and no intervention control) were examined for 3 months. For acupuncture, 12 sessions were applied during 6 weeks, at 30 minutes each by a trained acupuncturist. Acupoints used included ST-9, LU-7, LI-4, K-6, and CV-23. Significant improvement in vocal function was found, as indicated by the maximum fundamental frequency produced, and also perceived quality of life, for both the genuine and sham acupuncture groups but not in the control no treatment group. In addition, the genuine acupuncture group demonstrated a significant reduction in the size of vocal fold lesions. This group also evaluated salivary cortisol levels as a surrogate for emotional stress in subjects with phonotraumatic injuries. Eighteen female subjects, all with phonotraumatic injuries, were randomized to either genuine or sham acupuncture during a 30 minute session. Saliva samples were collected from each subject before, during, and after acupuncture. The findings showed that the subjects' salivary cortisol concentration did not decrease after acupuncture, and while the authors surmised that acupuncture may not be able to reduce the emotional stress level in female dysphonic speakers,[27] a validated quality of life questionnaire would likely have been a better measurement tool.

Stress and a history of extensive voice use have been associated with the onset of another voice disorder: spasmodic dysphonia (SD), a rare focal laryngeal dystonia affecting more women than men, with age of onset after 40 years and an estimated prevalence of 1 in 100,000. One mechanism for this may be related to painful stimuli causing neural plasticity changes in the basal ganglia, which could lead to the development of dystonia.[28] Two small studies have looked at using acupuncture for SD. In a 1997 case-control report, 2 men with adductor SD were treated: with botulinum toxin injection in one, whereas the other received acupuncture therapy. Using fundamental frequency, acoustic perturbation measurements, durational measurements of voice and speech, and spectrographic analysis, acupuncture was comparable to botulinum toxin injection at up to 1 year follow-up.[29] A slightly larger study of 10 patients with SD was reported on in 2003. Patients were evaluated pretreatment and posttreatment using the CSL (computerized speech lab) Motor Speech Profile (MSP), Unified Spasmodic Dysphonia Rating Scale, and Voice Handicap Index (VHI). Significant differences were found for some MSP measures as well as all 3 subtests of the VHI, with an average score difference of 17 points.[30]

In 2021, 2 separate groups performed systematic reviews and meta-analyses of acupuncture for poststroke dysphagia. Zhong and colleagues analyzed 35 RCTs (randomized controlled trials) involving 3024 patients and found that acupuncture combined with other interventions was better than that of the control group for the standardized swallowing assessment score (mean difference [MD] = -3.78, 95% CI: -4.64 to -2.91, $P < .00001$), Ichiro Fujishima rating scale score (MD = 1.68, 95% CI: 1.16–2.20, $P < .00001$), videofluoroscopic swallowing study (VFSS) score (MD = 2.26, 95% CI: 1.77–2.74, $P < .00001$), and water swallowing test score (MD = -1.21, 95% CI: -1.85 to -0.57, $P = .0002$). No serious adverse events were reported.[31] Similarly, Lu and colleagues reviewed 39 RCTs and confirmed the effectiveness of the experimental group was higher than that of the control group (relative risk [RR] = 1.23, 95% confidence interval [CI]: 1.19–1.27, $P < .00001$). The drinking test grading score of patients in the experimental group was lower than that of the control group (MD = -0.75, 95% CI: -1.11 to -0.41, $P < .0001$), the swallowing scores of patients in the experimental group were lower than those in the control group (MD = -4.63, 95% CI: -5.68 to -3.59, $P < .00001$), Fujishima eating–swallowing rating score of the experimental group was higher than that of the control group (standardized mean difference [SMD] = 1.92, 95% CI: 1.30 to 2.54, $P < .00001$), the score of the dysphagia-specific quality of life scale of the experimental group was higher than that of the control group (SMD = 2.02, 95% CI: 0.82–3.22, P = .0001), and finally VFSS of the experimental group was higher than that of the control group (MD = 2.53, 95% CI: 1.89–3.17, P < .00001).[32] Both groups concluded that current evidence supports acupuncture to facilitate improvement in the swallowing function of patients with poststroke dysphagia.

OTOLOGIC APPLICATIONS

In 2014, the American Academy of Otolaryngology-Head and Neck Surgery (AAO-HNS) published a clinical practice guideline (CPG) on tinnitus.[33] No recommendation was given on the use of acupuncture for tinnitus based on Grade C evidence. A systematic review conducted in 2012 found an insufficient size and quality of RCTs to make any definitive conclusions about the effectiveness of acupuncture for the treatment of tinnitus.[34] Earlier research suggested a connection between tinnitus and chronic pain, and hypothesized tinnitus to be a form of phantom auditory pain, considering both are subjective sensations that may change in quality and character over time, have the potential to be masked, and are under the control of the central nervous system with limited success in efforts to treat both.[35]

More recently, a systematic review and meta-analysis of 8 RCTs among 504 patients showed no significant differences in the visual analog score (VAS) changes (MD = −1.81, 95% CI = −3.69–0.07; P = .06) between acupuncture and control groups but favorable effects of acupuncture on tinnitus handicap inventory score (MD = −10.11, 95% CI = −12.74 to −7.48; P < .001) and tinnitus severity index score (MD = −8.36, 95% CI = −8.87 to −7.86; P < .001).[36] However, the authors concluded that due to small numbers of patients and lower quality studies, no firm recommendation could be made. This echoes a previous report describing methodological flaws, risk of bias, and heterogeneity of studies in this regard.[37] Given promising research suggesting benefit for some patients and because Western medicine has remained largely unsuccessful at treating tinnitus, Luetzenberg and colleagues discussed that treatment may be worth trying because it is both noninvasive and well tolerated.[38]

Cervical vertigo (CV) is a clinical syndrome causing dizziness, blurred vision, headache, nausea, vomiting, and even fainting. Symptoms can be induced and aggravated by head turning or lateral bending of the neck. It is thought to arise from hyperostosis of cervical vertebra and degeneration of cervical intervertebral discs, leading to narrowing and insufficient blood supply from the vertebral artery. This may lead to indirect compression of the vertebral artery and the sympathetic nerve with certain movement of the vertebral body. Atherosclerosis and decreased vascular elasticity may also contribute. The adult incidence of the disease is estimated at 10%. Hou and colleagues performed a systematic review and meta-analysis of the efficacy of acupuncture for CV.[39] Ten RCTs involving 914 patients were analyzed and found that acupuncture was overall significantly more effective than conventional medication (RR: 1.27; 95% CI: 1.19–1.34; P < .00001), including improvement rate of vertigo (RR: 1.15; 95% CI: 1.03–1.28; P = .009) and headache (RR: 1.30; 95% CI: 1.1–1.53; P = .001). Three studies detected improvement of blood supply to the vertebral arteries: left vertebral artery (MD: 2.86; 95% CI: 1.25–4.46; P = .0005), right vertebral artery (MD: 3.52; 95% CI: 1.52–5.51; P = .0006), and basilar artery (MD: 2.60; 95% CI: 1.42–3.79; P < .0001) compared with medication. Possible mechanisms for the effects of acupuncture were postulated to be release of cervical fascial tissue and improved perfusion via vasodilation. Chosen points often included Fengchi (GB 20), Baihui (GV 20), and Lieque (LU 7). Only mild adverse events were reported. However, the authors note that many studies were of low quality, thus limiting generalizability.

Sudden sensorineural hearing loss (SSNHL) is defined as an abrupt decrease in hearing of 30 dB in 3 contiguous frequencies during 72 hours and is more often unilateral. Its annual incidence ranges from 5 to 20 per 100,000 persons to as high as 160 cases per 100,000. Potential causes are viral infection, vascular perturbance, and autoimmune but most cases remain idiopathic. Currently used therapies include systemic and intratympanic steroids, antiviral agents, vasodilators, and hyperbaric oxygen. A 2015 systematic review and meta-analysis examined acupuncture in SSNHL,[40] which included 12 RCTs involving 863 patients. One measure universally reported was the proportion of participants with absolute improvements in pure tone average of 15 dB and greater. Five studies used manual acupuncture combined with conventional Western medical treatment (WMCT), and 6 studies used electroacupuncture combined with WMCT. Manual acupuncture combined with WMCT was better than WMCT alone (RR 1.33, 95%CI 1.19–1.49; $P < .00001$), and the combination of electroacupuncture and WMCT was better than WMCT alone (RR 1.33, 95%CI 1.19–1.50; $P < .00001$). In half of these studies, WMCT included hyperbaric oxygen therapy. All studies were from China. Criticism of the studies were a high risk of bias, small sample sizes, lack of blinding, and unclear randomization protocols. Mechanisms of action of acupuncture were postulated to be improved blood flow and rheology, as well as anti-inflammatory effects.

Acupuncture in its various forms: body, ear, scalp, moxibustion, and injection has been studied in Meniere disease (MD). The first systematic report from Long and colleagues in 2011 included 27 studies, which demonstrated an overall beneficial effect of acupuncture for MD, in both acute (within 1–10 days of symptoms) and chronic phases. Most of the studies were done in China, and a common research theme in these articles used a graded outcome approach detailing 4 categories: 1. Cured—dizziness and other symptoms absent without recurrence with ability to return to work/resume normal activities, 2. Markedly effective—with occasional recurrence of symptoms, 3. Effective—relief of symptoms, or 4. Not effective.[41] An updated systematic review from 2016 focused on 12 RCTs with 993 patients.[42] Common acupoints chosen were Baihui (DU20), Tinggong (SI19), and Fengchi (GB20). Four studies compared acupuncture alone versus WMCT. Acupuncture was more effective (RR = 0.21; 95% CI, 1.03–1.42; Z = 2.27; $P = .02$), although with significant heterogeneity (I 2 = 65%, $P = .04$). Three trials combined acupuncture plus WMCT versus WMCT, with the former found to be significantly better (I 2 = 47%, $P = .15$, RR = 1.26; 95% CI, 1.10–1.44; Z = 3.34; $P = .0008$). Analysis of vertigo specifically showed that acupuncture combined with WMCT had a better effect than WMCT alone (RR = 1.15; 95% CI, 1.06–1.24; Z = 3.56; $P = .0004$). However, when comparing hearing improvement between these same groups, no significant difference was found. The dizziness handicap inventory was the main outcome studied in 2 trials. Compared with the WMCT group, acupuncture was not found to have a significant advantage (MD = −21.26; 95% CI, −55.36, 12.84; $P = .22$).

A 2010 Cochrane review was conducted on acupuncture for Bell's palsy. The primary endpoints examined were the efficacy of acupuncture in hastening recovery and reducing long-term morbidity from Bell's palsy. Six RCTs were included with 537 participants. Five used acupuncture and one used acupuncture plus medication. Unfortunately, no trial reported on the outcomes specified for the review. The authors felt the quality of the included trials was inadequate to allow any conclusion to be made about the efficacy of acupuncture.[43] Similarly, a CPG published by the AAO-HNS in 2013 made no recommendation on the use of acupuncture, citing Grade B evidence, and concerns regarding the cost and duration of treatment, potential side effects, and delay in instituting oral steroids.[44] In 2015, a systematic review and meta-analysis was done. Fourteen RCTs involving 1541 individuals were included. In this meta-analysis, acupuncture had a higher effective response rate for Bell's palsy (RR, 1.14; 95% CI, 1.04–1.25; P = .005) but there was significant heterogeneity among studies (I2 = 87%). In the authors' assessment, acupuncture seemed to be an effective therapy for Bell's palsy but there was insufficient evidence to support efficacy due to issues of bias and incomplete reporting on safety of acupuncture.[45] More recently, 2 additional meta-analyses in 2019 and 2021 have reached similar conclusions.[46,47]

RHINOLOGY APPLICATIONS

There have been several systematic reviews and meta-analyses on acupuncture for the treatment of allergic rhinitis (AR). The first, published in 2008, reviewed 7 RCTs and concluded that there was insufficient evidence to support or refute the use of acupuncture in patients with AR, given the high level of heterogeneity and low methodological rigor.[48] A 2009 systematic review had mixed results, demonstrating that acupuncture was superior to placebo on rhinitis and nasal symptom scores for perennial AR but not for seasonal AR.[49] A meta-analysis in 2015, which included 13 studies and 2365 participants, showed a significant improvement for the group receiving true acupuncture on nasal symptom scores (weighted mean difference [WMD]: −4.42, 95% CI: −8.42 to −0.43, P = .03) and medication scores (WMD: 1.39, 95% CI: −2.18 to −0.61, P = .0005), as well as efficacy in improving the quality of life as found on the Rhinoconjunctivitis Quality of Life Questionnaire (RQLQ) and 36-item short-form (SF-36).[50] In 2020, 2 systematic reviews were published. One included 15 RCTs and found acupuncture to have a moderate-to-high Grading of Recommendations, Assessment, Development, and Evaluations rating.[51] The other reviewed 39 studies, including several from China, and showed that true acupuncture was superior to sham acupuncture with improvement in nasal symptom and RQLQ scores.[52] However, there have been very few studies comparing acupuncture to standard conventional AR medication, emphasizing the paramount importance of comparative effectiveness research, as prioritized by the National Academy of Medicine.[53]

Jung and colleagues reported on the effects of acupuncture and moxibustion on a mouse model of AR.[54] Moxibustion is a warming treatment that involves burning the herb, Artemisia vulgaris, above the skin at acupuncture points. A point corresponding to LI20 was used between the medial canthus and nostril. The experimental group received daily treatment for 7 days. Their hypothesis was that acupuncture and moxibustion stimulation would inhibit Th2 cell differentiation through decreases in the intramural substance P, STAT6 (signal transducer and activator of transcription), NFκB (nuclear factor kappa-light-chain-enhancer of activated B cells), and iNOS (inducible nitric oxide synthase) levels. Substance P, a neuropeptide, is found in nerve fiber tissue of the nasal mucosa and secreted from neuroterminals if histamine is secreted from mast cells. STAT6 is a transcription factor for IL-4, which is essential for Th2 cell differentiation. Similarly, NFκB is another transcription factor important in immune regulation especially as an inhibitor of GATA-3 (part of a family of zinc finger proteins that bind the consensus DNA sequence (T/A)GATA(A/G)), which suppresses allergic inflammation. Nitric oxide plays a role in inflammatory lung disease such as asthma. The experimental groups showed significant reductions in the STAT6 level, whereas expression of NFκB and iNOS was markedly inhibited. Substance P was suppressed. Eosinophil production in blood was markedly suppressed following acupuncture and moxibustion stimulation.

The sphenopalatine ganglion (SPG) acupoint, in the area of the notch formed by the mandibular coronoid process and the lower edge of the zygomatic arch, has been evaluated for its efficacy in perennial AR.[55] Mi and colleagues recruited 120 patients with PAR in an RCT comparing SPG acupuncture to traditional acupoints (bilateral Yingxiang [LI 20] and Hegu [LI 4] points, and Yintang [Ex-HN 3]) and medical therapy alone (budesonide nasal spray). They used the Total Nasal Symptom Score (TNSS) and Rhinoconjunctivitis Quality of Life Questionnaire (RQLQ) as endpoints after treatment and up to 16 weeks posttreatment. They found no significant differences in reductions in symptoms and improvements in TNSS between the SPG-acupuncture group and the drug-treatment group at each follow-up timepoint ($P > .05$). Moreover, for the RQLQ, no significant differences were found between the SPG-acupuncture group and the traditional-acupuncture group or the drug-treatment group at week 16 ($P = .036$ and $P = .635$, respectively).

In the 2015 AAO-HNS CPGs for AR, the expert panel following clinical review stated "clinicians may offer acupuncture, or refer to a clinician who can offer acupuncture, for patients with AR who are interested in nonpharmacologic therapy."[56] This was based on RCTs with limitations, observational studies with consistent effects, and a preponderance of benefit over harm. A middle of the road conclusion was reached by an international consensus group statement on AR who felt that the evidence was inconclusive but that acupuncture could be appropriate for some patients as an adjunct therapy, especially in those who wish to avoid medications.[57] However, a more recent review of practice parameters for AR and non-AR in The Journal of Allergy and clinical immunology differed, instead finding "neither acupuncture nor herbal products have adequate studies to support their use for AR."[58]

Nasal congestion can be a primary complaint in both rhinitis and sinusitis. Researchers from Heidelberg, Germany studied 24 patients with nasal congestion secondary to inferior turbinate hypertrophy or chronic sinusitis without polyposis in a pilot RCT. Patients scored the severity of their nasal congestion on a visual analog scale (VAS), and nasal airflow (NAF) was measured by using active anterior rhinomanometry. True acupoints according to TCM tenets were tested against nonspecific control acupoints. VAS and NAF were taken before and 15 and 30 minutes after acupuncture. Results showed sham acupuncture to have a significant improvement in VAS but a deterioration of NAF, whereas true acupuncture showed highly significant improvements in both VAS and NAF.[59] Jin and Chin looked at the evidence for acupuncture in reducing overall symptomatology in chronic rhinosinusitis.[60] They concluded there is insufficient evidence to support its use in CRS (chronic rhinosinusitis) currently. Although there is data to show it is useful as an adjunct to conventional therapy,[61] limited data from published studies have not shown a significant advantage over conventional medical therapy. They found the existing literature to be limited by small sample sizes, lack of standardization in acupuncture techniques, and poorly defined CRS diagnostic criteria.

CHALLENGES

To better evaluate studies on acupuncture, it is important to understand some of the inherent challenges involved. First, acupuncture protocols in research trials are typically quite different from what is used in real-world clinical practice settings. Research is often driven by "standardization" of the intervention with predetermined fixed acupoints, whereas, in the clinic, acupuncture points are selected based on TCM "pattern differentiation" diagnoses that lead to "individualization" of treatment. There can be variations in study design including the style of acupuncture, frequency/duration of treatment sessions, intensity/type of stimulation and variability with blinding. Experience and training of acupuncturists also play key roles but often go unmentioned in studies.[62] Moreover, there is controversy surrounding whether sham acupuncture can actually serve as an appropriate control or placebo. Sham acupuncture that penetrates the skin likely elicits nonspecific physiologic effects and, therefore, may not be truly inert. Finally, clinical trials should aim to study acupuncture in a manner that best reflects real-world practice, such as through pragmatic trials and whole-system research. An acupuncture visit seldom involves needling alone but also incorporates other tenets of TCM such as dietary and lifestyle counseling, an exhortation to exercise/practice Tai Chi, and prescription of herbal medicine. More questions remain to be answered, including the individual attributes, which may impact the effect size of acupuncture, as well as the optimal timing and specific regimen for its application.

CLINICS CARE POINTS

- Interventions that improved postoperative tonsillectomy pain were paracetamol, nonsteroidal anti–inflammatory drugs, intravenous dexamethasone, ketamine (only assessed in children), gabapentinoids, dexmedetomidine, honey, and acupuncture in a 2021 guideline.
- Current evidence supports acupuncture to facilitate improvement in the swallowing function of patients with post stroke dysphagia.
- For cervical vertigo, the most recent systematic review found that acupuncture is overall significantly more effective than conventional medication.
- Acupuncture may be helpful for patients with allergic rhinitis who are interested in nonpharmacologic therapy.

DISCLOSURE

The authors have no relevant financial interests pertaining to this article.

REFERENCES

1. National Health Statistics Reports, Number 95, June, 2016 (cdc.gov).
2. Shakeel M, Trinidade A, Ah-See KW. Complementary and alternative medicine use by otolaryngology patients: a paradigm for practitioners in all surgical specialties. Eur Arch Otorhinolaryngol 2010;267(6):961–71.
3. White E Ernst. A brief history of acupuncture. Rheumatology 2004;43(Issue 5): 662–3. https://doi.org/10.1093/rheumatology/keg005.
4. Yap L, Pothula VB, Warner J, et al. The root and development of otorhinolaryngology in traditional Chinese medicine. Eur Arch Otorhinolaryngol 2009;266(9): 1353–9.
5. Lundeberg T. To be or not to be: the needling sensation (de qi) in acupuncture. Acupunct Med 2013;31:129–31.
6. Available at: https://www.news-medical.net/health/Acupuncture-Theories.aspx. Accessed February 11 2022.
7. Johnson M. Transcutaneous Electrical Nerve Stimulation: Mechanisms, Clinical Application and Evidence. Rev Pain 2007;1(1):7–11.
8. Hui KK, Napadow V, Liu J, et al. Monitoring acupuncture effects on human brain by FMRI. J Vis Exp 2010;38:1190.
9. Pomeranz B, Chiu D. Naloxone blockade of acupuncture analgesia: endorphin implicated. Life Sci 1976;19(11):1757–62.
10. Tsuchiya M, Sato EF, Inoue M, et al. Acupuncture enhances generation of nitric oxide and increases local circulation. Anesth Analg 2007;104(2):301–7.

11. Goldman N, Chen M, Fujita T, et al. Adenosine A1 receptors mediate local anti-nociceptive effects of acupuncture. Nat Neurosci 2010;13(7):883–8.
12. Musial F, Tao I, Dobos G. Ist die analgetische Wirkung der Akupunktur ein Place-boeffekt? [Is the analgesic effect of acupuncture a placebo effect?]. Schmerz 2009;23(4):341–6. German.
13. Kahn CI, Huestis MJ, Cohen MB, et al. Evaluation of Acupuncture's Efficacy Within Otolaryngology. Ann Otol Rhinol Laryngol 2020;129(7):727–36.
14. Golianu B, Yeh AM, Brooks M. Acupuncture for Pediatric Pain. Children (Basel) 2014;1(2):134–48.
15. Volkow ND, McLellan TA, Cotto JH, et al. Characteristics of opioid prescriptions in 2009. JAMA 2011;305(13):1299–301.
16. Kuehn BM. FDA: No Codeine After Tonsillectomy for Children. JAMA 2013; 309(11):1100.
17. Ochi JW. Acupuncture instead of codeine for tonsillectomy pain in children. Int J Pediatr Otorhinolaryngol 2013;77(12):2058–62. Epub 2013 Oct 20. PMID: 24210291.
18. Tsao GJ, Messner AH, Seybold J, et al. Intraoperative acupuncture for posttonsil-lectomy pain: a randomized, double-blind, placebo-controlled trial. Laryngo-scope 2015;125(8):1972–8. Epub 2015 Apr 7. PMID: 25851423.
19. Dingemann J, Plewig B, Baumann I, et al. Acupuncture in posttonsillectomy pain : A prospective, double-blinded, randomized, controlled trial. HNO 2017;65(Suppl 1):73–9. English.
20. Keefe KR, Byrne KJ, Levi JR. Treating pediatric post-tonsillectomy pain and nausea with complementary and alternative medicine. Laryngoscope 2018; 128(11):2625–34. Epub 2018 May 4. PMID: 29729030.
21. Ochi JW, Richardson AC. Intraoperative pediatric acupuncture is widely accepted by parents. Int J Pediatr Otorhinolaryngol 2018;110:12–5. Epub 2018 Apr 19. PMID: 29859572.
22. Adams D, Cheng F, Jou H, et al. The safety of pediatric acupuncture: a system-atic review. Pediatrics 2011;128(6):e1575–87. Epub 2011 Nov 21. PMID: 22106073.
23. Shah AN, Moore CB, Brigger MT. Auricular acupuncture for adult tonsillectomy. Laryngoscope 2020;130(8):1907–12. Epub 2019 Oct 11. PMID: 31603582.
24. Aldamluji N, Burgess A, Pogatzki-Zahn E, et al. PROSPECT Working Group col-laborators*. PROSPECT guideline for tonsillectomy: systematic review and procedure-specific postoperative pain management recommendations. Anaes-thesia 2021;76(7):947–61.
25. Yiu EM, Chan KM, Li NY, et al. Wound-healing effect of acupuncture for treating phonotraumatic vocal pathologies: A cytokine study. Laryngoscope 2016;126(1): E18–22.
26. Yiu EM, Chan KM, Kwong E, et al. Is Acupuncture Efficacious for Treating Phono-traumatic Vocal Pathologies? A Randomized Control Trial. J Voice 2016;30(5): 611–20.
27. Kwong EY, Yiu EM. A preliminary study of the effect of acupuncture on emotional stress in female dysphonic speakers. J Voice 2010;24(6):719–23. Epub 2010 Jan 18. PMID: 20083382.
28. Hintze JM, Ludlow CL, Bansberg SF, et al. Spasmodic Dysphonia: A Review. Part 1: Pathogenic Factors. Otolaryngology–Head Neck Surg 2017;157(4):551–7.
29. Crevier-Buchman L, Laccourreye O, Papon JF, et al. Adductor spasmodic dysphonia: case reports with acoustic analysis following botulinum toxin injection and acupuncture. J Voice 1997;11(2):232–7.

30. Lee L, Daughton S, Scheer S, et al. Use of acupuncture for the treatment of adductor spasmodic dysphonia: a preliminary investigation. J Voice 2003; 17(3):411–24. PMID: 14513964.

31. Zhong L, Wang J, Li F, et al. The Effectiveness of Acupuncture for Dysphagia after Stroke: A Systematic Review and Meta-Analysis. Evid Based Complement Alternat Med 2021;19:8837625.

32. Lu Y, Chen Y, Huang D, et al. Efficacy of acupuncture for dysphagia after stroke: a systematic review and meta-analysis. Ann Palliat Med 2021;10(3):3410–22.

33. Tunkel DE, Bauer CA, Sun GH, et al. Clinical Practice Guideline: Tinnitus Executive Summary. Otolaryngology–Head Neck Surg 2014;151(4):533–41.

34. Kim JI, Choi JY, Lee DH, et al. Acupuncture for the treatment of tinnitus: a systematic review of randomized clinical trials. BMC Complement Altern Med 2012; 12:97.

35. Folmer RL, Griest SE, Martin WH. Chronic Tinnitus as Phantom Auditory Pain. Otolaryngology–Head Neck Surg 2001;124(4):394–400.

36. Huang K, Liang S, Chen L, et al. Acupuncture for tinnitus: a systematic review and meta-analysis of randomized controlled trials. Acupunct Med 2021;39(4): 264–71. PMID: 32772848.

37. Liu F, Han X, Li Y, et al. Acupuncture in the treatment of tinnitus: a systematic review and meta-analysis. Eur Arch Otorhinolaryngol 2016;273(2):285–94.

38. Luetzenberg FS, Babu S, Seidman MD. Alternative Treatments of Tinnitus: Alternative Medicine. Otolaryngol Clin North Am 2020;53(4):637–50. Epub 2020 Apr 30. PMID: 32362562.

39. Hou Z, Xu S, Li Q, et al. The Efficacy of Acupuncture for the Treatment of Cervical Vertigo: A Systematic Review and Meta-Analysis. Evid Based Complement Alternat Med 2017;2017:7597363.

40. Zhang XC, Xu XP, Xu WT, et al. Acupuncture therapy for sudden sensorineural hearing loss: a systematic review and meta-analysis of randomized controlled trials [published correction appears in PLoS One 2015;10(6):e0131031. 2015;10(4):e0125240. Published 2015 Apr 28.

41. Long AF, Xing M, Morgan K, et al. Exploring the Evidence Base for Acupuncture in the Treatment of Ménière's Syndrome-A Systematic Review. Evid Based Complement Alternat Med 2011;2011:429102.

42. He J, Jiang L, Peng T, et al. Acupuncture Points Stimulation for Meniere's Disease/Syndrome: A Promising Therapeutic Approach. Evid Based Complement Alternat Med 2016;2016:6404197.

43. Chen N, Zhou M, He L, et al. Acupuncture for Bell's palsy. Cochrane Database Syst Rev 2010;2010(8):CD002914.

44. Baugh RF, Basura GJ, Ishii LE, et al. Clinical practice guideline: Bell's palsy. Otolaryngol Head Neck Surg 2013;149(3 Suppl):S1–27.

45. Li P, Qiu T, Qin C. Efficacy of Acupuncture for Bell's Palsy: A Systematic Review and Meta-Analysis of Randomized Controlled Trials. PLoS One 2015;10(5):e0121880.

46. Zhang R, Wu T, Wang R, et al. Compare the efficacy of acupuncture with drugs in the treatment of Bell's palsy: A systematic review and meta-analysis of RCTs. Medicine (Baltimore) 2019;98(19):e15566.

47. Zou Z. Comparison of Efficacy and Safety of Acupuncture and Moxibustion in Acute Phase and Non-acute Phase of Bell's Palsy: a meta-analysis. Neuro Endocrinol Lett 2021;42(7). Epub ahead of print. PMID: 34847316.

48. Roberts J, Huissoon A, Dretzke J, et al. A systematic review of the clinical effectiveness of acupuncture for allergic rhinitis. BMC Complement Altern Med 2008;8:13.

49. Lee MS, Pittler MH, Shin BC, et al. Acupuncture for allergic rhinitis: a systematic review. Ann Allergy Asthma Immunol 2009;102(4):269–79.
50. Feng S, Han M, Fan Y, et al. Acupuncture for the treatment of allergic rhinitis: A systematic review and meta-analysis. Am J Rhinol Allergy 2015;29:57–62.
51. Wu AW, Gettelfinger JD, Ting JY, et al. Alternative therapies for sinusitis and rhinitis: a systematic review utilizing a modified Delphi method. Int Forum Allergy Rhinol 2020;10:496–505.
52. Yin Z, Geng G, Xu G, et al. Acupuncture methods for allergic rhinitis: a systematic review and bayesian meta-analysis of randomized controlled trials. Chin Med 2020;15:109.
53. Taw MB, Reddy WD, Omole FS, et al. Acupuncture and allergic rhinitis. Curr Opin Otolaryngol Head Neck Surg 2015;23(3):216–20.
54. Jung D, Lee S, Hong S. Effects of Acupuncture and Moxibustion in a Mouse Model of Allergic Rhinitis. Otolaryngology–Head Neck Surg 2012;146(1):19–25.
55. Mi JP, He P, Shen F, et al. Efficacy of Acupuncture at the Sphenopalatine Ganglion in the Treatment of Persistent Allergic Rhinitis. Med Acupunct 2020;32(2):90–8. Epub 2020 Apr 16. PMID: 32351662; PMCID: PMC7187981.
56. Seidman MD, Gurgel RK, Lin SY, et al. Clinical Practice Guideline: Allergic Rhinitis. Otolaryngology–Head Neck Surg 2015;152(1_suppl):S1–43.
57. Wise SK, Lin SY, Toskala E, et al. International Consensus Statement on Allergy and Rhinology: Allergic Rhinitis. Int Forum Allergy Rhinol 2018;8(2):108–352.
58. Dykewicz MS, Wallace DV, Amrol DJ, et al. Rhinitis 2020: A practice parameter update. J Allergy Clin Immunol 2020;146(4):721–67.
59. Sertel S, Bergmann Z, Ratzlaff K, et al. Acupuncture for Nasal Congestion: A Prospective, Randomized, Double-Blind, Placebo-Controlled Clinical Pilot Study. Am J Rhinology Allergy 2009;23(6):e23–8.
60. Jin AJ, Chin CJ. Is acupuncture effective in reducing overall symptomatology in chronic rhinosinusitis? Laryngoscope 2019;129:1727–8. https://doi.org/10.1002/lary.27708.
61. Suh JD, Wu AW, Taw MB, et al. Treatment of recalcitrant chronic rhinosinusitis with integrative East-West medicine: a pilot study. Arch Otolaryngol Head Neck Surg 2012;138(3):294–300.
62. Acupuncture – UpToDate. Available at: www.uptodate.com. Accessed March 2, 2022.

Endocannabinoid System and the Otolaryngologist

Brandon Tapasak, BS[a,*], Luke Edelmayer, MD[b], Michael D. Seidman, MD[a,b,c]

KEYWORDS

- Endocannabinoid system • Cannabinoid drugs • Cannabis • Head and neck cancer
- Obstructive sleep apnea • Tinnitus • Vertigo • Dizziness

KEY POINTS

- The endocannabinoid system has a role in the practice of otolaryngology, particularly when addressing inflammatory pain and the vestibular system.
- Cannabinoids may be a useful treatment option when treating patients with head and neck cancer for chronic pain, nausea, and vomiting.
- The use of cannabinoids for the treatment of obstructive sleep apnea, tinnitus, and dizziness/vertigo is hotly debated and should be considered on a case-by-case basis.
- Otolaryngologists should be aware of the potential complications of cannabinoid use to include tinnitus, vertigo, and hearing loss.
- More research is needed in the role of cannabinoids in otolaryngologic pathology.

INTRODUCTION
Significance of the Endocannabinoid System

There are three broad classes or cannabinoids: phytocannabinoids (plant-based, ie, *Cannabis*), synthetic cannabinoids, and endocannabinoids (cannabinoids produced by the human body). The primary psychoactive component of *Cannabis* Δ^9-tetrahydrocannabinol (THC) and cannabidiol (CBD) were isolated in the 1960s, thus kick-starting the research which revealed the effects of these chemicals on the brain and body.

The endocannabinoid system refers to cannabinoid receptors (CB1 and CB2) that are acted on by cannabinoid ligands. The CB1 receptors in the central nervous system (CNS) function as presynaptic terminals of γ-Aminobutyric acid (GABA)ergic neurons to curtail release of neurotransmitters.[1] They are abundant in the cerebral cortex,

[a] University of Central Florida College of Medicine, 6850 Lake Nona Boulevard, Orlando, FL 32827, USA; [b] Advent Health Celebration, 400 Celebration Place, Kissimmee, FL 34747, USA; [c] University of South Florida Morsani College of Medicine, 12901 Bruce B Downs Boulevard, Tampa, FL 33612, USA
* Corresponding author. 6850 Lake Nona Boulevard, Orlando, FL 32827.
E-mail address: btapasak@knights.ucf.edu

Otolaryngol Clin N Am 55 (2022) 1101–1110
https://doi.org/10.1016/j.otc.2022.06.012
0030-6665/22/© 2022 Elsevier Inc. All rights reserved.

basal ganglia, hippocampus, and cerebellum.[2] The CB1 receptors are also present on plasma membranes, endosomes, and mitochondria, regulating neuronal energy metabolism. Astrocytes, oligodendrocytes, and their precursors also possess CB1 receptors, impairing working memory. Acute cannabinoids impair working memory through astroglial CB1 receptor modulation of hippocampal long-term potentiation. But of the utmost clinical relevance, CB1 peripheral receptors located in the heart, lung, prostate, liver, uterus, ovary, testis, vas deferens, and bone mediate physiologic processes such as gastrointestinal motility and energy balance, reproduction and fertility, pain, and skeletal muscle energy metabolism. Expression of central and peripheral cannabinoid receptors have also been found in human immune tissues and leukocyte subpopulations.[3,4]

The CB2 receptors are similar to CB1 receptors. Research is ongoing to develop specific CB2 agonists as these drugs produce antinociceptive actions without cannabimimetic side effects. The CB2 receptors predominate peripherally within immune regulatory tissues such as B cells and natural killer cells. In this way, CB2 regulates inflammatory responses. Unlike CB1, CB2 seems to decrease reactive oxygen species.[5,6]

History of Medical Cannabinoid Use

Proponents of medicinal cannabis argue that there is evidence to support its use in the treatment of conditions which are refractory to other therapies. These proponents also argue that cannabis is relatively safe and inexpensive compared with pharmaceutical agents.[7] Opponents instead argue that medicinal cannabis has not been subjected to the US Food and Drug Administration approval process. They surmise that because there is no standardization of pharmacologically active constituents, its use could lead to adverse health effects, such as unmasking of mental health disorders, impaired coordination and judgment, and potential for addiction and abuse.[8]

Select states have passed laws allowing medicinal cannabis use for the treatment of Alzheimer's disease, human immunodeficiency virus/acquired immunodeficiency syndrome (HIV/AIDS), amyotrophic lateral sclerosis, cancer, inflammatory bowel disease, multiple sclerosis (MS), Parkinson's disease, and post-traumatic stress disorder. Many symptoms indicated in the use of medicinal cannabis include cachexia, severe or chronic pain, severe or chronic nausea, seizure disorders, and skeletal muscle spasticity.[9]

Recent clinical practice guidelines issued a weak recommendation for using medicinal cannabis for treating chronic pain because of the balance between benefit and harm. The guidelines reflect small improvements in self-reported pain intensity, physical functioning, and sleep quality with willingness to accept a small to moderate risk of self-limited and transient harm.[10]

This article identifies common otolaryngologic pathologies that may be managed with cannabinoids. The discussion also includes debate of the potential benefits and drawbacks to cannabinoid use and suggests future directions for more research into the use of medicinal cannabinoids.

CANNABINOID CONSIDERATIONS IN HEAD AND NECK CANCER
Approach to Cannabinoid Use in Patients with Cancer (Head and Neck)

The main route of marijuana exposure continues to be through smoke inhalation.[11] Marijuana smoke and tobacco smoke share carcinogens and polycyclic aromatic hydrocarbons which are 20 times higher in unfiltered marijuana than cigarette smoke. Marijuana use is associated with histopathological bronchial inflammatory changes like those observed with smoking tobacco.[12] THC may have adverse immunomodulatory effects associated with cancer. Two proto-oncogenes are overexpressed in the bronchial epithelium of marijuana-only smokers with higher gene expression than tobacco-only smokers.[13] Conversely, several animal studies have found cannabinoids inhibit proliferation of some cancer cell types, impede angiogenesis, and reduce cancer growth.[4,14]

Compared with nonsmokers, those who ever used marijuana had a similar risk of developing head and neck squamous cell carcinoma. Findings among heavier users were mixed. Studies have revealed no association between ever using marijuana and oral cancer. The data are mixed on the association between laryngeal, pharyngeal, and esophageal cancer. There are few reliable studies which have investigated this association. According to a recent meta-analysis by Ghasemiesfe and colleagues, there are insufficient data to conclude there is any association between marijuana smoking and head and neck cancer.[15]

On a molecular scale, there are increased cannabinoid receptors in a variety of tumor cell types. The antineoplastic mechanisms of endocannabinoids include increased reactive oxygen species, inhibition of angiogenesis, arrest of cell-cycle progression, and induction of autophagy and apoptosis. Data have shown that oropharyngeal and tongue cancer, thyroid cancer, lymphoma, basal cell, squamous cell, and melanoma are potentially affected by the antineoplastic effects of cannabinoids. Other promising studies have shown a strong antitumoral effect on anaplastic thyroid cancer cells in mice as well as a synergistic mechanism of induced apoptosis when used with paclitaxel.[16]

Patients with head and neck cancer who use marijuana report an improved quality of life. Studies have reported statistically lower scores for pain, anxiety, and depression and statistically higher scores for general well-being reported by patients with cancer who use marijuana. However, these studies identify the need for determining if these effects are maintained throughout treatment and among long-term survivors.[17]

Chronic refractory pain has recently been recognized as an indication for cannabinoid use. Cannabis is a moderate analgesic which may function synergistically with opioids for pain control. With the opioid epidemic still raging, the use of cannabis for chronic pain, cancer related or not, may be a solution. There has been a nearly 25% decrease in opioid-related mortality rates in states which have enacted a medical marijuana program.[18]

Furthermore, studies have shown the addition of oral THC:CBD with antiemetics to be associated with less nausea and vomiting with an improvement in response from 14% to 25%. However, there were additional unintended adverse effects including sedation, dizziness, and disorientation. Nonetheless, 83% of participants preferred cannabis to the placebo.[19–21]

Complications/Concerns in Patients with Cancer

Although primarily in favor of cannabinoids functioning in an antineoplastic manner, there are reports of cannabinoids functioning as carcinogenic depending on their concentration. Many older studies identified a possible link between smoking marijuana and the development of head and neck carcinoma, but most of these were case reports.[22,23] However, there may be a link between cannabinoid use and progression of human papillomavirus (HPV) positive head and neck squamous cell carcinoma. Cell lines and animal models showed CB1 and CB2 as well as nonselective cannabinoid receptor activation promoting cell growth, migration, and apoptosis through p38 mitogen-activated protein kinase (MAPK) pathway activation.[24]

CANNABINOID USE IN GENERAL OTOLARYNGOLOGY
Approach to Cannabinoid Use for Obstructive Sleep Apnea

Obstructive sleep apnea (OSA) is a common ailment treated by the otolaryngologist. A 2015 study reported 50% of men and 23% of women had at least moderate OSA.[25] There are estimations that 82% of men and 93% of women in the United States with OSA are undiagnosed.[26] Patients with moderate-to-severe OSA are at a higher risk for stroke, myocardial infarction, hypertension, hyperlipemia, glucose intolerance, diabetes, arrhythmias, pulmonary hypertension, congestive heart failure, and depression. Those with cardiovascular disease such as hypertension, heart failure, arrhythmias, stroke, and coronary artery disease have a very high prevalence of OSA.[27]

Increased awareness and earlier treatment are essential to reduce the cardiovascular disease burden. The American Academy of Sleep Medicine (AASM) released a statement recommending medical cannabis and/or synthetic extracts not to be used for the treatment of OSA because of unreliable delivery methods and insufficient evidence of effectiveness, tolerability, and safety. They also recommended OSA to be excluded from the list of chronic medical conditions made by state medical cannabis programs. However, the AASM stated that there are signs of potential benefit from dronabinol and cannabis extract use in patients with OSA, but more research is needed before recommending them as treatments.[28,29]

This stance has been hotly debated. Proponents of cannabis use for OSA state there are placebo-controlled randomized clinical trials that show significant evidence for decreased sleepiness with no significant evidence for increased adverse effects. They maintain that the argument against cannabis because of the "lack of long-term research" is short-sided and harms patients. They claim that the gold standard of treatment of OSA, continuous positive airway pressure machines (CPAP machines) are expensive and encourage noncompliance due to discomfort.[30,31]

Regardless, trials have shown that the use of dronabinol presents a greater benefit than placebo regarding the Apnea–Hypopnea index (AHI), with a mean difference from baseline of -19.64 in patients with OSA. The use of 2.5 to 10 mg doses of dronabinol resulted in a significant reduction in the short-term AHI, as well as improved self-reported sleepiness, and patients reported greater overall treatment satisfaction. This is thought to be due to three pathways: THC stabilization of autonomic output during sleep, reduction of spontaneous sleep-disordered breathing, and blocking of serotonin-induced exacerbation of sleep apnea. Nevertheless, these articles recommend that larger scale clinical trials are needed to confirm the aforementioned results.[32–34]

The mechanism of cannabinoid treatment in OSA is thought to suppress apnea facilitated by peripheral rather than central nervous system activity. Higher concentrations of the endocannabinoid oleoylethanolamide (OEA) but not anandamide or 2-arachidonoylglycerol were found in patients with OSA, associated with difficulty breathing. This suggested endocannabinoids, specifically OEA, may protect the brain from the symptoms of sleep apnea.[35,36]

In the end, we are hopeful for the future of sleep apnea treatment, as CPAP is not always sufficient as a single modality of treatment of OSA, because of its high rates of noncompliance. Therefore, more research is needed to confirm the benefits of endocannabinoids in the treatment of OSA. It is important that every otolaryngologist is aware of the literature and have an informed discussion with their patients on alternative treatments for OSA.

Approach to Cannabinoid Use for Tinnitus

Tinnitus is a common and frustrating problem to manage for the neurotologist and the patient. The most recent epidemiologic study of tinnitus was performed in 2018 and reported that 9.6% of American adults had experienced tinnitus in the past 12 months. Among these tinnitus sufferers, 27% had symptoms greater than 15 years and 7.2% reported their tinnitus as a "big" or "very big" problem. Despite this, only 49.4% had discussed their tinnitus with their physician.[37]

Tinnitus itself is the perception of sound in the absence on an external stimulus. If persistently bothersome, tinnitus can impair thought processing, emotional stability, subjective hearing, sleep, and concentration. The enthusiasm for cannabinoids for the treatment of chronic pain and epilepsy raises the question whether they could be used for other abnormal neuronal activity such as tinnitus. Tinnitus has been theorized to be the result of neuronal hyperactivity or epilepsy of the cochlear nucleus. Although cannabinoids have been shown to decrease neuronal hyperactivity in the brain, evidence shows that they have the potential to facilitate hyperactivity in the dorsal cochlear nucleus, exacerbating tinnitus. In animal models, cannabinoids have been shown to not affect or even worsen tinnitus. These studies focused on neural CB1 receptor-based responses.[38,39]

Proponents have suggested that the pharmacology of cannabinoids is more complex, and they maintain the possibility that some cannabinoids may reduce tinnitus, similar to the treatment of anxiety (ie, to worsen or improve). In particular, CBD is an anti-inflammatory and acts on the pathways involved in cochlear damage protection. With tinnitus being a result of neuronal inflammation, theoretically CBD would improve tinnitus.[40]

However, according to larger literature reviews, there is not enough evidence to determine an association between cannabis use and tinnitus. Ultimately, we do not understand enough about the pathophysiology of tinnitus at this point to make a recommendation on the use of cannabinoids as treatment. Otolaryngologists should consider the research which primarily indicates cannabinoids do not affect or may even worsen tinnitus when treating patients for this frustrating problem.

Approach to Cannabinoid Use for Vertigo/Dizziness

There is evidence of a high burden of dizziness and vertigo in the community. Large population-based studies show that dizziness (including vertigo) affects 15% to 20% of adults yearly. Vestibular vertigo is the cause of 25% of dizziness complaints. Vestibular vertigo has a 12-month prevalence of 5% and an annual incidence of 1.4%.[41]

As there is evidence that cannabinoid CB1 receptors are expressed in the vestibular nucleus complex, CB1 receptors and endogenous cannabinoids could be important in central vestibular function. This could explain the reported adverse effects of cannabinoids including dizziness and vertigo.[42–44]

Unfortunately, what little research there is on the association of cannabinoids and the vestibular system is dated, and new research is needed. Of these older studies, dated techniques such as gaze nystagmus, tracking a pendulum, spontaneous nystagmus, and torsion swing rotation were objective measurements of vestibular function. Even so, it was found that acute cannabis use did not significantly change any of the measurements compared with the control groups. However, chronic cannabis use showed a significant decrease in maximum amplitude on torsion swing, increase in incidence of nystagmus in two or more supine positions, and decrease in speed of slow component on caloric tests.[45,46]

In a recent meta-analysis of cannabis-induced otolaryngologic side effects, vestibular dysfunction, with a particular emphasis on vertigo, was found to be the second most common side effect.[47] In clinical trials of cannabis used to treat MS, dizziness was found to be a common side effect. Upward of 14.6% of patients experienced this unwanted side effect. However, these studies concluded the side effects were manageable in the long-term treatment of MS.[48,49]

The effect of cannabinoids on dizziness and vertigo remains a mystery. Although there are some promising signs for cannabinoids as a treatment option, not enough research has been performed to confirm the efficacy. In fact, biochemically there is evidence cannabinoids may cause dizziness and vertigo. Therefore, until more substantial research is performed, there are no indications or possible contraindications to the treatment of vestibular-induced dizziness and vertigo with cannabinoids.

Cannabinoid Complications/Concerns in Otolaryngology

The potential use for cannabinoids in otolaryngologic pathologies is not without concern. Although uncommon, cannabis toxicity can affect many different organ systems in adults. Acute poisoning can cause neurologic symptoms (to include dizziness), ocular symptoms, gastrointestinal symptoms (to include nausea and vomiting), and cardiovascular symptoms. Children and users with preexisting cardiac, pulmonary, or psychiatric diseases are at higher risk for cannabis toxicity.[50]

A recent review of cannabis-related side effects in the practice of otolaryngology reports the most common side effect was tinnitus, followed by vertigo, hearing loss, infection, malignancy, sinusitis, allergic rhinitis, thyroid dysfunction, and dyspnea. Of the 48 studies analyzed, 32 were head and neck and 8 were otology. More than half (54.1%) of studies showed increased side effects or no change in symptoms following cannabis use.[47]

Disquietingly, however, are the number of studies indicating an association between cannabis smoking and neurotoxicity of the auditory system. In these smaller population studies, male smokers had significantly poorer distortion product otoacoustic emissions than male nonsmokers in the low frequencies. These were mostly long-term smokers. Still, the results indicate that cannabis smoking may negatively alter the function of outer hair cells in young men. In addition, when investigating electrophysiological outcomes such as auditory brainstem responses, a significant neurotoxic effect on the auditory system was suggested. These studies warrant further investigation with larger confirmatory studies.[51,52]

FUTURE DIRECTIONS
Recommendations for Clinical Practice

There continues to be great debate in the consideration of cannabinoids as treatment options in the world of Otolaryngology—Head and Neck Surgery. A systematic review of randomized clinical trials of cannabinoid use in medicine was conducted to determine its role. Cannabinoids were associated with a greater average number of patients showing a complete nausea and vomiting response, reduction in pain, and average reduction in spasticity. These indicate moderate evidence to support the use of cannabinoids for chronic pain and spasticity treatment but low evidence to suggest cannabinoids improved nausea and vomiting, weight gain, sleep disorder, and Tourette syndrome. Cannabinoids were also associated with an increased risk of short-term adverse effects. These included dizziness, dry mouth, nausea, fatigue, somnolence, euphoria, vomiting, confusion, and loss of balance.[32]

Substantial evidence is needed to determine a place for cannabinoids in practice of Otolaryngology—Head and Neck Surgery, but studies have been promising. Otolaryngologists should initiate an informed discussion with their patients when considering cannabinoids for treatment. Although there are many benefits, there are many unknowns and drawbacks that may influence the decision for cannabinoid use. Balancing these pros and cons is essential to determine how to improve the lives of our patients.

SUMMARY

This article shares information to help the otolaryngologist better understand the mechanisms of the endocannabinoid system and how this system can be used in the clinical setting. Treatment with cannabinoids is a rapidly evolving topic, especially with the increasing status of legalization in the United States. High-quality research on medical cannabinoids has been difficult to complete because of federal restrictions. However, otolaryngologists should be familiar with the evidence for management of common pathologies, potential complications, and the unknowns. Understanding these fundamental aspects will allow otolaryngologists to make informed recommendations to patients who have questions regarding medical cannabinoid use.

CLINICS CARE POINTS

- The use of cannabinoids in otolaryngology is hotly debated for the treatment of common pathology.
- The range of effects of cannabinoids on pain, inflammation, and the vestibular system is still undergoing research.
- Otolaryngologists should weigh the benefits, drawbacks, and unknowns before discussing cannabinoids as a treatment option.
- The literature while controversial seems to support the use of medicinal cannabinoids for pain control, nausea and vomiting, obstructive sleep apnea, and tinnitus, but additional research is required before consideration as a viable treatment option.

FUNDING

The authors received no financial support for the research, authorship, and/or publication of this article.

DISCLOSURE

The authors have nothing relevant to disclose.

REFERENCES

1. Schurman LD, Lu D, Kendall DA, et al. Molecular mechanism and cannabinoid pharmacology. Handb Exp Pharmacol 2020;258:323–53.
2. Lu HC, Mackie K. An Introduction to the Endogenous Cannabinoid System. Biol Psychiatry 2016;79(7):516–25.
3. Donvito G, Nass SR, Wilkerson JL, et al. The endogenous cannabinoid system: a budding source of targets for treating inflammatory and neuropathic pain. Neuropsychopharmacology 2018;43:52–79.
4. Bryant LM, Daniels KE, Cognetti DM, et al. Therapeutic Cannabis and Endocannabinoid Signaling System Modulator Use in Otolaryngology Patients. Laryngoscope Investig Otolaryngol 2018;3(3):169–77.
5. Pacher P, Mechoulam R. Is lipid signaling through cannabinoid 2 receptors part of a protective system? Prog Lipid Res 2011;50(2):193–211.
6. Han KH, Lim S, Ryu J, et al. CB1 and CB2 cannabinoid receptors differentially regulate the production of reactive oxygen species by macrophages. Cardiovasc Res 2009;84(3):378–86.

7. Clark PA, Capuzzi K, Fick C. Medical marijuana: medical necessity versus political agenda. Med Sci Monit 2011;17(12):RA249–61. https://doi.org/10.12659/msm.882116.

8. MacDonald K, Pappas K. WHY NOT POT?: a review of the brain-based risks of cannabis. Innov Clin Neurosci 2016;13(3–4):13–22. Published 2016 Apr 1.

9. Bridgeman MB, Abazia DT. Medicinal cannabis: history, pharmacology, and implications for the acute care setting. P T 2017;42(3):180–8.

10. Busse JW, Vankrunkelsven P, Zeng L, et al. Medical cannabis or cannabinoids for chronic pain: a clinical practice guideline. BMJ 2021;374:n2040.

11. Steigerwald S, Wong PO, Cohen BE, et al. Smoking, vaping, and use of edibles and other forms of marijuana among US adults. Ann Intern Med 2018;169(12): 890–2.

12. Tashkin DP, Baldwin GC, Sarafian T, et al. Respiratory and immunologic consequences of marijuana smoking. J Clin Pharmacol 2002;42(S1):71S–81S.

13. Barsky SH, Roth MD, Kleerup EC, et al. Histopathologic and molecular alterations in bronchial epithelium in habitual smokers of marijuana, cocaine, and/or tobacco. J Natl Cancer Inst 1998;90(16):1198–205.

14. Pellati F, Borgonetti V, Brighenti V, et al. *Cannabis sativa* L. and nonpsychoactive cannabinoids: their chemistry and role against oxidative stress, inflammation, and cancer. Biomed Res Int 2018;2018:1691428.

15. Ghasemiesfe M, Barrow B, Leonard S, et al. Association between marijuana use and risk of cancer: a systematic review and meta-analysis. JAMA Netw Open 2019;2(11):e1916318. https://doi.org/10.1001/jamanetworkopen.2019.16318.

16. Zhang H, Xie M, Archibald SD, et al. Association of marijuana use with psychosocial and quality of life outcomes among patients with head and neck cancer. JAMA Otolaryngol Head Neck Surg 2018;144(11):1017–22. https://doi.org/10.1001/jamaoto.2018.0486.

17. Shi Y, Zou M, Baitei EY, et al. Cannabinoid 2 receptor induction by IL-12 and its potential as a therapeutic target for the treatment of anaplastic thyroid carcinoma. Cancer Gene Ther 2008;15(2):101–7. https://doi.org/10.1038/sj.cgt.7701101.

18. Bachhuber MA, Saloner B, Cunningham CO, et al. Medical cannabis laws and opioid analgesic overdose mortality in the United States, 1999-2010 [published correction appears in JAMA Intern Med. 2014 Nov;174(11):1875. JAMA Intern Med 2014;174(10):1668–73.

19. VanDolah HJ, Bauer BA, Mauck KF. Clinicians' Guide to Cannabidiol and Hemp Oils. Mayo Clin Proc 2019;94(9):1840–51.

20. Grimison P, Mersiades A, Kirby A, et al. Oral THC:CBD cannabis extract for refractory chemotherapy-induced nausea and vomiting: a randomised, placebo-controlled, phase II crossover trial. Ann Oncol 2020;31(11):1553–60.

21. Blake A, Wan BA, Malek L, et al. A selective review of medical cannabis in cancer pain management. Ann Palliat Med 2017;6(Suppl 2):S215–22.

22. Donald PJ. Marijuana smoking–possible cause of head and neck carcinoma in young patients. Otolaryngol Head Neck Surg 1986;94(4):517–21.

23. Donald PJ. Advanced malignancy in the young marijuana smoker. Adv Exp Med Biol 1991;288:33–46. https://doi.org/10.1007/978-1-4684-5925-8_4.

24. Liu C, Sadat SH, Ebisumoto K, et al. Cannabinoids promote progression of HPV-positive head and neck squamous cell carcinoma via p38 MAPK activation. Clin Cancer Res 2020;26(11):2693–703.

25. Heinzer R, Vat S, Marques-Vidal P, et al. Prevalence of sleep-disordered breathing in the general population: the HypnoLaus study. Lancet Respir Med 2015; 3(4):310–8.

26. Young T, Evans L, Finn L, et al. Estimation of the clinically diagnosed proportion of sleep apnea syndrome in middle-aged men and women. Sleep 1997;20(9): 705–6.

27. Rundo JV. Obstructive sleep apnea basics. Cleve Clin J Med 2019;86(9 Suppl 1): 2–9. https://doi.org/10.3949/ccjm.86.s1.02.

28. Ramar K, Rosen IM, Kirsch DB, et al. Medical Cannabis and the Treatment of Obstructive Sleep Apnea: An American Academy of Sleep Medicine Position Statement. J Clin Sleep Med 2018;14(4):679–81. https://doi.org/10.5664/jcsm. 7070. Published 2018 Apr 15.

29. Ramar K, Kirsch DB, Carden KA, et al. Medical cannabis, synthetic marijuana extracts, and obstructive sleep apnea. J Clin Sleep Med 2018;14(10):1815–6. Published 2018 Oct 15.

30. Schears RM, Fischer AC, Hodge WA. Medical Cannabis and AASM Position Statement: The Don't Ask, Don't Tell Wishing Well. J Clin Sleep Med 2018; 14(10):1811.

31. Takakuwa KM. Stop the Attack on Minnesota's Courageous Stance to Allow Its Residents to Sleep Safely. J Clin Sleep Med 2018;14(10):1813.

32. Whiting PF, Wolff RF, Deshpande S, et al. Cannabinoids for Medical Use: A Systematic Review and Meta-analysis. JAMA 2015;313(24):2456–73. https://doi.org/ 10.1001/jama.2015.6358.

33. Carley DW, Prasad B, Reid KJ, et al. Pharmacotherapy of Apnea by Cannabimimetic Enhancement, the PACE Clinical Trial: Effects of Dronabinol in Obstructive Sleep Apnea. Sleep 2018;41(1):zsx184. https://doi.org/10.1093/sleep/zsx184.

34. Prasad B, Radulovacki MG, Carley DW. Proof of concept trial of dronabinol in obstructive sleep apnea. Front Psychiatry 2013;4:1.

35. Calik MW, Carley DW. Intracerebroventricular injections of dronabinol, a cannabinoid receptor agonist, does not attenuate serotonin-induced apnea in Sprague-Dawley rats. J Negat Results Biomed 2016;15:8.

36. Jumpertz R, Wiesner T, Blüher M, et al. Circulating endocannabinoids and N-acyl-ethanolamides in patients with sleep apnea–specific role of oleoylethanolamide. Exp Clin Endocrinol Diabetes 2010;118(9):591–5. https://doi.org/10.1055/ s-0030-1253344.

37. Bhatt JM, Lin HW, Bhattacharyya N. Prevalence, Severity, Exposures, and Treatment Patterns of Tinnitus in the United States. JAMA Otolaryngol Head Neck Surg 2016;142(10):959–65. https://doi.org/10.1001/jamaoto.2016.1700.

38. Zheng Y, Smith PF. Cannabinoid drugs: will they relieve or exacerbate tinnitus? Curr Opin Neurol 2019;32(1):131–6. https://doi.org/10.1097/WCO. 0000000000000631.

39. Smith PF, Zheng Y. Cannabinoids, cannabinoid receptors and tinnitus. Hear Res 2016;332:210–6. https://doi.org/10.1016/j.heares.2015.09.014.

40. Perin P, Mabou Tagne A, Enrico P, et al. Cannabinoids, Inner Ear, Hearing, and Tinnitus: A Neuroimmunological Perspective. Front Neurol 2020;11:505995. https://doi.org/10.3389/fneur.2020.505995. Published 2020 Nov 23.

41. Neuhauser HK. The epidemiology of dizziness and vertigo. Handb Clin Neurol 2016;137:67–82. https://doi.org/10.1016/B978-0-444-63437-5.00005-4.

42. Smith PF, Ashton JC, Darlington CL. The endocannabinoid system: A new player in the neurochemical control of vestibular function? Audiol Neurootol 2006;11(4): 207–12. https://doi.org/10.1159/000092588.

43. Newsham-West D, Darlington CL, Smith PF. Potent effects of a selective cannabinoid receptor agonist on some guinea pig medial vestibular nucleus neurons.

Eur J Pharmacol 1998;348(1):R1–2. https://doi.org/10.1016/s0014-2999(98)
00237-4.

44. Smith PF. New approaches in the management of spasticity in multiple sclerosis patients: role of cannabinoids. Ther Clin Risk Manag 2010;6:59–63. https://doi.org/10.2147/tcrm.s5974. Published 2010 Mar 3.

45. Spector M. Acute vestibular effects of marijuana. J Clin Pharmacol 1973;13(5):214–7. https://doi.org/10.1002/j.1552-4604.1973.tb00210.x.

46. Spector M. Chronic vestibular and auditory effects of marijuana. Laryngoscope 1974;84(5):816–20. https://doi.org/10.1288/00005537-197405000-00012.

47. Phulka JS, Howlett JW, Hu A. Cannabis related side effects in otolaryngology: a scoping review. J Otolaryngol Head Neck Surg 2021;50(1):56.

48. Wade DT, Makela PM, House H, et al. Long-term use of a cannabis-based medicine in the treatment of spasticity and other symptoms in multiple sclerosis. Mult Scler 2006;12(5):639–45. https://doi.org/10.1177/1352458505070618.

49. Aragona M, Onesti E, Tomassini V, et al. Psychopathological and cognitive effects of therapeutic cannabinoids in multiple sclerosis: a double-blind, placebo controlled, crossover study. Clin Neuropharmacol 2009;32(1):41–7.

50. Breijyeh Z, Jubeh B, Bufo SA, et al. Cannabis: a toxin-producing plant with potential therapeutic uses. Toxins (Basel) 2021;13(2):117.

51. Brumbach S, Goodman SS, Baiduc RR. Behavioral hearing thresholds and distortion product otoacoustic emissions in cannabis smokers. J Speech Lang Hear Res 2019;62(9):3500–15.

52. Baiduc RR, Mullervy S, Berry CM, et al. An Exploratory Study of Early Auditory Evoked Potentials in Cannabis Smokers. Am J Audiol 2020;29(3):303–17.

Establishing Healthy Lifestyle Choices Early

How to Counsel Children and Their Parents

Laith Mukdad, MD, Nina L. Shapiro, MD*

KEYWORDS

- Preventative health • Foreign body • Noise exposure • Upper respiratory infection
- Aural hygiene • Secondhand smoke

KEY POINTS

- Parents should recognize the symptoms and signs of foreign body ingestion and aspiration. A witnessed foreign body aspiration or ingestion may require an immediate emergency department consultation. In addition, identification of nasal and aural foreign bodies will be addressed.
- Use of noise-canceling headphones, avoidance of events and concerts where noise levels are likely to be excessively high, and utilization of smart devices to measure noise exposure are important in reducing the risk of noise-induced hearing loss in children and adolescents.
- Parents and children should be counseled on avoidance of cotton tip applicators in cerumen removal.
- Parents should be advised on the risks of secondhand smoke exposure, which include adverse health outcomes such as neurobehavioral disorders, obesity, upper respiratory infections, disrupted lung development, and cardiovascular complications. Parents and children should be able to recognize and discuss risks of tobacco use and electronic nicotine delivery systems.
- Maintaining good sleep hygiene includes following a nighttime routine, maintaining a consistent sleep schedule, keeping the sleeping environment cool (68°F–72°F) and free from noise, and avoiding disruptors of sleep, such as light and screen time.

Promoting childhood and adolescent health and long-term well-being requires an emphasis on preventative care and anticipatory guidance. In this review, the authors will focus on pertinent ear, nose, and throat preventative health in children, providing clinicians with pertinent and succinct information to counsel children and their parents on the following essential subjects: foreign body aspiration and ingestion, upper respiratory infection prevention, noise exposure risks, aural hygiene, risks of primary and secondhand smoke exposure, and sleep hygiene.

Department of Head and Neck Surgery, David Geffen School of Medicine at UCLA, 200 UCLA Medical Plaza, Suite 550, Los Angeles, CA 90095, USA
* Corresponding author.
E-mail address: Nshapiro@mednet.ucla.edu

Otolaryngol Clin N Am 55 (2022) 1111–1124
https://doi.org/10.1016/j.otc.2022.06.013
0030-6665/22/© 2022 Elsevier Inc. All rights reserved.
oto.theclinics.com

FOREIGN BODY ASPIRATION AND INGESTION

Ingested and aspirated foreign bodies are common in children and are important causes of morbidity and mortality, particularly among children between the ages of 6 months and 3 years.[1] These children are most vulnerable due to less developed dentition and immature swallowing coordination.[1,2] Ninety-eight percent of foreign body ingestions in children are accidental and involve common objects found in the home environment, such as coins, toys, jewelry, magnets, and button batteries (BBs).[1,2]

Aspiration

When the aspiration episode is witnessed, the clinical presentation is clear: parents or caregivers may note a brief period of coughing and choking, which may be associated with dysphonia. As the foreign body passes through the vocal cords, trachea, and into the bronchi, a relative asymptomatic period may begin. During this time, the diagnosis may be more difficult to ascertain, particularly if the initial event was unwitnessed. Indeed, bronchial foreign body symptoms include cough, wheezing, and decreased breath sounds. The resulting symptoms may mimic bronchitis, pneumonia, or asthma.[1] These children may be treated with antibiotics and steroids, which may mask symptoms and further delay the diagnosis.[1,2] For this reason, in children with atypical or prolonged pulmonary symptoms, the possibility of a foreign body should be raised. Delayed complications associated with a retained foreign body include pneumonia, emphysema, and bronchiectasis. The most common objects aspirated by young children are food products (most are peanuts, but seeds and other nuts are common as well). In older children, foods such as hotdogs, popcorn kernels, hard candy, and large chunks of raw vegetables are more common sources of aspiration events. There are approximately 10,000 emergency room visits annually in the United States alone due to food choking events, and one child dies every 3 to 5 days in the United States from choking on food.[3]

Ingestion

Esophageal foreign bodies usually are considered less serious than aspirated foreign bodies, yet a report by Webb and colleagues indicated about 1500 people die per year from complications from esophageal foreign body ingestions.[4] The most common symptoms may be laryngeal irritation, coughing, choking, or drooling caused by the highly compliant membranous wall between the trachea and the esophagus in the child.[1,4] Dysphagia is a later finding, and its absence may lead to a low level of suspicion concerning this diagnosis. Coins are the most frequent esophageal foreign body in children, although undigested food, fish bones, and safety pins also are common.[4]

Parents should be counseled about the importance of recognizing foreign body aspiration and ingestion red flag symptoms noted above and should know that they constitute an emergency that requires immediate attention at the nearest hospital emergency department. Imaging plays an important role in both diagnosing ingested and aspirated foreign bodies and guiding clinical management.[5,6] Clinicians should be familiar with the characteristic "halo" or "double-ring" sign appearance of BBs on anterior–posterior X-ray imaging (**Fig. 1**), which indicate the need for emergent removal.[6] Indeed, BB ingestion is associated with high morbidity and mortality because studies indicate significant esophageal injury within 2 hours via liquefaction necrosis, which may lead to perforation, tracheoesophageal fistula, or fistulization into major vessels.[1,5,6] Chao and colleagues demonstrated that use of common household tape (Scotch/clear, masking tape, black electrical tape) to cover button (watch) batteries reduce the incidence of BB-related esophageal injuries.[5,6] Thus, parents should be counseled to cover BBs immediately after removal from a device for either recycling or disposal and to not allow them to be within reach of their toddlers.[5,6] For witnessed or suspected early-stage BB ingestions, mitigation protocols with protective pH-neutralizing viscous solutions such as honey in a home setting or Carafate in the clinical setting have the potential to significantly slow the rate of esophageal injury before endoscopic removal, and should be considered in the algorithm for BB management.[7] According to Anfang and colleagues, the risk associated with the rapidly progressing button battery injury outweigh that of aspiration-related anesthetic complications in a child with a full stomach proceeding to surgery.[7]

Reducing risk of button battery ingestion has gained nationwide attention because the US Consumer Product Safety Commission enacted a new mandatory standard in 2017 to include use of warning labels and instructions of BB risks for BB-requiring toys, as well as new testing requirements to ensure child-resistant toy packaging with locked BBs.[6] More recently, Duracell(R) released 3 new BBs with nontoxic bitter coating in a measure to deter accidental ingestions.[6]

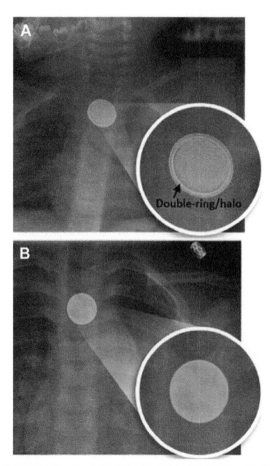

Fig. 1. The following 2 images are chest X-ray images of toddlers with foreign body ingestions. (*A*) Portrays a double ring or halo sign, which indicates a button battery, whereas (*B*) is characteristic of an esophageal coin. (Reproduced with permission from Kris Jatana, MD.)

Aural and Nasal Foreign Bodies

Although generally not life-threatening, aural and nasal foreign bodies cause morbidity and are important to recognize. Common aural and nasal foreign bodies include jewelry, paper products, beads, and food matter.[8] The most common presenting symptom of a nasal foreign body is unilateral foul-smelling nasal discharge, whereas the most common presenting symptoms of aural foreign bodies include ear pain and bleeding.[8] The highest-risk foreign bodies in these locations are BBs, which should be removed immediately. In the nose, BBs may lead to necrosis of the nasal mucosa and septal perforation.[9] In the external ear canal, BBs may cause skin and bony canal necrosis, tympanic membrane perforation, and even facial nerve injury.[8]

The "parent's kiss" technique has been described as a physically and emotionally nontraumatic way of removing nasal foreign bodies, with a reported 64.5% success rate according to Purohit and colleagues.[10] The technique involves the parent exhaling while covering their mouth over the child's mouth and occluding the unaffected nostril (**Fig. 2**).[10] This technique delivers a puff of air through the nasopharynx, out through the affected nostril, and if successful, results in expulsion of the foreign body.

HYGIENE AND UPPER RESPIRATORY INFECTION PREVENTION

Upper respiratory tract infections (URIs) including nasopharyngitis, pharyngitis, tonsillitis, and otitis media constitute 87.5% of the total episodes of respiratory infections.[11] The burden of URIs in pediatrics is high within both industrialized and developing countries. Because causative therapies of recurrent respiratory tract infections (RTIs) bear substantial limits, preventive measures deserve priority.

Breastfeeding has been shown to be associated with lowering the risk of URIs,[12] including acute and recurrent otitis media, in the first year of life.[11,12] In a study by Duijts and colleagues, examining more than 4000 infants in the Netherlands, infants who were breastfed exclusively until the age of 4 months and partially thereafter had lower risks of upper and lower RTIs in the first 6 months after birth.[12] Their team advocated for health-policy strategies to promote exclusive breastfeeding for at least 4 months in industrialized countries.[12] This is due to oligosaccharides and IgA present within human milk, which interfere with the binding of *Streptococcus pneumoniae* and *Haemophilus influenzae* to nasopharynx and oropharynx, thus

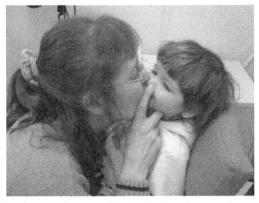

Fig. 2. Mother performing the "parent's kiss" technique in removing a nasal foreign body. (Reproduced with permission from Neeraj Purohit, MD.)

reducing colonization and infections.[13,14] Additionally, lactoferrin has broad antimicrobial properties including disruption of the bacterial outer membrane.[13] However, an important confounder to keep in mind when examining data associating breastfeeding with reduced URIs is that women of lower socioeconomic status (SES) are less likely to breastfeed as they tend to have more obstacles to breastfeeding at work, whereas women of higher SES generally have more supportive workplaces and/or home environments for breastfeeding/pumping.[15]

Following infancy, parents should be counseled that the best method for preventing transmission of URIs include hygiene, frequent handwashing, and avoiding touching one's mouth, nose, and eyes.[16] Viruses can be transmitted from the hands to objects in the environment or to other people. Parents should also be counseled on the importance of virucidal and bactericidal disinfectants (phenol and alcohol) for decontamination of environmental surfaces.[17]

Although not one immunization prevents all URIs, clinicians should recommend yearly influenza vaccination for all children older than age 6 months to prevent influenza infection and its complications. Additionally, parents with high-risk children (prematurity with bronchopulmonary dysplasia, congenital heart disease, neuromuscular disorders, immunocompromised hosts, and so forth) should confer with their pediatrician regarding the use of palivizumab as a preventive measure against respiratory syncytial virus infections.[18] Parents may also discuss with their pediatrician the possibility of using OM-85, a lysate of 21 common bacterial respiratory pathogens, for children aged 1 to 6 years with recurrent URIs (greater than 6 per year) because recent clinical trials demonstrated reduction of risk of recurrent RTIs in this population.[19,20]

Many other preventive measures have been studied with conflicting reports. Probiotics may be beneficial for preventing upper respiratory infections; however, the quality of the current evidence is low.[21] Vitamins A and C, herbal products, and honeybee products (honey, bee-pollen, beeswax, propolis) have all not demonstrated efficacy in preventing URIs in studies.[19] Vitamin D deficiency could play a role in children with recurrent RTIs, although further studies are needed to clarify the lowest minimum vitamin D serum level associated with an increased risk of respiratory infections, the most effective dosage, schedule of administration, and duration of treatment.[19] Parents should be made aware that the American Academy of Pediatrics recommends that exclusively or partially breastfed infants receive at least 400 IU of daily vitamin D supplementation in order to support healthy bone development.[22]

NOISE EXPOSURE RISKS

Portable music players (PMPs), including mobile phones and tablets, in combination with headphones, are embedded in daily life and serve educational purposes in schools.[23,24] Approximately 93% of children and adolescents between ages 12 and 19 years are reported to use PMPs on a daily basis.[25] Moreover, more than half of adolescent PMP users exceed the recommended maximum noise dose.[26] Attention for noise-induced hearing loss (NIHL) has risen and prevention programs have been launched.[27]

According to the National Institute of Occupational Health and Safety (NIOSH), exposure to noise levels more than 85 dB for no more than 8 hours is the federal threshold for hearing protection.[28] For parents, a sometimes-overlooked source of noise exposure to their toddlers and preschoolers is toys. The Sight and Hearing Association screens all loud toys (>85 dB) and publishes a yearly "Noisy Toys List" at http://www.sightandhearing.org/Services/NoisyToysList%C2%A9.aspx, naming the loudest toys that reach the 85 dB threshold.[29] We encourage providers to share this list with parents on an annual basis in order to encourage purchase of toys that are safe for hearing preservation.

A report from a large-scale US national health survey indicated that 12% to 15% of school-aged children have audiometric confirmed hearing deficits attributable to noise exposure,[30] suggesting children are being exposed to hazardous levels of noise. NIHL is strongly related to noise dose, which includes both level of exposure and duration of exposure. Jiang and colleagues found that adolescents were more likely to exceed the 100% daily noise dose in the presence of high-level background noise (61–80 dB) compared with those in the presence of low-level background noise (40–60 dBA).[26] Therefore, the World Health Organization (WHO) encourages the use of noise-canceling headphones to help block noise from the general environment so that the listener does not have to increase the volume of their personal listening devices (PLDs) to overcome interference from background noise.[27] This is of special importance when children are planning on traveling by plane where at cruising altitudes the engine noise is approximately 85 dB.[27]

Additionally, parents should seek to use smart devices to measure noise exposure of venues and activities to determine if noise exceeds 85 dB, and adjust exposure as needed. The WHO encourages the use of the NIOSH sponsored Sound Level Meter application (available on iOS and Android devices) and the Soundmeter (available on Android devices), both of which have demonstrated efficacy in measurements.[27,31] It should be noted that there are several variables that influence the accuracy of these measurements, so an end user should only use these devices for general guidance and educational purposes.[31]

Parents should be encouraged to limit their children's participation in sporting events, concerts, and other activities where noise levels are likely to be excessively high. Although the duration of exposure from these locations is generally lower than that of PLDs, the levels of noise can be much higher, ranging from 79 to 130 dB.[27] Sound levels at music concerts are often greater than 85 dB, with certain reports suggesting intensity reaching up to 122 dB.[32] Furthermore, according to Opperman and colleagues, sound pressure levels seemed equally hazardous in all parts of the concert hall, regardless of the type of music played. Thus, when these types of events are attended, hearing protection (such as sound attenuation earplugs) should be worn regardless of distance to the stage.[32]

Finally, it should be noted that whenever parents are concerned about a potential hearing loss, they should seek hearing evaluation for their children by a licensed audiologist or other qualified professional.

AURAL HYGIENE

Aural hygiene is commonly performed and is often incorporated into a person's daily hygienic routine. Specific measures used to clean the ears range from washing the outer ear with soap and water to inserting objects into the external ear canal such as cotton-tipped applicators (CTAs; most commonly), paper clips, and bobby pins.[33] Consensus opinion from clinicians is that cerumen impaction may be exacerbated by CTAs, and a higher incidence of cerumen has been reported in children whose ears were cleaned with CTAs.[34]

Although objects for cleaning are ubiquitous, parents should be counseled not to insert any foreign objects into their children's ear canals because these objects can cause injuries such as bleeding, laceration, tympanic membrane perforation, or worsen cerumen impaction by pushing cerumen deeper into the canal.[33,34] Moreover, external ear canal injuries secondary to CTAs have been linked with increased risk of otitis externa, also known as "swimmer's ear," an inflammation or infection of the external ear canal.[35] In a study by Nussinovitch and colleagues, more than 70% of children aged 3 to 12 years had their ears cleaned with a CTA during the 10 days preceding the diagnosis of otitis externa.[35]

Another popular form of ear cleaning is the use of ear candling, in which a hollow candle that is burned with one end is placed within the external ear canal, with the intent of displacing cerumen. This is also known as "ear coning" or "thermo-auricular therapy."[33,36] Studies have shown that this method of ear cleaning is not only ineffective but also potentially dangerous with complications such as ear canal burn, tympanic membrane perforation, and otitis externa.[36] Clinicians should thus strongly recommend against ear candling for treating or preventing cerumen impaction.[33,36]

Parents should be advised that cerumen is part of the ear's self-cleaning mechanism and is usually naturally expelled from the ear canal without issues. When this mechanism fails, however, cerumen is retained in the canal and may become impacted; interventions to encourage its removal may then be needed. Application of ear drops is one of these methods.[33,37] In a clinical trial by Soy and colleagues examining 1243 pediatric patients with total or nearly total occlusive cerumen, the best cerumenolytic solution was found to be a mixture of glycerine 10 cc + 3% hydrogen peroxide 10 cc + 10% sodium bicarbonate 10 cc + distilled water 10 cc, which provided ease in terms of pain for the patient and in terms of time and comfort for the physician during the removal procedure.[37]

Most importantly, clinicians should identify at-risk children with obstructing cerumen in the ear canal who may not be able to express symptoms (developmentally delayed, nonverbal patients with behavioral challenges, children with fevers, children with parental concerns, or children with speech delay) and promptly refer them to an otolaryngologist for further workup with an audiogram, and treatment with cerumenolytic agents and/or manual removal requiring instrumentation.[33] Clinicians should also be aware that children with hearing aids and/or frequent use of in-the-ear headphones or ear buds are at increased risk of cerumen impaction.

RISKS OF SECONDHAND AND PRIMARY SMOKE EXPOSURE

Secondhand smoke (SHS) is a mixture of gases and fine particles that release from a burning tobacco product or from smoke that has been exhaled by an actively smoking individual.[38,39] The scope of SHS exposure can span the life cycle, beginning in utero with exposure to maternal direct smoking or maternal SHS.[38] A recent review concluded that any active maternal smoking was associated with increased risks of fetal loss, neonatal death, and perinatal death, and these increased with the amount smoked by the mother.[39] Additionally, maternal cigarette smoking is an established cause of in utero telomere shortening and is associated with several adverse health outcomes including neurobehavioral disorders, obesity, upper respiratory infections, disrupted lung development, and cardiovascular complications.[40,41]

It is also important to note that the respiratory flora of smokers contains fewer aerobic and anaerobic organisms with interfering activity against bacterial pathogens and therefore harbor more potential pathogens as compared with the flora of non-smokers.[42] As a result, parents who smoke may serve as a source of pathogens that can colonize and/or infect their children. The reduction in the numbers of normal respiratory flora that interfere with the growth of pathogens and the greater adherence of bacterial pathogens to the oral mucosa are associated with the greater frequency of respiratory infections.[42] Moreover, SHS causes irritation of the respiratory tract in household contacts.[43] Unsurprisingly, studies have indicated that children exposed to smoke have more episodes of otitis media, which is a form of a respiratory infection, than children in smoke-free environments.[43]

Although the respiratory consequences of SHS exposure are clinically apparent in childhood, the cardiovascular effects of SHS exposure are occult but significant. Evidence suggests that SHS exposure in children and youth persist into adult life. Compelling animal and human evidence shows that SHS exposure during childhood results in premature atherosclerosis and its cardiovascular consequences.[44] Childhood SHS exposure is also related to impaired cardiac autonomic function and changes in heart rate variability.[44] Moreover, childhood SHS exposure is associated with cardiometabolic risk factors such as obesity, dyslipidemia, and insulin resistance. As a result, broad-based governmental policy initiatives have taken place including community smoking bans and increased taxation.[44]

Additionally, smoking exposure has been associated with neurobehavioral disorders. Epidemiologic studies show an association between in utero tobacco smoke exposure and an elevated risk of attention-deficit/hyperactivity disorder.[45] A recent study in overweight and obese children found an association between plasma nicotine levels and poorer cognitive scores, suggesting that SHS exposure during childhood may affect brain development.[45] Additionally, Jacob and colleagues indicated a positive association between SHS exposure and depressive symptoms among adolescents from low-income and middle-income countries in a recent report.[46]

Prenatal and postnatal exposure to SHS also results in disrupted lung development, resulting in reduced lung function in children (reductions in forced expiratory volume and midexpiratory flow).[47] Studies indicate an inverse dose–response relationship between the number of cigarettes smoked per day by the mother prenatally and a variety of measures of lung functionality in newborns (after accounting for maternal smoking after pregnancy).[47,48]

Since their introduction to the US market in the mid-2000s, electronic nicotine delivery systems (ENDS) have become widely popular among adolescents, with an estimated 20.8% of high school students and 4.9% of middle school students being current users, a prevalence that has been described by the FDA as an epidemic.[49] ENDS companies, most of which are owned by the tobacco industry, target children and adolescents by promoting flavors such as strawberry melon, cotton candy, chocolate milk, and mango and using a wide array of advertising including television platforms and social media.[49] To counteract this, in 2019, CBS, WarnerMedia, and Viacom banned EC advertisements and legislation HR 4249 "Stop Vaping Ads Act" was introduced to Congress. Additionally, as of September 2021, all 50 states have passed legislation to prohibit sale of ENDS to individuals aged younger than 18 to 21 years, depending on the state.

The liquid solution within ENDS contains propylene glycol mixed with aldehydes, metals, and polycyclic aromatic hydrocarbons, which are known carcinogens and respiratory irritants (Jensen RP).[50] Although long-term respiratory effects of ENDS are yet to be established, reports suggest adolescent ENDS users are at increased risk of cough, wheeze, and asthma exacerbations.[51] Indeed, in a study by Lerner and colleagues, human lung cells exposed to ENDS aerosolized liquids demonstrated higher levels of inflammatory cytokines such as interleukin (IL)-6 and IL-8, which are known to contribute to chronic inflammatory diseases of the respiratory tract, making individuals more susceptible to chronic bronchitis and pneumonia.[52] Additionally, several well-designed studies show that adolescents who use ENDS are at higher risk of transitioning to traditional cigarettes.[53]

SLEEP HYGIENE

Although a variety of important sleep disorders may disrupt quality of sleep in children and adolescents, such as restless leg syndrome, obstructive sleep apnea, and narcolepsy, this article will focus on common disorders that affect the quantity of sleep, such as poor sleep hygiene, circadian rhythm disorders, and insomnia.

First, it is important to note that according to the American Academy of Sleep Medicine, the following sleep durations are recommended in order to optimize health: Infants 4 months to 12 months should sleep 12 to 16 hours per 24 hours (including naps). Children 1 to 2 years of age should sleep 11 to 14 hours per 24 hours (including naps). Children 3 to 5 years of age should sleep 10 to 13 hours per 24 hours (including naps). Children 6 to 12 years of age should sleep 9 to 12 hours per 24 hours. Teenagers 13 to 18 years of age should sleep 8 to 10 hours per 24 hours.[54]

Parents and children should be counseled on the importance of sleeping the above number of recommended hours on a regular basis, due to the association of nightly sleep duration with better health outcomes, including improved attention, learning, emotional regulation, quality of life, and mental and physical health.[54] On the contrary, sleep deprivation is associated with poor attention, disruptive behavior, and learning difficulties. Insufficient sleep in teenagers is associated with increased risk of self-harm, suicidal thoughts, and suicide attempts.[45,54,55]

Poor sleep-hygiene practices seem to be a major contributor to sleep disruption in children and adolescents.[55,56] Parents and children should be counseled on the importance of maintaining good sleep hygiene which include following a regular night-time routine, maintaining a consistent sleep schedule, keeping the sleeping environment cool (68°F–72°F) and free from noise, and avoiding disruptors of sleep, such as light and screen time.[56–58] Caffeine consumption is problematic, with an associated decrease in quality of sleep observed as doses increase.[58]

A common sleep disorder in adolescents is delayed sleep–wake phase disorder. Pubertal onset corresponds with a biologically mediated shift in sleep timing with a predisposition to a later sleep–wake cycle. This shift is mediated by 2 distinct processes. First, the homeostatic drive to sleep, which increases with increased wake time, accumulates more slowly during adolescence, which leads to a longer time to fall asleep and an increased ability to stay awake at night compared with prepubertal teenagers.[56,58,59] Second, melatonin secretion shifts to a later time, causing a delay in the circadian rhythm.[56] Management of this condition relies on melatonin supplementation and timing of light exposure.[56]

Delayed sleep phase syndrome (DSPS) should be distinguished from psycho-physiological insomnia (PI), which is also common among adolescents. PI is defined as the inability to fall asleep or stay asleep due to the intrusion of anxious or stressful thoughts while in bed.[56] Those with PI often sleep better in new settings, such as hotel rooms. Negative associations with sleep can lead to progressive anxiety with the propagation of insomnia.[57] Querying patients regarding intrusive thoughts and anxiety in bed is important in differentiating PI from DSPS. Parents should be counseled on the importance of cognitive behavioral therapy in treating insomnia. Some of the common components of cognitive behavioral treatment including stimulus control therapy (if unable to fall asleep after approximately 20 minutes, leave the bed until feeling drowsy), journaling (writing a "worry list" for ~5 minutes every day), and paradoxic intent (thinking about remaining awake instead of actively attempting to sleep to reduce anxiety around bedtime).

SUMMARY

In this article, the authors review pertinent ear, nose, and throat preventative health in children. First, the symptoms and signs of ingested and foreign body are summarized, and key points in identifying nasal and aural foreign bodies are addressed. Second, ways to reduce the risk of RTIs are elucidated, including frequent hand washing and the use of bactericidal and virucidal disinfectants for decontamination of environmental surfaces. Third, methods to reduce the risk of noise-induced hearing loss are identified, which include the use of noise-canceling headphones, avoidance of concerts where noise levels are excessively high, and utilization of smart devices to measure noise exposure. Fourth, the troubling consequences of cotton tip applicator use are described and effective management of cerumen impaction is explained. Fifth, adverse events associated with secondhand smoke exposure are detailed, which include neurobehavioral disorders, obesity, upper respiratory infections, disrupted lung development, and cardiovascular complications. The troubling consequences of ENDS use, which have become more popular among high school students, are examined. Finally, common sleep disorders are reviewed and maintenance of good sleep hygiene (which includes following a nighttime routine, keeping the sleeping environment cool (68°F–72°F) and free from noise, and avoiding disruptors of sleep, such as light and screen time) is accentuated.

CLINICS CARE POINTS

- Clinicians should counsel parents on the symptoms and signs of ingested and aspirated foreign bodies.
- Utilization of noise-canceling headphones and smart devices that measure noise exposure should be encouraged in order to reduce noise-induced hearing loss.
- Cotton–tip applicators should be avoided in cerumen removal.
- Children and their parents should be counseled on the adverse events associated with tobacco use and electronic nicotine delivery systems.
- Maintenance of good sleep hygiene should be encouraged.

DISCLOSURE

The authors have no conflicts of interest, no sponsorships, and no funding sources for this article.

REFERENCES

1. Ellen M. Friedman, Tracheobronchial foreign bodies. Otolaryngol Clin North Am 2000;33(Issue 1):179–85.
2. Sink JR, Kitsko DJ, Mehta DK, et al. Diagnosis of Pediatric Foreign Body Ingestion: Clinical Presentation, Physical Examination, and Radiologic Findings. Ann Otol Rhinol Laryngol 2016;125(4):342–50.
3. Committee on Injury, Violence, and Poison Prevention. Prevention of choking among children. Pediatrics 2010;125(3):601–7.
4. Webb WA. Management of foreign bodies of the upper gastrointestinal tract: update. Gastrointest Endosc 1995;41(1):39–51.

5. Chao S, Gibbs H, Rhoades K, et al. Button battery taping and disposal: Risk reduction strategies for the household setting. Int J Pediatr Otorhinolaryngol 2021;153:111008.
6. Sethia R, Gibbs H, Jacobs IN, et al. Current management of button battery injuries. Laryngoscope Invest Otolaryngol 2021;6:549–63.
7. Anfang RR, Jatana KR, Linn RL, et al. pH-neutralizing esophageal irrigations as a novel mitigation strategy for button battery injury. Laryngoscope 2019;129:49–57.
8. Mackle T, Conlon B. Foreign bodies of the nose and ears in children. Should these be managed in the accident and emergency setting? Int J Pediatr Otorhinolaryngol 2006;70(3):425–8.
9. Cetinkaya EA, Arslan İB, Cukurova İ. Nasal foreign bodies in children: Types, locations, complications and removal. Int J Pediatr Otorhinolaryngol 2015;79(11): 1881–5.
10. Purohit N, Ray S, Wilson T, et al. The 'parent's kiss': an effective way to remove paediatric nasal foreign bodies. Ann R Coll Surg Engl 2008;90(5):420–2.
11. Jain N, Lodha R, Kabra SK. Upper respiratory tract infections. Indian J Pediatr 2001;68(12):1135–8.
12. Duijts L, Jaddoe VWV, Hofman A, et al. Moll; Prolonged and Exclusive Breastfeeding Reduces the Risk of Infectious Diseases in Infancy. Pediatr July 2010; 126(1):e18–25.
13. Duncan B, Ey J, Holberg CJ, et al. Exclusive breast-feeding for at least 4 months protects against otitis media. Pediatrics 1993;91(5):867–72.
14. Andersson B, Porras O, Lars Å. Hanson, Teresa Lagergård, Catharina Svanborg-Edén, Inhibition of Attachment of Streptococcus pneumoniae and Haemophilus influenzae by Human Milk and Receptor Oligosaccharides. J Infect Dis 1986; 153(Issue 2):232–7.
15. Heck KE, Braveman P, Cubbin C, et al. Socioeconomic status and breastfeeding initiation among California mothers. Public Health Rep 2006;121(1):51–9.
16. Hanson LA, Korotkova M, Haversen L, et al. Breast-feeding, a complex support system for the offspring. Pediatr Int 2002;44(4):347–52.
17. Ashraf S, Islam M, Unicomb L, et al. Effect of Improved Water Quality, Sanitation, Hygiene and Nutrition Interventions on Respiratory Illness in Young Children in Rural Bangladesh: A Multi-Arm Cluster-Randomized Controlled Trial. Am J Trop Med Hyg 2020;102(5):1124–30.
18. Brady MT, Byington CL, Davies HD, et al. Updated Guidance for Palivizumab Prophylaxis Among Infants and Young Children at Increased Risk of Hospitalization for Respiratory Syncytial Virus Infection. Pediatr 2014;134(2):415–20.
19. Esposito S, Bianchini S, Bosis S, et al. A randomized, placebo-controlled, double-blinded, single-centre, phase IV trial to assess the efficacy and safety of OM-85 in children suffering from recurrent respiratory tract infections. J Transl Med 2019; 17(1):284.
20. Schaad UB. Prevention of pediatric respiratory tract inections: emphasis on the role of OM-85. Eur Respir Rev 2005;14(95):74–7.
21. Hao Q, Dong BR, Wu T. Probiotics for preventing acute upper respiratory tract infections. Cochrane Database Syst Rev 2015;(2):CD006895.
22. Wagner CL, Greer FR. American Academy of Pediatrics Section on Breastfeeding; American Academy of Pediatrics Committee on Nutrition. Prevention of rickets and vitamin D deficiency in infants, children, and adolescents. Pediatrics 2008;122(5):1142–52 [Erratum in: Pediatrics. 2009;123(1):197].
23. Harrison RV. Noise-induced hearing loss in children: A 'less than silent' environmental danger. Paediatrics Child Health 2008;13(5):377–82.

24. le Clercq C, Goedegebure A, Jaddoe V, et al. Association Between Portable Music Player Use and Hearing Loss Among Children of School Age in the Netherlands. JAMA Otolaryngol Head Neck Surg 2018;144(8):668–75.

25. Vogel I, Verschuure H, van der Ploeg CP, et al. Estimating adolescent risk for hearing loss based on data from a large school-based survey. Am J Public Health 2010;100(6):1095–100.

26. Jiang W, Zhao F, Guderley N, et al. Daily music exposure dose and hearing problems using personal listening devices in adolescents and young adults: A systematic review. Int J Audiol 2016;55(4):197–205.

27. Noise exposure limit for children in recreational settings: review of available evidence (PDF), World Health Organization, February 1, 2018. Available at: https://cdn.who.int/media/docs/default-source/documents/health-topics/deafness-and-hearing-loss/monograph-on-noise-exposure-limit-for-children-in-recreational-settings.pdf?sfvrsn=a5dcde0d_5.

28. Hearing Conservation Amendment, In: Occupational safety and health administration: occupational noise exposure. Federal register, Part III, 1981, Department of Labor, 37773-37778. Available at: https://www.osha.gov/sites/default/files/laws-regs/federalregister/1981-01-16_0.pdf

29. "Noisy Toys List." Sight & Hearing Association. Available at: http://www.sightandhearing.org/Services/NoisyToysList%C2%A9.aspx. Accessed February 1, 2022.

30. Niskar AS, Kieszak SM, Holmes AE, et al. Estimated prevalence of noise induced threshold shifts among children 6 to 19 years of age: The third National Health and Nutrition Examination Survey, 1998–1994, United States. Pediatrics 2001;108:40–3. Available at: https://pubmed.ncbi.nlm.nih.gov/11433052/.

31. Kardous CA, Shaw PB. Evaluation of smartphone sound measurement applications. J Acoust Soc Am 2014;135(4):EL186–92.

32. Opperman, Reifman, Schlauch. Levine "Incidence of spontaneous hearing threshold shifts during modern concert performances. Otol-HNS 2006;134(4):667–73.

33. Schwartz SR, Magit AE, Rosenfeld RM, et al. Clinical Practice Guideline (Update): Earwax (Cerumen Impaction). Otolaryngol Head Neck Surg 2017;156(1_suppl):S1–29.

34. Baxter P. Association between use of cotton tipped swabs and cerumen plugs. Br Med J 1983;287:1260.

35. Nussinovitch M, Rimon A, Volovitz B, et al. Cotton-tip applicators as a leading cause of otitis externa. Int J Pediatr Otorhinolaryngol 2004;68(Issue 4):433–5.

36. Seely DR, Quigley SM, Langman AW. Ear candles: efficacy and safety. Laryngoscope 1996;106:1226–9.

37. Soy FK, Ozbay C, Kulduk E, et al. A new approach for cerumenolytic treatment in children: In vivo and in vitro study. Int J Pediatr Otorhinolaryngol 2015;79(7):1096–100.

38. Peterson LA, Hecht SS. Tobacco, e-cigarettes, and child health. Curr Opin Pediatr 2017;29(2):225–30.

39. U.S. Department of Health and Human Services. A report of the surgeon general. Atlanta, GA: U.S. Dept. of Health and Human Services, Centers for Disease Control and Prevention, Coordinating Center for Health Promotion, National Center for Chronic Disease Prevention and Health Promotion, Office on Smoking and Health; 2014. The Health Consequences of Smoking: 50 Years of Progress.

40. Pineles BL, Hsu S, Park E, et al. Systematic review and meta-analyses of perinatal death and maternal exposure to tobacco smoke during pregnancy. Am J Epidemiol 2016;184:87–97.

41. Ip P, Chung BH, Ho FK, et al. Nicotine Tob Res 2017;19(1):111–8.

42. Brook I. The Impact of Smoking on Oral and Nasopharyngeal Bacterial Flora. J Dent Res 2011;90(6):704–10.

43. Klein JO. MD Nonimmune strategies for prevention of otitis media. Pediatr Infect Dis J 2000;19(5):S89–92.

44. Raghuveer G, White DA, Hayman LL, et al, American Heart Association Committee on Atherosclerosis, Hypertension, and Obesity in the Young of the Council on Cardiovascular Disease in the Young; Behavior Change for Improving Health Factors Committee of the Council on Lifestyle and Cardiometabolic Health and Council on Epidemiology and Prevention; and Stroke Council. Cardiovascular Consequences of Childhood Secondhand Tobacco Smoke Exposure: Prevailing Evidence, Burden, and Racial and Socioeconomic Disparities: A Scientific Statement From the American Heart Association. Circulation 2016;134(16):e336–59.

45. Davis CL, Tingen MS, Jia J, et al. Passive Smoke Exposure and Its Effects on Cognition, Sleep, and Health Outcomes in Overweight and Obese Children. Child Obes 2016;12:119–25. This study in overweight and obese children found an association between plasma cotinine levels and poorer cognitive scores, suggesting that environmental tobacco smoke exposure during childhood can impact brain development.

46. Jacob L, Lee S, Jackson SE, et al. Secondhand Smoking and Depressive Symptoms Among In-School Adolescents. Am J Prev Med 2020;58(Issue 5):613–21.

47. Gibbs K, Collaco JM, McGrath-Morrow SA. Impact of Tobacco Smoke and Nicotine Exposure on Lung Development. Chest 2016;149:552–61.

48. Hayatbakhsh MR, Sadasivam S, Mamun AA. Maternal smoking during and after pregnancy and lung function in early adulthood: a prospective study. Thorax 2009;64(9):810–4.

49. Jenssen BP, Walley SC. SECTION ON TOBACCO CONTROL, Judith A. Groner, Maria Rahmandar, Rachel Boykan, Bryan Mih, Jyothi N. Marbin, Alice Little Caldwell; E-Cigarettes and Similar Devices. Pediatrics 2019;143(2):e20183652.

50. Jensen RP, Luo W, Pankow JF, et al. Hidden formaldehyde in e-cigarette aerosols. N Engl J Med 2015;372(4):392–4.

51. National Academies of Sciences, Engineering, and Medicine. Public health consequences of E-cigarettes. Washington, DC: The National Academies Press; 2018.

52. Lerner CA, Sundar IK, Yao H, et al. Vapors Produced by Electronic Cigarettes and E-Juices with Flavorings Induce Toxicity, Oxidative Stress, and Inflammatory Response in Lung Epithelial Cells and in Mouse Lung. PLoS One 2015;10(2): e0116732.

53. Soneji S, Barrington-Trimis JL, Wills TA, et al. Association between initial use of e-cigarettes and subsequent cigarette smoking among adolescents and young adults: a systematic review and meta-analysis. JAMA Pediatr 2017;171(8): 788–97.

54. Paruthi S, Brooks LJ, D'Ambrosio C, et al. Consensus Statement of the American Academy of Sleep Medicine on the Recommended Amount of Sleep for Healthy Children: Methodology and Discussion. J Clin Sleep Med 2016;12(11):1549–61.

55. Mindell JA, Meltzer LJ, Carskadon MA, et al. Developmental aspects of sleep hygiene: findings from the 2004 National Sleep Foundation Sleep in America Poll. Sleep Med 2009;10(7):771–9.

56. Kansagra S. Sleep Disorders in Adolescents. Pediatrics 2020; 145(Supplement_2):S204–9.
57. Levenson JC, Shensa A, Sidani JE, et al. Social media use before bed and sleep disturbance among young adults in the United States: a nationally representative study. Sleep 2017;40(9).
58. Troynikov O, Watson CG, Nawaz N. Sleep environments and sleep physiology: a review. J Therm Biol 2018;78:192–203.
59. Pollak CP, Bright D. Caffeine consumption and weekly sleep patterns in US seventh-, eighth-, and ninth-graders. Pediatrics 2003;111(1):42–6.

Recent Advancements in Understanding the Gut Microbiome and the Inner Ear Axis

Alexa J. Denton, BS[a,1], Dimitri A. Godur, MS[a,1], Jeenu Mittal, MSc[a],
Nathalie B. Bencie, BS[a], Rahul Mittal, PhD[a],
Adrien A. Eshraghi, MD, MSc[a,b,c,d],*

KEYWORDS

- Gut–microbiome–inner ear axis • Blood labyrinth barrier • Cochlea • Gut–brain axis
- Sensorineural hearing loss

KEY POINTS

- The gut microbiome fosters a symbiotic relationship with the gastrointestinal tract by facilitating in maintaining homeostasis, metabolizing fuel, and protecting the body from pathogenic microorganisms.
- Gut dysbiosis has been associated with disorders of the gastrointestinal (GI) tract, such as inflammatory bowel disease (IBD) and celiac disease (CD), as well as with conditions in other organ systems, such as neurodegenerative disorders due to the change in blood–brain barrier (BBB) permeability.
- Studies have highlighted the similarities in structure and function between the BBB and the blood labyrinth barrier (BLB), a key regulator in endolymph and perilymph ionic concentration, emphasizing the potential for an association between the gastrointestinal microbiome and inner ear disorders.
- IBD has been found to be commonly associated with sensorineural hearing loss (SNHL) via changes in the BLB, the mechanism of which is still under further study.
- Noise exposure has also been observed to compromise the BLB and increase the levels of proinflammatory cytokines as well as reactive oxygen species (ROS), leading to downstream gut dysbiosis and further promoting the hypothesis of bidirectional communication in the gut–inner ear axis.

[a] Department of Otolaryngology, Hearing Research and Cochlear Implant Laboratory, University of Miami Miller School of Medicine, Miami, FL, USA; [b] Department of Neurological Surgery, University of Miami Miller School of Medicine, Miami, FL, USA; [c] Department of Biomedical Engineering, University of Miami, Coral Gables, FL, USA; [d] Department of Pediatrics, University of Miami Miller School of Medicine, Miami, FL, USA
[1] Contributed equally to this work.
* Corresponding author. Department of Otolaryngology, Neurological Surgery, Biomedical Engineering, and Pediatrics, University of Miami Miller School of Medicine, 1600 Northwest 10th Avenue, Miami, FL 33136.
E-mail address: aeshraghi@med.miami.edu

Otolaryngol Clin N Am 55 (2022) 1125–1137
https://doi.org/10.1016/j.otc.2022.07.002
0030-6665/22/© 2022 Elsevier Inc. All rights reserved.
oto.theclinics.com

INTRODUCTION

The gut–brain axis has been widely studied with a special focus placed on the microbiota as a primary regulator of gut–brain function. The gut microbiota and brain communicate via several routes such as through neurotransmitters, the immune system, the enteric nervous system, and the vagus nerve.[1–5] Gut dysbiosis, defined as an imbalance in the microbiota of the gut, serves as a predisposing factor for several neurologic disorders such as Alzheimer's disease, Parkinson's disease, multiple sclerosis, depression, anxiety, and autism spectrum disorder (ASD).[6–11] The inner ear resembles the brain in several ways that may make it equally susceptible to influences from the gut, potentially leading to hearing loss. One such resemblance is that there are similarities between the blood–brain barrier (BBB) and the blood labyrinth barrier (BLB).[12] It is thus hypothesized that there is bidirectional communication between the gut and the inner ear; however, investigation into this association has not been widely examined.

Sensorineural hearing loss (SNHL) is one of the most common neurosensory disorders affecting humans. There are approximately 66,000 new cases annually in the United States alone. SNHL has been linked to several genetic and acquired factors such as chronic noise exposure, ototoxic medications, consumption of diets high in fat, and obesity.[12–14] Hearing loss is also commonly attributed to autoimmune inner ear disease (AIED), referred to as primary AIED when acting alone, or secondary AIED when observed to be working in conjunction with another disease.[15] SNHL has also been reported to be the most common inner ear disorder that positively correlates with gastrointestinal (GI) conditions such as inflammatory bowel diseases (IBD), including ulcerative colitis and Crohn's disease.[16] Each of these conditions has also been implicated in gut dysbiosis; however, the link between dysbiosis and inner ear pathology has not been clearly outlined.

A bidirectional relationship between the inner ear and the GI tract is suggested by the fact that chronic noise exposure affects the composition of gut microbiota and inflammation in the GI tract[17] (**Fig. 1**). In this review, we discuss recent advancements that enhance our understanding of the relationship between the gut microflora and the inner ear in order to introduce the concept of the gut microbiome–inner ear axis (see **Fig. 1**). We aim to summarize pathophysiological processes that lead to inflammation in both the GI tract and the inner ear while linking inner ear pathology to gut dysbiosis, and vice-versa (see **Fig. 1**).

GUT MICROSTRUCTURE AND MICROBIOME
Overview of Gastrointestinal Cellular Biology

The GI tract contains structural and physiologic properties that allow it to both function as a protective barrier between the lumen and the bloodstream as well as carry out its role in nutrient absorption and transportation.[18] The epithelial layer of the GI tract is highly specialized and serves as a chemical and physical barrier to direct exposure from the external environment. In addition to the actual cells comprising the mucosal layer, there is also a robust immune system component that assists in regulating GI homeostasis.[18] Ultimately, inflammation, pathogens, and other external insults can disrupt this system and lead to systemic effects.

At a microscopic level, the cells of the GI tract are organized into villi and crypts that are lined by multiple types of intestinal epithelial cells.[19] Most of the intestinal epithelial cells are enterocytes, which function in digestion and contain transport proteins that facilitate the absorptive processes. However, there are also specialized cells that function to maintain and regulate the various functions of the GI tract.[18,19] These

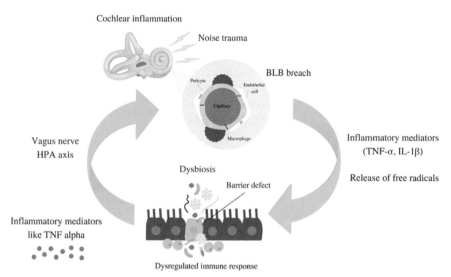

Fig. 1. Schematic representation of bidirectional communication between the Gut Microbiome and the Inner Ear Axis.

include enteroendocrine cells which regulate the hormonal secretions of the GI tract, Paneth cells which secrete lysozyme and defensins to regulate the microbiota contents, goblet cells which secrete mucin for lubricating and cytoprotective effects, and microfold (M) cells which endocytose pathogens to generate an immune response.[18–20] Apical and basal extracellular components also play a large role in the GI tract barrier system. Tight junctions, comprised of claudin and occludin proteins, and desmosomes, comprised of desmoglein proteins, contribute to the regulation of paracellular transport and provide a scaffolding for the mechanical barriers between cells. Disruptions in tight junction proteins have been implicated in gastrointestinal diseases and can lead to hyperpermeability and inflammatory diseases.[21–23]

Additionally, the GI tract contains immunomodulatory factors that contribute to its protective function and serve as another line of defense against external insults. Components of both the innate and acquired immune systems are represented in the GI tract.[18] Epithelial cells contain pattern recognition receptors (PRRs) that function to sense pathogenic microbes in the environment and trigger a cytokine release and a resultant immune response if needed. Toll-like receptors (TLRs) are examples of PRRs that recognize conserved patterns on pathogens and lead to a specific inflammatory response, depending on the detected microbe or toxin.[18] Following endocytosis of a pathogen by M cells, antigens are presented to B and T cells in the underlying lymphoid tissue of the small intestine submucosa, also known as Peyer's patches. The presentation of antigens to B cells in Peyer's patches leads to the generation of immunoglobulin A (IgA) via B cells for that specific pathogen. IgA, the predominant antibody of mucosal surfaces, functions to neutralize insulting microbial pathogens and toxins and is noted to be at elevated levels when an immune response is needed.[24] This immune system works in conjunction with the epithelium and extracellular components of the GI tract to regulate homeostasis of the gut and its microbiome.[18]

The Gut Microbiome

The gut microflora consists of a dynamic combination of commensal bacteria, viruses, protozoa, and fungi that create a symbiotic relationship with the human GI tract. It has been estimated that nearly one trillion microorganisms inhabit the small and large intestines, with around 2000 different bacterial species making up this functional unit of the bowel.[25,26] Most of these bacteria are part of 5 phyla: Verrucomicrobia, Proteobacteria, Firmicutes, Actinobacteria, and Bacteroidetes; however, the microbiome varies widely from person to person and can change in an individual over time. This disparity depends on the mode of fetal birth, infections, use of antibiotics, genetics, diet, and stressors in the environment.[2] There is also a variation in the composition of the gut microbiome along the GI tract itself, which depends on the function that region serves.[26]

The anti-inflammatory inhabitants of the microbiota, such as *Akkermansia muciniphila,* serve many beneficial functions to assist the cellular and extracellular components of the GI tract maintain homeostasis, metabolize fuel, and protect the rest of the body from pathogenic microorganisms.[12] These include generating nutrients such as vitamins K and B12, producing necessary carbohydrate metabolites for biochemical processes such as short-chain fatty acids (SCFAs), neutralizing toxins, and reinforcing the integrity of the epithelial barrier.[26] An important immunomodulatory function of the microbiome is fostering the expansion of helper T cells via the response generated by PRRs.[26] These dynamic microbial contents can change according to the environment introduced to the GI tract, including diet, medications, and toxins.[12] All of these vital processes are carried out when the microbiome is in a healthy steady state, or eubiosis. In dysbiosis, there is inadequate regulation of proinflammatory and pathogenic microorganisms. Notably, gram-negative microbes produce substances such as lipopolysaccharides (LPS) which can lead to oxidative stress, induce a robust systemic inflammatory response, and increase gut epithelium permeability.[12]

Gut Microbiome Dysbiosis and Pathology

It is critical to understand the relationships that have already been thoroughly studied between the GI microbiome and other systems to understand the possible association that it has with the inner ear. The dysregulation of the gut microbiome has been proven to play a crucial role in the pathophysiology of disorders associated with both the GI tract and distant organs. Evidence suggests that a proinflammatory microbiome plays a role in the pathogenesis of both Crohn's disease and ulcerative colitis in genetically susceptible individuals.[27] Although the current evidence is heterogeneous, some studies have also concluded that the composition of the gut microbiome may play a role in the disease initiation of Celiac disease (CD), a condition associated with a hypersensitivity to gluten.[28] It is hypothesized that the increased gut permeability in all 3 of these conditions mediated by proinflammatory microbes leads to pathogenic extrusion into the bloodstream, initiating the extraintestinal immune response associated with these conditions.[27,28]

Recently, there has been an emphasis on the association of the GI microbiome with other organ systems, such as the cardiovascular system. Metabolites produced by microorganisms are implicated in either protective or causal correlations with atherosclerosis, hypertension, and heart failure. For example, SCFAs have a protective effect, with decreased levels associated with increased incidence of these conditions. However, increased trimethylamine-N-oxide (TMAO) has been implicated as having a causal association.[29] Endotoxins produced by gram-negative bacteria have also been shown to exacerbate heart failure. Consequently, the association between microbial metabolites and cardiovascular disease has led to more investigation into possible treatment avenues for such conditions and further research on the associations of the GI microbiome beyond the GI tract.[29]

Studies have demonstrated the bidirectional relationship between the GI tract microbiota and the nervous system, defined as the gut–brain axis. The nervous system plays an important role in regulating the enteric nervous system of the GI tract.[2] The complex communication within the gut–brain axis is mediated by the metabolism of tryptophan, the transmission between the vagus nerve and enteric nervous system, the regulatory function of the immune system, and the metabolites produced by the microorganisms.[2] Chemical modulators, such as cytokines, hormones, and neurotransmitters, can be secreted into the bloodstream from both the nervous system via the BBB and the GI tract epithelium to maintain homeostasis in the body.[12] Dysregulation in the GI microbiome results in neurodegeneration and neuroinflammation, leading to pathologic conditions such as Alzheimer's disease, multiple sclerosis, ASD, and psychiatric conditions.[2,12]

With evidence outlining the association between gut microbial dysbiosis and pathologic conditions beyond the GI tract itself, this review will further examine the bidirectional relationship between the GI tract microbiome and the inner ear, termed the gut microbiome–inner ear axis[12]

GUT MICROBIOME–INNER EAR AXIS

As previously mentioned, the changes in the gut microbiome have been implicated in potentiating diseases in systems beyond the GI tract, such as the nervous system and the cardiovascular system. Studies have been conducted to investigate the association between GI tract disorders and SNHL and the effect of noise exposure on the gut microbiome. However, the idea of the gut microbiome–inner ear axis, as it relates to bidirectional communication, is relatively unexplored.

The Blood Labyrinth Barrier

The pathophysiology of inner ear damage caused by the GI microbiome can be linked to its effect on the BLB. The BLB is a semipermeable partition in between the intricate blood vessel capillaries and the fluid of the inner ear known as perilymph and endolymph.[30,31] This barrier is most notably located at the lateral wall of the cochlea adjacent to the stria vascularis and spiral ligament (**Fig. 2**).[12] Perilymph fills the structures of the bony labyrinth, the scala tympani, and scala vestibuli. Low in potassium and high in sodium, the perilymph's ionic concentration resembles that of the extracellular fluid and the cerebrospinal fluid (CSF). Conversely, the endolymph, which fills the scala media (cochlear duct) is low in sodium and high in potassium, similar to intracellular membranes. This difference in the concentration of sodium and potassium ions generates a positive endocochlear potential in the membranous labyrinth, leading to current transduction within cochlear hair cells, resulting in proper auditory and vestibular transmission.[32] Changes in this gradient have been associated with hearing loss.[33]

Studies have elucidated the analogous structures and functions between the BLB and the BBB, which has been a highlight of the connection between the gut microbiome and neurologic conditions.[12,34,35] Structurally, the BBB contains blood vessel endothelial cells, pericytes that assist with the permeability of the vessel, and astrocyte foot processes that maintain the environment of the BBB and brain parenchyma via their macrophage function. The BLB also contains blood vessel endothelial cells, pericytes, and perivascular resident macrophage-type melanocytes.[12,30] Similar to the BBB, the BLB regulates the passage of circulating fluids, cells, oxygen, metabolites, and ions into the inner ear. It also protects the inner ear structures from toxins, pathogens, and mediators of inflammation.[34] One of the most important functions

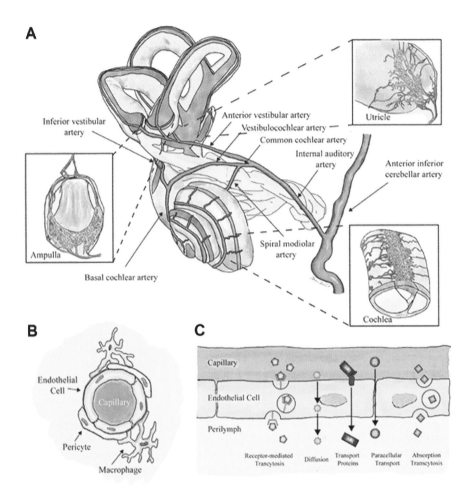

Fig. 2. Schematic showing the components of the blood–labyrinth barrier. (*A*) Blood supply to the labyrinth is shown, with insets showing capillary beds near the sensory epithelia of the ampullae, otoconial organs, and cochlea. (*B*) Capillaries of the blood–labyrinth barrier include endothelial cells with tight junctions, surrounded by pericytes and resident macrophages that regulate permeability. (*C*) Examples of hypothetical mechanisms by which molecules can transit across the barrier are shown. (*From* Song CI, Pogson JM, Andresen NS, Ward BK. MRI With Gadolinium as a Measure of Blood-Labyrinth Barrier Integrity in Patients With Inner Ear Symptoms: A Scoping Review. Front Neurol. 2021;12:662264. Published 2021 May 20. https://doi.org/10.3389/fneur.2021.662264, This is an open-access article distributed under the terms of the Creative Commons Attribution License (CC BY). The use, distribution, or reproduction in other forums is permitted, provided the original author(s) and the copyright owner(s) are credited and that the original publication in this journal is cited, in accordance with accepted academic practice.)

of this barrier system is the maintenance of the ion balance of the endolymph and perilymph for sensory hair cell transduction. Based on the functional and structural similarities between the BLB and BBB, it can be hypothesized that compromising this barrier can lead to changes in the inner ear fluid environment, leading to pathologies associated with SNHL, including noise-induced and age-related hearing loss, AIED, and genetic etiologies of hearing loss.[34,36]

Table 1
A summary of different mediators released during gut dysbiosis leading to increased blood labyrinth barrier permeability and cochlear inflammation

Class	Mediator (s)	Effect on Cochlea	References
Proinflammatory cytokines	• Tumor necrosis factor-α (TNF-α) • Interleukin-1β (IL-1β) • Interleukin-6 (IL-6)	• Increase vascular permeability • Attract leukocytes to promote inflammatory response	Kociszewska et al,[12] 2021
Free Radicals	• Reactive oxygen species (ROS) • Reactive nitrogen intermediates (RNI) • Nicotinamide adenine dinucleotide phosphate (NADPH) oxidase • Intracellular free calcium	• Activate perivascular macrophages • Decrease expression of tight junction proteins in the blood labyrinth barrier (BLB) • Direct damage to cochlear hair cells and intracellular components, such as DNA	Prasad & Bondy,[39] 2020
Endotoxins	• Lipopolysaccharide (LPS)	• Bind to toll-like receptors (TLR), stimulating proinflammatory intracellular pathways and cytokine release • Alter BLB permeability directly	Kociszewska et al,[12] 2021; Shi,[36] 2016

Abbreviations: IL-1β, interleukin-1β; IL-6, interleukin-6; NADPH, nicotinamide adenine dinucleotide phosphate; ROS, reactive oxygen species; TLRs, lipopolysaccharide, toll-like receptors; TNF-α, Tumor necrosis factor-α.

Cochlear Inflammation and Blood Labyrinth Barrier Permeability

Following infection or direct injury across the human body, the immune system responds locally by producing an inflammatory response. Proinflammatory cytokines, such as interleukin-1β (IL-1β), interleukin-6 (IL-6), and tumor necrosis factor-alpha (TNF-α) are stimulated to be released into the vascular system and attract leukocytes to the targeted location.[12] Though this response in the acute phase is a beneficial immune response, chronic inflammation with these cytokines can lead to the production of reactive oxygen species (ROS) and result in damage to healthy tissues.[12] The cochlea itself is directly prone to inflammatory damage from ototoxic medications, surgical trauma, overstimulation from noise exposure, endotoxemia, and degeneration with aging. Therefore, it is reasonable to speculate that various mediators generated during gut dysbiosis can lead to cochlear damage directly or via their impact on the BLB permeability, including proinflammatory cytokines, free radicals, and endotoxins (**Table 1**). On the other hand, SCFAs generated in gut eubiosis can be protective against these mediators of cochlear damage.

Although previously thought to be "immune-privileged," the cochlea itself has been shown to house its own population of leukocytes in the blood-rich stria vascularis and spiral ligament, dominated by macrophages.[37] Neutrophils and additional monocytes can be subsequently recruited to the cochlea to supplement the initial response; however, there is conflicting evidence to whether or not these extraneous cells infiltrate the tight junctions of the BLB.[37,38] In addition to an increase in leukocyte recruitment during the inflammatory response in the cochlea, an upregulation in immune-modulating receptors and enzymes has been found which propagates this response. These receptors and enzymes include cytokine receptors, complement cascade proteins, chemokine receptors, and TLRs.[37] The only location that is devoid of immune cells in the cochlea is the organ of Corti; however, cochlear macrophages have the capability to extend their processes to remove cellular debris from the hair cell region.[37]

The inflammation produced by acoustic trauma, autoimmune hearing loss, endotoxemia, and aging has been shown to alter the integrity of the layers of the BLB. Similar to the epithelium in the GI tract, the permeability of the BLB epithelial layer is dictated by tight junction proteins and the basement membrane. Noise-induced hearing loss results from direct damage to hair cells via ROS from acoustic trauma, which has also been proven to both activate the perivascular macrophages and decrease the expression of cadherin tight junction proteins.[39] Both age-related hearing loss and autoimmune hearing disorders have been associated with alterations in the blood vessel permeability via atrophy of the stria vascularis and immune complex deposition in the epithelium, respectively. This ultimately leads to the increased vascular permeability of the BLB and resulting endolymph ion concentration disruption.[36,40]

Another known cause of inflammation in the cochlea is endotoxemia from LPS. As previously mentioned, LPS is generally released into the bloodstream following infection with gram-negative bacteria. LPS triggers an inflammatory response by either binding to TLRs or inducing the nuclear factor kappa-light-chain enhancer of activated B cells (NF-κB), both of which stimulate the production of proinflammatory cytokines. As it relates to inner ear pathology, LPS has been shown to cause elevated cytokine levels within the cochlear blood vessels, leading to the increased vascular permeability associated with cochlear inflammation.[36] This has been corroborated by studies showing that LPS directly potentiates the trafficking of ototoxic substances beyond the BLB.[41,42]

Gastrointestinal Tract and Hearing Loss

Crohn's disease and ulcerative colitis, the 2 subsets of IBD, are known to have associations with both GI microbiome dysfunction and SNHL; however, the exact pathophysiology of these sequelae is not well understood.[43] Studies have hypothesized that the inner ear is targeted as part of a systemic autoimmune response from IBD, with histologic examination of cochleae showing loss of hair cells and spiral ganglion neurons accompanied by intracochlear fibrosis in patients with chronic IBD, postmortem.[15,16,43] Although no studies have been found that directly connect the GI gut dysbiosis and SNHL in patients with IBD, it has been hypothesized that the resultant leaky gut in IBD may give rise to extravasation by GI bacteria into the circulation. This extravasation leads to an inflammatory immune response that has the ability to travel to the inner ear blood supply.[43] Additionally, even with the pathophysiology of the systemic effects of IBD not being well known, studies have observed an increase in gram-negative bacteria and subsequent endotoxemia with LPS during this GI disorder.

Similarly, SNHL has been reported as a common extraintestinal effect of CD. The mechanism of pathophysiology has been a common topic of study, with disagreement among researchers. It was thought that the hearing loss experienced by patients with CD was part of a systemic autoimmune manifestation, similar to IBD. Other studies have elucidated causal associations with vasculitis, poor vitamin and nutrition absorption, lymphocytic invasion of the BLB, osteoprotegerin loss leading to bone remodeling, and immune complex deposition.[44] Although no studies have examined the composition of the GI tract microbiome of patients with CD who have experienced SNHL, a similar proposed mechanism of action of IBD gut microbiome and SNHL should be investigated.

Noise Exposure and Gut Dysbiosis

Chronic noise exposure has been proven to have a direct effect on the inner ear as it relates to inflammation, production of ROS, and changes in the BLB. One study found increased expression of "injury receptors" such as transient receptor potential vanilloid 1 (TRPV1) and inflammatory mediators such as TNF-α and inducible nitric oxide (iNOS) in rats from 48 hours to 21 days after exposure.[45] Other studies have shown that noise is known to decrease antioxidant levels, increase NADPH oxidase levels, and activate NF-κB, resulting in the production of proinflammatory cytokines.[39] The BLB is also directly affected by noise exposure due to the decrease in junction proteins such as claudin and occludin. Studies in guinea pigs have shown increased BLB permeability with a decrease in tight junction density.[46] Recently, there has been increased interest in how chronic noise exposure affects the gut microbiome, to determine the existence of the bidirectional communication within the gut microbiome–inner ear axis.

The noise acts as a stressor to the human body, activating the sympathetic nervous system and the hypothalamus–pituitary–adrenal axis. Overall, this response increases glucocorticoid and catecholamine levels and alters metabolic processes.[47] Although the mechanism is still unknown, this systemic response to exogenous stress alters the gut microbiota. One study showed that high levels of noise in mice resulted in an increased Firmicutes/Bacteroidetes ratio, a marker for gut dysbiosis, and decreased tight junction protein expression in the colon.[17] This study also concluded that increased noise exposure can cause an elevation in intestinal proinflammatory cytokines and IgA, suggesting an increase in both proinflammatory bacteria and the response to this change. Although a link between noise exposure and alterations in the commensal GI microbiome has been shown in the literature, more research is needed to evaluate the mechanism of action.[47]

SUMMARY

There is evidence that suggests bidirectional communication between the gut microbiome and the inner ear, similar to the gut–brain axis. Studies have shown that gut dysbiosis is accompanied by diseases of the GI tract, such as IBD and CD, and subsequently, these conditions have an increased incidence of hearing loss as an extraintestinal manifestation. Chronic noise exposure can also be linked to alterations in the GI tract microbiome due to its proinflammatory effects. Further studies are warranted to explore the role of the gut microbiome–inner ear axis in health and disease. Better knowledge about the gut microbiome–inner ear axis will pave the way for developing effective therapeutic interventions for auditory disorders such as SNHL.

CLINICS CARE POINTS

- The gut microbiome contains a combination of microorganisms that fosters a symbiotic relationship with the gastrointestinal tract and facilitates maintaining homeostasis, metabolizing fuel, and protecting the body from pathogenic microorganisms.

- Proinflammatory dysregulation in the gut microbiome has been associated with conditions of the GI tract, such as inflammatory bowel disease (IBD) and celiac disease (CD), as well as with conditions in other organ systems, such as neurodegenerative disease due to the change in blood–brain barrier permeability.
- Studies have highlighted the similarities in structure and function between the BBB and the blood labyrinth barrier (BLB), a key regulator in endolymph and perilymph ionic concentration, emphasizing the potential for an association between the gastrointestinal microbiome and inner ear disorders.
- Inflammatory bowel disease (IBD) has been found to be commonly associated with sensorineural hearing loss (SNHL) via changes in the BLB, the mechanism of which is still under further study.
- Noise exposure has also been found to compromise the BLB and increase reactive oxygen species (ROS), leading to downstream gut dysbiosis and further promoting the hypothesis of bidirectional communication in the gut–inner ear axis.

ACKNOWLEDGMENTS

The authors are grateful to Dr Valerie Gramling for her critical reading of the article.

DISCLOSURE

The authors declare no conflict of interest.

REFERENCES

1. Chakrabarti A, Geurts L, Hoyles L, et al. The microbiota-gut-brain axis: pathways to better brain health. perspectives on what we know, what we need to investigate and how to put knowledge into practice. Cell Mol Life Sci 2022;79(2):80.
2. Cryan JF, O'Riordan KJ, Cowan CSM, et al. The microbiota-gut-brain axis. Physiol Rev 2019;99(4):1877–2013. https://doi.org/10.1152/physrev.00018.2018.
3. Guerrero AC, Shah V, Mishra D, et al. Chapter 3: crosstalk between gut and brain via neurotransmitters. In: Eshraghi AA, editor. Gut–brain connection, myth or reality? Role of the microbiome in health and diseases. Hackensack, NJ: World Scientific Publishing Co; 2021. p. 49–70.
4. Mittal R, Debs LH, Patel AP, et al. Neurotransmitters: the critical modulators regulating gut-brain axis. J Cell Physiol 2017;232(9):2359–72.
5. Varanoske AN, McClung HL, Sepowitz JJ, et al. Stress and the gut-brain axis: Cognitive performance, mood state, and biomarkers of blood-brain barrier and intestinal permeability following severe physical and psychological stress. Brain Behav Immun 2022;101:383–93.
6. Belizário JE, Faintuch J. Microbiome and gut dysbiosis. Exp Suppl 2018;109: 459–76.
7. Davies C, Mishra D, Eshraghi RS, et al. Altering the gut microbiome to potentially modulate behavioral manifestations in autism spectrum disorders: A systematic review. Neurosci Biobehav Rev 2021;128:549–57.
8. Davies C, Bergman J, Eshraghi AA, et al. Chapter 9: the gut microbiome: potential clinical applications in disease management: novel approaches using diet and nutraceuticals to reduce manifestations of accelerated aging, obesity, type 2 diabetes, gastrointestinal disorders, neurological disorders, immunological disorders, anxiety, and depression. In: Eshraghi AA, editor. Gut–brain connection,

myth or reality? role of the microbiome in health and diseases. Hackensack, NJ: World Scientific Publishing Co; 2021. p. 195–236.

9. Eshraghi RS, Davies C, Iyengar R, et al. Gut-induced inflammation during development may compromise the blood-brain barrier and predispose to autism spectrum disorder. J Clin Med 2020;10(1):27.

10. Eshraghi RS, Deth RC, Mittal R, et al. Early Disruption of the Microbiome Leading to Decreased Antioxidant Capacity and Epigenetic Changes: Implications for the Rise in Autism. Front Cell Neurosci 2018;12:256.

11. Takahashi K, Nishiwaki H, Ito M, et al. Altered gut microbiota in Parkinson's disease patients with motor complications. Parkinsonism Relat Disord 2021;95:11–7.

12. Kociszewska D, Chan J, Thorne PR, et al. The Link between Gut Dysbiosis Caused by a High-Fat Diet and Hearing Loss. Int J Mol Sci 2021;22(24):13177. https://doi.org/10.3390/ijms222413177.

13. Alexander TH, Harris JP. Incidence of sudden sensorineural hearing loss. Otol Neurotol 2013;34(9):1586–9.

14. Tanna RJ, Lin JW, De Jesus O. Sensorineural hearing loss. StatPearls. Treasure Island (FL): StatPearls Publishing; 2021.

15. Fousekis FS, Saridi M, Albani E, et al. Ear involvement in inflammatory bowel disease: a review of the literature. J Clin Med Res 2018;10(8):609–14. https://doi.org/10.14740/jocmr3465w.

16. Karmody CS, Valdez TA, Desai U, et al. Sensorineural hearing loss in patients with inflammatory bowel disease. Am J Otolaryngol 2009;30(3):166–70. https://doi.org/10.1016/j.amjoto.2008.04.009.

17. Cui B, Su D, Li W, et al. Effects of chronic noise exposure on the microbiome-gut-brain axis in senescence-accelerated prone mice: implications for Alzheimer's disease. J Neuroinflammation 2018;15(1):190. https://doi.org/10.1186/s12974-018-1223-4.

18. Peterson LW, Artis D. Intestinal epithelial cells: regulators of barrier function and immune homeostasis. Nat Rev Immunol 2014;14(3):141–53. https://doi.org/10.1038/nri3608.

19. Volk N, Lacy B. Anatomy and physiology of the small bowel. Gastrointest Endosc Clin N Am 2017;27(1):1–13.

20. Gelberg HB. Comparative anatomy, physiology, and mechanisms of disease production of the esophagus, stomach, and small intestine. Toxicol Pathol 2014; 42(1):54–66.

21. Buckley A, Turner JR. Cell biology of tight junction barrier regulation and mucosal disease. Cold Spring Harb Perspect Biol 2018;10(1):a029314. https://doi.org/10.1101/cshperspect.a029314.

22. Ding Y, Wang K, Xu C, et al. Intestinal Claudin-7 deficiency impacts the intestinal microbiota in mice with colitis. BMC Gastroenterol 2022;22(1):24.

23. Huo J, Wu Z, Sun W, et al. Protective effects of natural polysaccharides on intestinal barrier injury: A review. J Agric Food Chem 2022;70(3):711–35.

24. Woof JM, Kerr MA. The function of immunoglobulin a in immunity. J Pathol 2006; 208(2):270–82. https://doi.org/10.1002/path.1877.

25. Eshraghi AA, Bergman J, Davies C. Chapter 1: the role of microbiome in health and neurosensory disorders: historical and clinical perspectives. In: Eshraghi AA, editor. Gut–brain connection, myth or reality? Role of the microbiome in health and diseases. Hackensack, NJ: World Scientific Publishing Co; 2021. p. 1–21.

26. Thursby E, Juge N. Introduction to the human gut microbiota. Biochem J 2017; 474(11):1823–36. https://doi.org/10.1042/BCJ20160510. Published 2017 May 16.

27. Glassner KL, Abraham BP, Quigley EMM. The microbiome and inflammatory bowel disease. J Allergy Clin Immunol 2020;145(1):16–27. https://doi.org/10.1016/j.jaci.2019.11.003.

28. Valitutti F, Cucchiara S, Fasano A. Celiac disease and the microbiome. Nutrients 2019;11(10):2403. https://doi.org/10.3390/nu11102403.

29. Peng J, Xiao X, Hu M, et al. Interaction between gut microbiome and cardiovascular disease. Life Sci 2018;214:153–7. https://doi.org/10.1016/j.lfs.2018.10.063.

30. Ishiyama G, Lopez IA, Ishiyama P, et al. The blood labyrinthine barrier in the human normal and Meniere's disease macula utricle. Sci Rep 2017;7(1):253. https://doi.org/10.1038/s41598-017-00330-5.

31. Salt AN, Hirose K. Communication pathways to and from the inner ear and their contributions to drug delivery. Hear Res 2018;362:25–37.

32. Ekdale EG. Form and function of the mammalian inner ear. J Anat 2016;228(2): 324–37. https://doi.org/10.1111/joa.12308.

33. Zdebik AA, Wangemann P, Jentsch TJ. Potassium ion movement in the inner ear: insights from genetic disease and mouse models. Physiology (Bethesda) 2009; 24:307–16. https://doi.org/10.1152/physiol.00018.2009.

34. Hirose K, Hartsock JJ, Johnson S, et al. Systemic lipopolysaccharide compromises the blood-labyrinth barrier and increases entry of serum fluorescein into the perilymph. J Assoc Res Otolaryngol 2014;15(5):707–19. https://doi.org/10.1007/s10162-014-0476-6.

35. Song CI, Pogson JM, Andresen NS, et al. MRI With Gadolinium as a Measure of Blood-Labyrinth Barrier Integrity in Patients With Inner Ear Symptoms: A Scoping Review. Front Neurol 2021;12:662264. https://doi.org/10.3389/fneur.2021.662264.

36. Shi X. Pathophysiology of the cochlear intrastrial fluid-blood barrier (review). Hear Res 2016;338:52–63. https://doi.org/10.1016/j.heares.2016.01.010.

37. Hu BH, Zhang C, Frye MD. Immune cells and non-immune cells with immune function in mammalian cochleae. Hear Res 2018;362:14–24. https://doi.org/10.1016/j.heares.2017.12.009.

38. Fujioka M, Okano H, Ogawa K. Inflammatory and immune responses in the cochlea: potential therapeutic targets for sensorineural hearing loss. Front Pharmacol 2014;5:287. https://doi.org/10.3389/fphar.2014.00287.

39. Prasad KN, Bondy SC. Increased oxidative stress, inflammation, and glutamate: potential preventive and therapeutic targets for hearing disorders. Mech Ageing Dev 2020;185:111191. https://doi.org/10.1016/j.mad.2019.111191.

40. Trune DR, Nguyen-Huynh A. Vascular pathophysiology in hearing disorders. Semin Hear 2012;33(3):242–50. https://doi.org/10.1055/s-0032-1315723.

41. Quintanilla-Dieck L, Larrain B, Trune D, et al. Effect of systemic lipopolysaccharide-induced inflammation on cytokine levels in the murine cochlea: a pilot study. Otolaryngol Head Neck Surg 2013;149(2):301–3.

42. Urdang ZD, Bills JL, Cahana DY, et al. Toll-like receptor 4 signaling and downstream neutrophilic inflammation mediate endotoxemia-enhanced blood-labyrinth barrier trafficking. Otol Neurotol 2020;41(1):123–32. https://doi.org/10.1097/MAO.0000000000002447.

43. Wengrower D, Koslowsky B, Peleg U, et al. Hearing loss in patients with inflammatory bowel disease. Dig Dis Sci 2016;61(7):2027–32.

44. Karunaratne D, Karunaratne N. ENT Manifestations of celiac disease: a scholarly review. Ear Nose Throat J 2020;145561320972604. https://doi.org/10.1177/0145561320972604 (in press).

45. Dhukhwa A, Bhatta P, Sheth S, et al. Targeting inflammatory processes mediated by TRPVI and TNF-α for treating noise-induced hearing loss. Front Cell Neurosci 2019;13:444.
46. Wu YX, Zhu GX, Liu XQ, et al. Noise alters guinea pig's blood-labyrinth barrier ultrastructure and permeability along with a decrease of cochlear Claudin-5 and Occludin. BMC Neurosci 2014;15:136. https://doi.org/10.1186/s12868-014-0136-0.
47. Karl JP, Hatch AM, Arcidiacono SM, et al. Effects of psychological, environmental and physical stressors on the gut microbiota. Front Microbiol 2018;9:2013. https://doi.org/10.3389/fmicb.2018.02013.

UNITED STATES POSTAL SERVICE® Statement of Ownership, Management, and Circulation
(All Periodicals Publications Except Requester Publications)

1. Publication Title	2. Publication Number	3. Filing Date
OTOLARYNGOLOGIC CLINICS	466 – 550	9/18/2022

4. Issue Frequency	5. Number of Issues Published Annually	6. Annual Subscription Price
FEB, APR, JUN, AUG, OCT, DEC	6	$450.00

7. Complete Mailing Address of Known Office of Publication (Not printer) (Street, city, county, state, and ZIP+4®)

ELSEVIER INC.
230 Park Avenue, Suite 800
New York, NY 10169

Contact Person
Malathi Samayan

Telephone (Include area code)
91-44-4299-4507

8. Complete Mailing Address of Headquarters or General Business Office of Publisher (Not printer)

ELSEVIER INC.
230 Park Avenue, Suite 800
New York, NY 10169

9. Full Names and Complete Mailing Addresses of Publisher, Editor, and Managing Editor (Do not leave blank)

Publisher (Name and complete mailing address)

DOLORES MELONI, ELSEVIER INC.
1600 JOHN F KENNEDY BLVD. SUITE 1800
PHILADELPHIA, PA 19103-2899

Editor (Name and complete mailing address)

Stacy Eastman, ELSEVIER INC.
1600 JOHN F KENNEDY BLVD. SUITE 1800
PHILADELPHIA, PA 19103-2899

Managing Editor (Name and complete mailing address)

PATRICK MANLEY, ELSEVIER INC.
1600 JOHN F KENNEDY BLVD. SUITE 1800
PHILADELPHIA, PA 19103-2899

10. Owner (Do not leave blank. If the publication is owned by a corporation, give the name and address of the corporation immediately followed by the names and addresses of all stockholders owning or holding 1 percent or more of the total amount of stock. If not owned by a corporation, give the names and addresses of the individual owners. If owned by a partnership or other unincorporated firm, give its name and address as well as those of each individual owner. If the publication is published by a nonprofit organization, give its name and address.)

Full Name	Complete Mailing Address
WHOLLY OWNED SUBSIDIARY OF REED/ELSEVIER, US HOLDINGS	1600 JOHN F KENNEDY BLVD. SUITE 1800 PHILADELPHIA, PA 19103-2899

11. Known Bondholders, Mortgagees, and Other Security Holders Owning or Holding 1 Percent or More of Total Amount of Bonds, Mortgages, or Other Securities. If none, check box. ► ☐ None

Full Name	Complete Mailing Address
N/A	

12. Tax Status (For completion by nonprofit organizations authorized to mail at nonprofit rates) (Check one)
The purpose, function, and nonprofit status of this organization and the exempt status for federal income tax purposes:
☒ Has Not Changed During Preceding 12 Months
☐ Has Changed During Preceding 12 Months (Publisher must submit explanation of change with this statement)

PS Form 3526, July 2014 [Page 1 of 4 (see instructions page 4)]   PSN: 7530-01-000-9931   PRIVACY NOTICE: See our privacy policy on www.usps.com.

13. Publication Title	14. Issue Date for Circulation Data Below
OTOLARYNGOLOGIC CLINICS	JUNE 2022

15. Extent and Nature of Circulation		Average No. Copies Each Issue During Preceding 12 Months	No. Copies of Single Issue Published Nearest to Filing Date
a. Total Number of Copies (Net press run)		287	230
b. Paid Circulation (By Mail and Outside the Mail)	(1) Mailed Outside-County Paid Subscriptions Stated on PS Form 3541 (Include paid distribution above nominal rate, advertiser's proof copies, and exchange copies)	144	113
	(2) Mailed In-County Paid Subscriptions Stated on PS Form 3541 (Include paid distribution above nominal rate, advertiser's proof copies, and exchange copies)	0	0
	(3) Paid Distribution Outside the Mails Including Sales Through Dealers and Carriers, Street Vendors, Counter Sales, and Other Paid Distribution Outside USPS®	101	69
	(4) Paid Distribution by Other Classes of Mail Through the USPS (e.g., First-Class Mail®)	0	0
c. Total Paid Distribution (Sum of 15b (1), (2), (3), and (4))		245	182
d. Free or Nominal Rate Distribution (By Mail and Outside the Mail)	(1) Free or Nominal Rate Outside-County Copies included on PS Form 3541	22	28
	(2) Free or Nominal Rate In-County Copies Included on PS Form 3541	0	0
	(3) Free or Nominal Rate Copies Mailed at Other Classes Through the USPS (e.g., First-Class Mail)	0	0
	(4) Free or Nominal Rate Distribution Outside the Mail (Carriers or other means)	0	0
e. Total Free or Nominal Rate Distribution (Sum of 15d (1), (2), (3) and (4))		22	28
f. Total Distribution (Sum of 15c and 15e)		267	210
g. Copies not Distributed (See Instructions to Publishers #4 (page 3))		20	20
h. Total (Sum of 15f and g)		287	230
i. Percent Paid (15c divided by 15f times 100)		91.76%	86.66%

* If you are claiming electronic copies, go to line 16 on page 3. If you are not claiming electronic copies, skip to line 17 on page 3.

16. Electronic Copy Circulation	Average No. Copies Each Issue During Preceding 12 Months	No. Copies of Single Issue Published Nearest to Filing Date
a. Paid Electronic Copies ►		
b. Total Paid Print Copies (Line 15c) + Paid Electronic Copies (Line 16a) ►		
c. Total Print Distribution (Line 15f) + Paid Electronic Copies (Line 16a) ►		
d. Percent Paid (Both Print & Electronic Copies) (16b divided by 16c × 100) ►		

☒ I certify that 50% of all my distributed copies (electronic and print) are paid above a nominal price.

17. Publication of Statement of Ownership

☒ If the publication is a general publication, publication of this statement is required. Will be printed   ☐ Publication not required.
in the   October 2022   issue of this publication.

18. Signature and Title of Editor, Publisher, Business Manager, or Owner	Date
Malathi Samayan *Malathi Samayan* - Distribution Controller	9/18/2022

I certify that all information furnished on this form is true and complete. I understand that anyone who furnishes false or misleading information on this form or who omits material or information requested on the form may be subject to criminal sanctions (including civil penalties).

PS Form 3526, July 2014 (Page 3 of 4)   PRIVACY NOTICE: See our privacy policy on www.usps.com

Moving?

Make sure your subscription moves with you!

To notify us of your new address, find your **Clinics Account Number** (located on your mailing label above your name), and contact customer service at:

Email: journalscustomerservice-usa@elsevier.com

800-654-2452 (subscribers in the U.S. & Canada)
314-447-8871 (subscribers outside of the U.S. & Canada)

Fax number: 314-447-8029

Elsevier Health Sciences Division
Subscription Customer Service
3251 Riverport Lane
Maryland Heights, MO 63043

*To ensure uninterrupted delivery of your subscription, please notify us at least 4 weeks in advance of move.

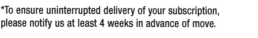

Printed and bound by CPI Group (UK) Ltd, Croydon, CR0 4YY

03/10/2024

01040476-0019